Clinics in Developmental Medicine
DISORDERS OF THE SPINAL CORD IN CHILDREN

Clinics in Developmental Medicine

Disorders of the Spinal Cord in Children

Edited by

MICHAEL PIKE
Children's Hospital,
Oxford University Hospitals NHS Trust,
Oxford, UK

2013
Mac Keith Press

© 2013 Mac Keith Press
6 Market Road, London N7 9PW

Editor: Hilary Hart
Managing Director: Ann-Marie Halligan
Production Manager: Udoka Ohuonu
Project Manager: Chris Purdon
Indexer: Laurence Errington

First published in this edition in 2013

British Library Cataloguing-in-Publication data
A catalogue record for this book is available from the British Library

ISBN 978 1 908316-80-6

Typeset by Toppan Best-Set Premedia Limited, Hong Kong and The Clyvedon Press Ltd, Cardiff, UK
Printed by Latimer Trend & Company, Plymouth, Devon, UK

Mac Keith Press is supported by Scope

For
Jess and Joe

CONTENTS

AUTHORS' APPOINTMENTS

Michael Absoud Consultant in Paediatric Neurodisability, Evelina Children's Hospital, Children's Neurosciences Centre, Kings's Health Partners Academic Health Science Centre; Newcomen Centre at St Thomas', St Thomas' Hospital, London, UK

Saleel R Chandratre Consultant Paediatric Neurologist, Children's Hospital, Oxford University Hospitals NHS Trust, Oxford, UK

David A Chesler Research Fellow, Departments of Neurosurgery and Oncology, Johns Hopkins School of Medicine, Baltimore, MD; Chief Resident, Department of Neurosurgery, University of Maryland Medical Center, Baltimore, MD, USA

Allison Graham Consultant Physician in Spinal Injuries, Stoke Mandeville Hospital, Buckinghamshire Healthcare NHS Trust, UK

John Houten Chief, Division of Spinal Neurosurgery, Department of Neurosurgery, Montefiore Medical Center; Associate Professor of Neurological Surgery, Leo M. Davidoff Department of Neurological Surgery, Albert Einstein College of Medicine, New York, NY, USA

George I Jallo Professor of Neurological Surgery, Pediatrics and Oncology, Departments of Neurosurgery and Pediatrics, Johns Hopkins School of Medicine, Baltimore, MD, USA

Sandeep Jayawant Consultant Paediatric Neurologist, Children's Hospital, Oxford University Hospitals NHS Trust, Oxford, UK

Roger Keynes Professor of Neuroscience, Department of Physiology, Development and Neuroscience, University of Cambridge, UK

John-Paul Kilday	Chief Neuro-Oncology Fellow/Brain Tumour Program, Division of Haematology/Oncology, The Hospital for Sick Children, University of Toronto, Toronto, Ontario, Canada
Ravi Knight	Consultant in Clinical Neurophysiology, John Radcliffe Hospital, Oxford University Hospitals NHS Trust, Oxford, UK
Abhaya V Kulkarni	Consultant Paediatric Neurosurgeon, Associate Professor, Division of Neurosurgery, Hospital for Sick Children, University of Toronto, Toronto, Ontario, Canada
Ming J Lim	Consultant Paediatric Neurologist, Evelina Children's Hospital, Children's Neurosciences Centre, Kings's Health Partners Academic Health Science Centre; Newcomen Centre at St Thomas', St Thomas' Hospital, London, UK
Elizabeth Muir	Research Associate, Department of Physiology, Development and Neuroscience, University of Cambridge, UK
Gary Nicolin	Consultant Paediatric Oncologist, Department of Paediatric Oncology, University Hospital Southampton NHS Foundation Trust, Southampton, UK
Joseph Noggle	Medical Student, Departments of Neurosurgery and Pediatrics, Johns Hopkins School of Medicine, Baltimore, MD, USA
Michael Pike	Consultant Paediatric Neurologist, Children's Hospital, Oxford University Hospitals NHS Trust, Oxford, UK
Gerardine Quaghebeur	Consultant Neuroradiologist, John Radcliffe Hospital, Oxford University Hospitals NHS Trust, Oxford, UK

Authors' Appointments

Lawrence Vogel   Professor of Pediatrics, Rush Medical College;
Assistant Chief of Staff, Medicine Chief of
Pediatrics, Shriners Hospitals for Children, Chicago,
IL, USA

Evangeline Wassmer   Consultant Paediatric Neurologist, Birmingham
Children's Hospital, Birmingham, UK

Reza Yassari   Assistant Professor of Clinical Neurosurgery,
Montefiore Medical Center, Albert Einstein
College of Medicine, Department of
Neurosurgery, New York, NY, USA

Michel Zerah   Professor of Neurosurgery, Department of
Paediatric Neurosurgery, Hôpital Necker-Enfants
Malades, Paris, France

FOREWORD

The spinal cord is a component of the nervous system that is too easy to take for granted. Primary spinal conditions in children are rare, and one can be forgiven for not putting impairments of spinal cord function high on a list of differential considerations when assessing childhood impairments. Now, at last, comes an excellent and comprehensive book on *Disorders of the Spinal Cord in Children*, brought together under the editorial leadership of Dr Michael Pike, consultant paediatric neurologist at the Oxford Children's Hospital. Dr Pike has assembled an international group of experts who together have created a comprehensive and detailed account of the spinal cord: its structure, functions, vulnerabilities, and strategies for management of the resultant functional challenges associated with impairments.

The book starts with the clinical assessment of the child or adolescent with a disorder of the spinal cord (Chapter 1), and progresses to discussions of how to image the cord (Chapter 2). Chapter 3 presents an accessible account of developmental neurobiology and spine physiology.

The next several chapters systematically present what is known about malformations of the spinal cord (Chapter 4), acute insults such as abscesses, haemorrhage and trauma (Chapter 5), tumours that affect the spinal cord either intrinsically or extrinsically (Chapter 6), and discussion of a host of other pathological processes (inflammatory, metabolic, vascular, and demyelinating) that can have devastating effects on the developing young person (Chapter 7).

Chapter 8 provides a broad, comprehensive, and 'developmentally based' overview of the challenges and opportunities associated with management of children and adolescents with impaired spinal cord function. The discussion addresses these issues by exploring, among other considerations, the implications of the ages of children and youth when their impairments occur, and of course takes the discussion forward into the adult years.

Finally, Chapter 9 presents what I found to be both an exciting and sobering account of the prospects for spinal cord repair. At the leading edge of current research are the huge strides that the field has made in understanding the physiology and pathophysiology of the impaired spinal cord, and the systematic efforts of people around the world to extend the frontiers of this amazing programme of scientific and clinical development. The sobering reality, however, is that even 85 years after Cajal's pioneering work we remain stymied by so many elements of this tangled web of complexity, and it would appear that any headline-grabbing reports of cures remain a somewhat distant dream

It had always been my impression that the spinal cord (especially in children) played the role of 'country cousin' to the worldly and sophisticated brain! The brain receives most of the attention, most of the time, while the spinal cord seems to linger at the fringes of many people's consciousness about the 'nervous system'. The cerebellum has recently been the focus of a book in the Mac Keith Press *Clinics in Developmental Medicine* series, as have brain tumours and sonographic imaging techniques used to reveal the secrets of the infant brain. In the past decade, this book series also published a text on the clinical management of craniosynostosis. The current text by Dr Pike and his colleagues now adds importantly to this excellent collection of text on a less-understood component of the nervous system.

The good news about spinal cord impairment in children is that, compared with many neurodisabilities in the Western world, most of the causes are rare. The converse of this fact is that few people have a large and comprehensive experience of these conditions. I was heartened to see how many collaborative efforts are underway across the world to bring people's experience together, to strive for order in the classification and assessment of outcomes, and to highlight the essential role of expertise in addressing the clinical challenges that often accompany both diagnostic and management puzzles.

We are indebted to Dr Pike and his generous colleagues for sharing a wealth of experience, perspective, advice, and encouragement to work together to solve the mysteries of the country cousin, and to bring it appropriately into the light of childhood disability.

Professor Peter Rosenbaum
McMaster University, Canada

PREFACE

Peter Rosenbaum's vivid characterization, in his excellent Foreword, of the cord as the marginal and apologetic country cousin to the more prominent and influential brain will have resonance with many clinicians. The spine features less both in undergraduate and postgraduate paediatric training than it might, and less than the devastating impact of a spinal cord lesion might justify.

But the country cousin is not without guile. Examples of the often enigmatic role of the cord in a spectrum of clinical situations might include the unidentified cord lesion in a sick and floppy neonate, or in a ventilated child recovering from severe pneumococcal meningitis, the incipient cord compression underlying a strikingly 'non-organic' gait disorder in a teenager, and the increasing awareness of cord involvement in shaken impact syndrome.

The range of subject matter, the complexity of many of the clinical issues, and the variety of expertise engaged in paediatric spinal cord disease were all persuasive reasons for taking up the challenge of editing this book. It was a delight to collaborate with the distinguished and diverse group of clinicians and academics who generously agreed to contribute. Our fascinating, often humorous, and occasionally surreal e-mail traffic over a substantial gestational period could produce a worthy chapter in itself!

I have received kindness, support, and forbearance in equal measure from everyone at Mac Keith Press and am grateful in particular to Peter Baxter, Hilary Hart, Ann-Marie Halligan, Udoka Ohuonu, and Alessy Beaver. Chris Purdon of The Clyvedon Press has been a perceptive and kindly copy-editor, Laurence Errington a precise and rigorous indexer, and Karl Hunt an imaginative cover designer.

Finally, I am most grateful of all to my wife Claire who has been a source of love, support, and perceptive comment throughout the genesis of this book.

Michael Pike
Children's Hospital, Oxford, UK
May 2013

1
THE NEUROLOGICAL EXAMINATION OF CHILDREN WITH SPINAL CORD DISORDERS

Saleel R Chandratre and Sandeep Jayawant

In this chapter we present an approach to the clinical assessment of children who have symptoms and signs suggestive of spinal cord dysfunction, with a view to formulating a differential diagnosis and management strategy. The spinal cord is involved in many complex neurological disorders, either in isolation or as part of a multisystem disorder. This warrants a thorough clinical history and both a general systems and neurological examination in addition to a focused assessment of the functions of the spinal cord itself.

History of present illness
The history narrows the differential diagnosis and focuses the examination. Spinal cord dysfunction may present with motor, sensory, or a combination of motor and sensory symptoms, sphincter disturbances, autonomic dysfunction, and/or pain. The most common symptoms are gait abnormality (in an ambulant child), paucity of limb movement (in the pre-ambulant infant), sensory disturbance including reduced sensation and dysaesthesia, sphincter disturbance, and neck, back, or truncal pain.

The age at onset of symptoms, the nature of the initial symptoms, and their evolution over time will influence the clinical approach. Preceding events including identifiable triggers, concurrent infection and trauma, and the pace of progression may identify a static, progressive, or episodic process with implications for focused examination and investigation.

The causes of myelopathy are myriad and extensively described in other chapters. To set the background to the clinical approach, Table 1.1 lists selected categories of acute myelopathy and Table 1.2 selected causes of chronic myelopathy. Table 1.3 lists characteristic presenting symptoms and signs of childhood spinal pathology. Table 1.4 highlights some salient features that should be specifically sought when eliciting the history of a suspected myelopathy.

Clinical examination
The identification and localization of cord pathology is dependent on a familiarity with its anatomy and physiology. Figures 1.1–1.4 illustrate the anatomy of the spinal cord in section, the dermatomal distribution of sensory nerves, and the reflex arc.

TABLE 1.1
Selected categories of acute myelopathy

1. Infections: discitis, epidural abscess, tuberculosis, Herpes simplex virus
2. Trauma: birth-related trauma, accidental and non-accidental injury, acute disc prolapse
3. Vascular: thromboembolic events (paediatric intensive care unit) or haemorrhage (spinal epidural haematoma)
4. Neoplastic: neuroblastoma, lymphoma, intrinsic spinal cord tumours
5. Toxins: lathyrism (e.g. caused by ingesting legumes of the genus *Lathyrus* or similar), chemotherapeutic drugs
6. Demyelinating: acute disseminated encephalomyelitis, neuromyelitis optica, multiple sclerosis

TABLE 1.2
Selected causes of chronic myelopathy

1. Degenerative/metabolic: bone pathology with compression, chronic disc prolapse, adrenomyeloneuropathy, sub-acute combined degeneration
2. Neoplastic: indolent tumours, neurofibromas
3. Genetic: spinocerebellar ataxias, hereditary spastic paraplegia

Salient features in the examination of suspected myelopathy through observation or formal examination are highlighted in the following paragraphs. In addition, depending on the age at presentation, certain aetiologies are more likely; therefore the following section focuses on some specific age and aetiology-based examination findings that need to be actively elicited.

OBSERVATION
An accurate description of pain or sensory impairment is often not obtained. It is therefore vital to observe the child's reaction to gauge this. Engagement with surroundings, visual attention and exploration, physical interaction with toys, the nature of play, paucity, and symmetry of movement, and response to sensory stimulus may be the primary examination tool in a young or fretful child.
    Observation of the following features is particularly important:

• Consciousness may be impaired in situations where the cord lesion is accompanied by other pathology. This may occur in traumatic injury, meningitis or demyelinating disorders (acute disseminated encephalomyelitis, neuromyelitis optica)
• Interaction with carer or parent
• Visual attention and strabismus
• Facial expression, weakness, and drooling
• Ability to weight bear and ambulate in an independently ambulant child
• Gait: paraplegic, spastic, antalgic, high stepping
• Ability to rise from the floor or climb stairs
• Paucity of use of limbs and antigravity movement especially in a pre-ambulant child
• Breathing pattern: pattern of diaphragmatic and intercostal muscle use.

TABLE 1.3

Characteristic presenting symptoms and signs of childhood spinal pathology

Motor symptoms and signs
  Hypotonia in the acute stage and at the level of cord involvement
  Weakness: may be static or progressive
  Ataxia: progressive (Friedreich ataxia, other spinocerebellar ataxias)
  Hypertonia
  Gait abnormality: toe walking, foot drop, hemiplegic, scissoring (hereditary spastic paraplegia)
  Frequent falls
  Torticollis or scoliosis
  Arthrogryposis

Sensory symptoms and signs
  Pain or segmental paraesthesiae: localized at the level of cord involvement and/or radiating (cervical, to
    the arms; thoracic, circumferential to the chest or abdomen; lumbar or sacral, to the legs or saddle
    area)
  Loss of ipsilateral discriminative sensation (position, vibration, discriminative touch, pressure touch,
    two-point discrimination, stereognosis, and shape and movement awareness).
  Loss of contralateral light touch (two or three segments below cord involvement)
  Loss of contralateral pain and temperature sensation (two or three segments below cord involvement)
  Sensory level (alteration of sensation to pinprick at and below a segmental level)
  Sensory ataxia

Sphincter disturbance
  It is extremely important to take a sphincter history even in the pre-toilet-trained infant including
  (1) Change in pattern of voiding and/or defaecation
  (2) Is there intermittent wet and/or soiled nappy with a dry one between, or is the nappy always wet
    and/or dirty suggesting continuing incontinence?
  (3) When the nappy is off for a period, is a normal voiding of urine with a good stream seen with full
    continence before and after?
  (4) Does the perianal area remain clean once wiped or is there a continuous faecal leak?

In the previously toilet-trained child:
  (1) Bladder (change in pattern and/or urinary urgency, hesitancy, retention or incontinence)
  (2) Bowel (change in pattern and/or constipation and/or faecal incontinence)

Other autonomic symptoms and signs
  Tachy-/bradycardia
  Orthostatic hypotension/labile blood pressure
  Sweating or lack thereof
  Impaired temperature control and vasomotor instability below the level of the lesion
  Ipsilateral Horner syndrome (cervico-thoracic cord lesion)
  Sexual dysfunction after puberty

Other symptoms that may be associated with cord pathology
  Raised intracranial pressure (due to cranio-cervical junction abnormalities)
  Eye movement abnormalities (for example in spinocerebellar ataxias)
  Respiratory distress (diaphragmatic breathing due to intercostal muscle weakness)

TABLE 1.4
Salient features when eliciting the history of a suspected myelopathy

1. Presentation history
   - Time frame of presentation and progression (distinguishing acute from chronic myelopathy)
   - Sensory, motor, autonomic, or associated symptoms as in Table 1.1
   - History of trauma
   - Intercurrent or preceding illness, for example upper respiratory tract infection, cold sores, gastroenteritis (e.g. in acute disseminated encephalomyelitis)
   - Medication history (see section 6 below)
   - Systemic disease (other autoimmune conditions if suspecting neuromyelitis optica, systemic lupus erythematosus, other autoimmune disorders)
   - Contact with infectious adults or children, particularly tuberculosis and herpes simplex virus
   - Contact with pets or animals, in particular exposure to ticks (Lyme disease)
   - Foreign travel (infectious pathology)
   - Diplopia, decreased visual acuity (neuromyelitis optica)
   - Encephalopathic features (acute disseminated encephalomyelitis, encephalitis)
   - Recent spinal surgery or period of intensive care including central vascular access (vascular, infectious)
   - Any risk factors for thromboembolism (ischaemic cord lesion)
2. Antenatal and birth history
   - Fetal movements in utero (congenital malformations, e.g. spina bifida)
   - Pregnancy: diabetes, antenatal bleeds, anomaly scan data, folate supplementation, medication use
   - Labour and delivery, for example shoulder dystocia, instrumental delivery, traumatic delivery
   - Arthrogryposis or talipes at birth
   - Neonatal intensive care including umbilical artery catheter placement
3. Developmental history and social history
   - Achievement of motor milestones (to elucidate congenital vs acquired and static vs progressive cord pathology)
   - Achievement of continence (and history of patterns of voiding in pre-toilet-trained child)
   - Social history, particularly where medically unexplained neurological symptoms are being considered or where there is a suspicion of non-accidental traumatic injury
4. Family history
   - First-degree relatives with demyelinating disorders
   - First-degree relatives with haemorrhage of the central nervous system (e.g. familial cavernomas)
   - First-degree relatives with neural tube defects
   - Genetic conditions, for example spinocerebellar ataxias, hereditary spastic paraparesis, neurofibromatosis
   - Family history of autoimmune disease
5. Immunization history (particularly recent vaccination): post vaccination demyelination
6. Medication and toxin exposure
   - Bronchodilators and steroids (Hopkin syndrome)
   - Chemotherapeutic agents, for example vincristine, methotrexate, cytosine
   - Contaminated dhal (lathyrism) and bitter cassava (konzo)
   - Out of date tetracyclines and quiniodochlor
   - Botulism presenting as flaccid paraplegia should be considered in the differential diagnosis of an acute myelopathy in an infant (prodromal constipation, rapidly progressive flaccid quadriparesis, cranial nerve involvement)

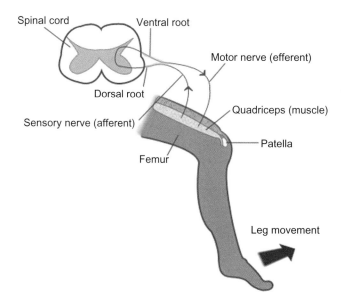

Fig. 1.1. Spinal reflex arc.

Spinal cord — Ventral root — Motor nerve (efferent) — Quadriceps (muscle) — Patella — Dorsal root — Sensory nerve (afferent) — Femur — Leg movement

GENERAL AND SYSTEMIC EXAMINATION

The general examination may reveal clinically relevant information either in terms of aetiology or of associated features requiring appropriate management.

For example neurocutaneous markers such as café au lait patches may suggest an underlying diagnosis of neurofibromatosis type 1 (NF1), or skin or retinal haemangiomas may suggest intracerebral and intraspinal haemangiomas. Spinal cord arteriovenous malformations have been reported in Klippel–Trenaunay–Weber syndrome, Osler–Weber–Rendu syndrome, and in NF1. Hemihypertrophy with or without hemimegalencephaly would suggest Klippel–Trenaunay–Weber syndrome with spinal cavernomas (Maher et al. 2008; Song et al. 2010).

Dysmorphic features may suggest an underlying genetic diagnosis and/or an identifiable syndrome diagnosis (achondroplasia, Down syndrome), which may warrant detailed assessment of other systems. Skeletal abnormalities, corneal clouding, coarse facial features, and organomegaly may suggest mucopolysaccharidoses with or without features of compressive myelopathy secondary to spinal stenosis or odontoid hypoplasia.

Scoliosis, kyphosis, and gibbus formation may indicate vertebral malformations or a bony destructive process with the possibility of underlying cord involvement.

Generalized lymphadenopathy may indicate infections such as tuberculosis or a leukaemia or lymphoma. Skin rashes and joint swelling raise the possibilities of Lyme disease or an autoimmune disorder. Pallor may be seen in lymphoproliferative disorders or vitamin B_{12} deficiency.

Cardiac examination, electrocardiography, and echocardiography may identify cardiac structural or rhythm disturbances as a source of cardioembolic anterior spinal artery stroke, or the cardiomyopathy of Friedreich ataxia.

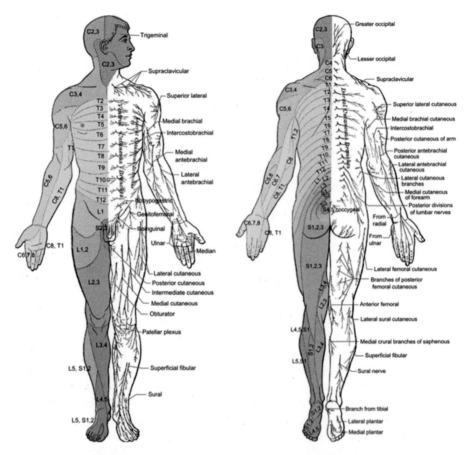

Fig. 1.2. Dermatomes: anterior aspect.   **Fig. 1.3.** Dermatomes: posterior aspect.

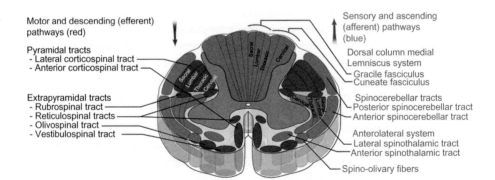

Fig. 1.4. Cross-section anatomy of spinal cord showing tracts within spinal cord. A colour version of this figure is available in the plate section at the end of the book.

Abdominal examination may reveal faecal loading due to anal sphincter disturbance. A painful or painless palpable bladder is an important early sign of urinary retention. Abdominal neuroblastoma or lymphoma may be palpated.

NEUROLOGICAL EXAMINATION

Neurological examination of a child with spinal cord dysfunction may be challenging because of the associated sensory symptoms, pain, and possible encephalopathy. Head circumference should be charted as a baseline measure and to monitor velocity of head growth over time using appropriate growth charts (compare with previous measurements if available). Macrocephaly is noted in achondroplasia and in chronic hydrocephalus.

Cranial nerve examination should focus on facial involvement (Guillain–Barré syndrome, neuromuscular disorders), hearing (a presenting feature in paediatric neurofibromatosis type 2 [NF2]), bulbar involvement (botulism, Guillain–Barré syndrome, high cervical pathology), Horner syndrome (may suggest a cervical or thoracic cord lesions) and vision (optic neuritis, multiple sclerosis, neuromyelitis optica), as well as ocular movements (foramen magnum lesions, spinocerebellar disorders).

The back needs to be carefully examined for the cutaneous markers of cord dysraphism and for kyposcoliosis and gibbus formation. The neck should be examined for torticollis.

Particular attention must be given to the assessment of skeletal abnormalities secondary to spinal cord dysfunction (congenital talipes, acquired bony deformities, dislocated hips, limb length discrepancy, scoliosis, and kyphosis)

Motor examination

This should start with a careful observation and characterization of the gait in an ambulant child. Gowers test will confirm proximal weakness if it is suspected on observation. In a non-ambulant child, opportunistic observation of posture, head and trunk control, and antigravity movement is a good guide to muscle strength. Careful assessment of distal power in hand muscles may point to a syrinx or a craniocervical junction anomaly such as a Chiari malformation. Distal weakness in the lower limbs points to a conus medullaris or cauda equina syndrome.

Wherever possible, formal muscle strength charting using the Medical Research Council grade from 0 to 5 or a more detailed grading used by physiotherapists using addition or subtraction signs in addition to whole numbers (e.g. 4− or 4+) helps ascertain the strength at baseline and aids the monitoring of recovery (Table 1.5).

Each muscle group or individual muscle strength needs to be charted depending on the nature (focal or diffuse) of spinal cord involvement to monitor improvement or deterioration. The Modified Ashworth scale (Table 1.6) and other muscle strength assessment scales are in practical usage. In non-organic symptomatology careful preliminary observation may demonstrate the inconsistencies suggestive of non-organic weakness. Mild weakness may be best detected by functional assessment, for example ability to walk on tiptoes and heels, standing on either leg, jumping, hopping, and supporting weight on hands in the wheelbarrow position.

TABLE 1.5
Medical Research Council grading of muscle power

Grade	Nature of movement
0	No muscle contraction visible
1	Trace or flicker of contraction, but no movement
2	Active joint movement when gravity is eliminated
3	Active movement against gravity
4	Active movement against gravity and resistance, but weaker than normal
5	Normal power

TABLE 1.6
Clinical scale for spastic hypertonia (Modified Ashworth Scale)

0	No increase in tone
1	Slight increase in muscle tone, manifested by a catch and release or minimal resistance at the end of the range of movement when the affected part(s) is moved in flexion or extension
1+	Slight increase in muscle tone, manifested by a catch, followed by minimal resistance throughout the remainder (less than half) of the range of movement
2	More marked increase in muscle tone through most of the range of movement, but affected part(s) easily moved
3	Considerable increase in muscle tone, passive movement difficult
4	Affected part(s) rigid in flexion or extension

Sensory examination

The sensory examination is challenging in an infant or young child and requires careful observation. The cooperative older child may be able to respond accurately to a formal 'adult' sensory examination.

Observation may suggest a difference in colour, temperature, perspiration, and the skin may be cooler and dry below the level of a spinal cord lesion.

The Romberg sign is positive in the sensory ataxia of spinal cord or peripheral nerve disorders, often with abnormal joint position sense and impaired vibration. In the upper limbs, sensory ataxia is assessed by asking the child to touch his nose with alternating fingers initially with eyes open and then with eyes closed. There is increased difficulty with eyes closed.

Neck flexion may elicit a sudden 'electric' sensation down the back or into the arms (Lhermitte sign), which is secondary to increased mechano-sensitivity of the dorsal columns and is seen in multiple sclerosis, compressive cord lesions, or after cervical cord irradiation.

Pain in spinal cord lesions

There are several types of pain that occur in spinal cord lesions. It is important to recognize this and manage it effectively: central pain, musculoskeletal pain, visceral pain and neuropathic pain.

Central pain is typically a burning, tingling, shooting, stinging, or 'pins and needles' sensation. Some individuals also complain of a stabbing, piercing, or lancinating pain. This type of pain usually occurs within days, weeks, or months of the injury and tends to decrease with time in both frequency and intensity. Central pain is diffuse and occurs most often in the legs, back, feet, thighs, and toes although it can also occur in the buttocks, hips, upper back, arms, fingers, abdomen, and neck. Young children may rub or simply scratch an affected area resulting in a mistaken assumption that the problem is dermatological. This type of pain is often exacerbated by noxious stimuli such as bladder and bowel distension, infection, and pressure sores. Management involves identifying triggers as well as addressing the pain itself.

Musculoskeletal pain is a dull aching sensation that occurs as result of muscle tension with increased frequency in the shoulder, hip and hand, although it also occurs in the lower back and buttock. Muscle tension is probably caused by a combination of factors including soft tissue inflammation and limb stretching in the setting of contractures owing to paralysis, spasticity, and disuse. Generally speaking, this pain is usually aggravated by activity and relieved by rest, analgesia, and anti-inflammatory drugs. Therapists involved in rehabilitation need to take account of this in planning mobilization programmes.

Visceral pain is a vague, dull, or diffuse abdominal sensation, or a feeling of discomfort or bloating, or sometimes a referred pain experienced, for example, in the shoulder. Visceral pain is caused by problems such as distension, perforation, inflammation, impaction, or constipation involving organs such as the stomach, kidney, gall bladder, urinary bladder, and intestines; immobility and autonomic dysfunction are often contributory. These problems may also cause associated symptoms such as nausea, fever, and malaise.

In children with an established cervical or high cord transection and a subsequent acute surgical abdomen, it is important to recognize that the expected abdominal and autonomic symptoms and signs, particularly pain and altered perfusion, may be modified by the pre-existing cord lesion.

Neuropathic pain, of varying type is a significant problem in some children with spinal cord disease. Nerve root pain is described as having a sharp or electric shock quality in a dermatomal distribution.

Specific spinal cord anatomical syndromes
Based on characteristic patterns of motor and sensory loss, various spinal cord syndromes affecting specific anatomical distributions and tracts within the spinal cord are described.

Figure 1.5 illustrates some common spinal cord syndromes. The signs and symptoms are a result of specific corresponding spinal tract involvement, as described below.

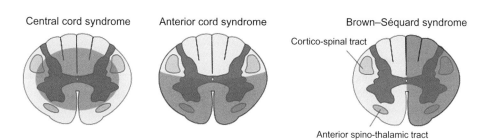

Fig. 1.5. Some common spinal cord syndromes.

1. Complete transection

   After complete spinal cord transection,
   - All sensory modalities (soft touch, position sense, vibration, temperature, and pain) are impaired below the level of the lesion
   - Loss of sharp/blunt sensation below a segmental level is most valuable in localizing the lesion. A sensory level may be easily missed unless carefully, and sometimes repeatedly, sought by gradually advancing from an area of normal sensation to where an alteration in sharpness is perceived. Specifically asking to distinguish sharp and dull sensation can also be used as adjunct to sharp/blunt testing
   - In incomplete lesions, particularly with extra-medullary pathology, the sensory level may be several segments below the level of the lesion as (1) axons of second-order neurons in the dorsal horns decussate over several segments through the ventral white commissure and (2) the lowest segments are represented more superficially in the lateral spinothalamic tract
   - Band-like radicular pain or segmental paresthesiae may occur at the level of the lesion. If the pain is cervical, it radiates to the arms; if thoracic in origin, it is circumferential to the chest or abdomen; and if lumbar or sacral, it radiates to the legs and/or saddle area
   - Localized vertebral pain, overlying the spinous process, worse on palpation or percussion may occur with destructive bony lesions e.g. tumours and infections.

2. Hemisection of the spinal cord (Brown–Séquard syndrome)

   Features of this syndrome are as follows:

   Unilateral interruption of the lateral corticospinal tracts:
   - Ipsilateral spastic weakness below the level of the lesion
   - Upgoing plantar ipsilateral to lesion
   - Abnormal reflexes and Babinski sign may not be present in acute injury.

   Unilateral interruption of the posterior column:
   - Ipsilateral loss of tactile discrimination, vibratory and position sensation below the level of the lesion.

   Unilateral interruption of lateral spinothalamic tracts:
   - Contralateral loss of pain and temperature sensation. This usually occurs two or three segments below the level of the lesion.

   Where the cord lesion is entirely unilateral, sphincter function tends to be preserved.

3. Central cord syndrome

   Lesions affecting the spinal cord centrally (syringomyelia, hydromyelia, haematomyelia, and intramedullary cord tumours) present with the following:
   - Dissociation of sensory loss (thermoanaesthesia and analgesia in a circumferential distribution with preservation of soft touch sensation and proprioception) because the decussating fibres of the spinothalamic tract conveying pain and temperature sensation are compromised initially

- Often sacral sensory sparing with relatively preserved dull and sharp pain and temperature sensation in the sacral dermatomal distribution because of the lamination of the spinothalamic tract (dorsomedial cervical sensation and ventrolateral sacral sensation)
- Syringomyelia may also occasionally result in a neuropathic arthropathy of the shoulder, elbow, and other joints
- Segmental neurogenic atrophy, paresis, and areflexia at the level of the lesion due to anterior extension of the disease process with anterior horn cell involvement.
- Bladder dysfunction (usually urinary retention) and patchy sensory loss below the level of the lesion with weakness more pronounced in the arms (distal more than proximal) is seen after severe hyperextension injuries of the neck. Strength in the legs may be regained in a matter of minutes or hours after the initial injury to the central grey matter and lateral corticospinal tract at the level of the cervical cord.

4. Anterior cord syndrome
   - Complete bilateral motor paralysis (flaccid tetraplegia or paraplegia) below the level of the lesion owing to interruption of the corticospinal tract
   - Loss of pain and temperature sensation at and below the level of the lesion owing to interruption of the spinothalamic tract
   Retained proprioception and vibratory sensation owing to intact dorsal columns
   - Areflexia, flaccid anal sphincter, urinary retention, and intestinal obstruction may also be present in individuals with anterior cord syndrome.

5. Conus medullaris and cauda equina (CES) syndromes
   Features of these are as follows:
   - Saddle anaesthesia (in cauda equina syndrome) and perianal anaesthesia (in conus medullaris syndrome)
   - Urinary retention followed by overflow
   - Loss of anal tone and sensation; constipation or incontinence
   - Often low back pain or 'sciatica'
   - Proximal and distal lower extremity motor weakness and loss of lower limb reflexes (cauda equina syndrome) or preserved knee jerks with symmetric distal weakness (conus medullaris syndrome). These motor features may be absent in low cord lesions (S2–S4).

REFLEXES

Deep tendon reflexes are reduced or absent during the acute 'spinal shock' phase of acute myelopathy. Spinal shock is a temporary physiological disorganization of spinal cord function below a total or near-total spinal cord lesion. This loss of neurological activity includes loss of motor, sensory, reflex, and autonomic function. It can start between 30 and 60 minutes after the onset of spinal cord pathology and can last up to 6 weeks.

Hyper-reflexia gradually sets in below the level of the lesion with associated hypertonia, spastic catch, and reflex spinal muscular spasms after a few days to weeks. In established or chronic myelopathy, hyper-reflexia is present below the level of the spinal cord lesion and hyporeflexia or areflexia at the level of the lesion.

In compressive myelopathy, there may be asymmetry of reflexes, with initial hyper-reflexia due to nerve root irritation followed by hypo- or areflexia at the level of the lesion and hyper-reflexia below the level.

Superficial reflexes, including the abdominal reflex (T8–T12), cremasteric reflex in males (L1–L2), and the plantar reflex (L5, S1), may help determine the level of the lesion.

- Absence of all abdominal reflexes suggests a level above T8
- Absence of abdominal reflexes below but presence above the umbilicus suggests a level at T10
- Presence of all abdominal reflexes suggests a level below T12
- Asymmetry of abdominal reflexes suggests hemi-spinal-cord syndrome
- The plantar reflex is equivocal or flexor during the early stages of acute myelopathy. During the recovery phase or with established myelopathy the plantar response is extensor in lesions at or above the conus medullaris. In cauda equina lesions the plantar reflex is diminished or absent
- Absence of the cremasteric reflex in males (gently stroking the superior medial thigh normally leads to immediate contraction of the ipsilateral cremaster muscle lifting the testis) localizes the lesion to L1–L2
- Anal sphincter involvement is manifested by a patulous anus, absence of contraction of the anal sphincter when the peri-anal skin is stimulated (anal wink), and by the lack of contraction of the anal sphincter during rectal examination. Faecal incontinence may occur with disorders of the sensory roots, conus, cauda equina, motor roots (S3–S4), or peripheral nerves and occasionally in high spinal lesions (better sphincter control than low spinal lesions).

CEREBELLAR EXAMINATION

Cerebellar signs are present in lesions at the foramen magnum and in the spinocerebellar ataxias. Cerebellar involvement leads to hypotonia, scanning dysarthria, downbeat, or pendular nystagmus, and decreased deep tendon reflexes. Gait ataxia is an early sign of Friedreich ataxia and is secondary to a combination of cerebellar and sensory ataxia.

SPINE EXAMINATION

Torticollis may be muscular but may indicate an underlying abnormality in the cervical vertebrae including craniocervical junction and posterior fossa abnormalities, or abnormalities of the intraspinal structures at the cervical level.

Scoliosis may be present in several spinal cord disorders including Chiari 1 malformation with associated syringomyelia, neural tube defects, Friedreich ataxia, and cord tumours

The skin over the spine may show evidence of an obvious neural tube defect either open (pre-surgical assessment) or repaired or have signs of occult dysraphism (tuft of hair, lipoma, dermal sinus). Kyphosis or scoliosis may suggest an underlying vertebral anomaly or a destructive process of the vertebrae.

Palpation of the spine may reveal tenderness, protective paraspinal muscle spasm in response to pain (neuropathic or musculoskeletal), or a 'step' indicative of a vertebral body fracture.

SPHINCTER ASSESSMENT
Sphincter assessment is a critical component of the assessment of spinal cord pathology and should always be performed even in infants. See under history above for a description of the relevant questions to be asked about the pre-toilet-trained child.
• The bladder is acontractile during the initial variable period of spinal shock
• Reflex detrusor activity returns in days to weeks and various types of bladder dysfunction may be noted.
  1. A hyperreflexic, uninhibited neurogenic bladder also called the spastic or upper motor neuron bladder (due to lesions above the bladder centre S2–S4, and usually above T12) results in urinary frequency, urgency, urge incontinence, and inability to initiate micturition voluntarily
  2. Detrusor-sphincter dyssynergia (reflex neurogenic bladder) sometimes occurs in lesions above the lower thoracic cord in which simultaneous contraction of the sphincter and the detrusor results in obstructed voiding, interrupted urinary stream, incomplete emptying and high intravesical pressures.
  3. An autonomous neurogenic bladder (detrusor areflexia) with loss of bladder sensation and overflow incontinence occurs with complete lesions below the T12 segment involving the conus medullaris and cauda equina including the bladder neurogenic centre at S2–S4 with associated saddle anaesthesia. This is also called a flaccid or lower motor neuron bladder
• Bladder muscle tone, residual urine volume, reflex bladder emptying and ureteric reflux are assessed by urodynamic studies.

Anal sphincter control is often similarly affected.
Spinal cord injury above the T12 level results in a reflex bowel. The ability to feel when the rectum is full may be lost. The anal sphincter muscle remains tight, however, and bowel movements will occur on a reflex basis. This means that when the rectum is full, the defaecation reflex will occur, emptying the bowel.
A spinal injury below the T12 level may damage the defaecation reflex and relax the anal sphincter muscle, resulting in a flaccid bowel with persistent faecal incontinence.
Faecal incontinence may also occur with disorders of the sensory roots, conus, or motor roots (S3–S4). The internal anal sphincter tone may be reduced on rectal examination (or more objectively using dynamic pressure studies) and there may be reduced perianal sensation and loss of the anal skin reflex (anal wink).

Important paediatric scenarios with myelopathy
In this section we discuss some specific issues and conditions that are age related and therefore need special mention.

NEONATAL PRESENTATION

The two main conditions that are seen in the newborn period are traumatic spinal cord lesions typically involving the cervical cord and spinal dysraphism (neural tube defects).

Less commonly, and usually in the neonatal intensive care setting, an ischaemic cord event may occur often in association with umbilical artery catheterization or major neonatal cardiac surgery; ischaemic events are usually thoracic or thoraco-lumbar rather than cervical (Ruggieri et al. 1999). The differential diagnosis in the neonatal period may also include neuromuscular disorders such as spinal muscular atrophy type 1.

Characteristic features in neural tube defects include the following:

- Spasticity may be predominant in a high lesion whereas a mixed or flaccid picture will be present in a lumbo-sacral lesion; in most cases, asymmetry is present, reflecting the complexity of the malformation which is not a transection
- There may be a history of decreased fetal movements and polyhydramnios; arthrogryposis, talipes, or hip dislocation may be evident
- The defect may be obvious or there may be markers for an occult dysraphism, but this is not invariably the case
- A spastic or flaccid bladder may result depending on the level of the defect. Early formal assessment of bladder function is vital
- Constipation may be significant
- Sensory level may be assessed using grimace to pinprick; superficial reflexes such as the abdominal, cremasteric, and anal wink reflexes may also help to determine the level of the lesion
- Hydrocephalus may be a comorbid feature
- Neurocutaneous markers and kyphoscoliosis may indicate an underlying occult dysraphism and a tethered cord (which may produce signs and symptoms as the child grows presenting with secondary disturbances of gait and sphincter dysfunction)
- Other systems may be involved such as renal, gastrointestinal, and cardiac as part of a dysmorphic syndrome and often caused by a shared embryological origin of neural and non-neural systems
- Small malformed paralysed legs, an abnormal natal cleft, and malformations of the rectum and genitourinary system point to the caudal regression syndrome.

Characteristic features in intra-partum spinal cord injury include the following:

- Most injuries involve the cervical cord and are associated with breech presentation (lower cervical and upper thoracic injury) or cephalic presentation (upper cervical segments). There is evidence of motor, sensory, and sphincter involvement
- Thoracic and lumbar vascular injury is rare and usually due to vascular embolism from umbilical catheters
- Lower cervical and high thoracic trauma presents with flaccid diplegia or quadriplegia and diaphragmatic breathing. There may be some proximal upper limb movement but the legs are flaccid and areflexic in the shock stage, later evolving to an upper motor neuron picture. Spinal reflexes will be evident as a withdrawal response to pinprick after

the shock phase has passed. The bladder distends and dribbles and priapism may be evident. Absence of sweating below the lesion may indicate level of injury
- Upper cervical injuries present with a flaccid, areflexic quadriplegia often with apnoea. Withdrawal to pinprick as a spinal reflex may be seen. There is lack of sweating over the entire body. Ventilatory requirement may be temporary or permanent
- A spinal injury above C4 paralyses the intercostals, abdominal wall muscles, and diaphragm. An injury between C4 and T6 produces weakness of intercostals and results in predominantly diaphragmatic breathing. Cough will be weak. Injuries between T6–T12 will not affect breathing but the cough will be weak
- Horner's syndrome (ptosis, miosis, and anhidrosis) may result from spinal injury between C8 and T4, interrupting neurons travelling from the hypothalamus down the spinal cord to synapse with secondary neurons which then ascend back up to the face and eye.

Features distinguishing neonatal neuromuscular disease from cord lesions include tongue fasciculation, an alert face, and normal sensation and sphincter function which distinguish spinal muscular atrophy type 1; a myopathic face with weakness, normal sensation, and normal sphincter function, suggest congenital myotonic dystrophy (often with an affected mother), or a congenital myopathy.

EARLY INFANCY AND CHILDHOOD
The main causes of myelopathy in this age group are trauma, infections (particularly discitis and epidural abscess), demyelination, and degenerative conditions such as Friedreich ataxia, copper deficiency myeloneuropathy, subacute combined degeneration of the spinal cord, spinal muscular atrophy, and hereditary spastic paraplegia.

It is important again to establish a timeline for the symptoms to distinguish acute, progressive, and static conditions. The early developmental history is essential in establishing whether the onset of the problem is recent or long-standing. Sometimes there are gradual and subtle changes in hand function, gait, school performance, and sphincter function, which need meticulous questioning to establish whether indeed the condition is static or slowly progressive.

Some important considerations in this age group are the following:

- Refusal to bear weight in a toddler or small child is often an indication of weakness, pain, or both. It is usually possible to localize hip, knee, ankle, and foot bone pain. Where pain is difficult to localize in toddlers, it is often in the lower back, a very characteristic feature of discitis in this age group
- Discitis typically occurs in toddlers with refusal to bear weight, limping, or sometimes discomfort in sitting as the initial presentation. There may loss of lumbar lordosis and resistance to flexion of the spine. Pain (abdominal or vertebral but often poorly localized) is an important feature sometimes with a low-grade temperature and raised inflammatory markers. Power, tone, reflexes, sensory examination, and sphincter function are normal. Diagnosis is by magnetic resonance spinal imaging, which demonstrates discitis often with adjacent oedema of the vertebral bodies

- Acutely developing scoliosis indicates a destructive bony process or a degenerative cord process and very occasionally can itself produce secondary cord compression
- Any acute presentation with weakness, pain, altered sensation, or sphincter dysfunction warrants meticulous neurological examination and urgent neuroimaging
- Acute inflammatory demyelinating polyneuropathy or Guillain–Barré syndrome and transverse myelitis may have overlapping clinical characteristics. Salient distinguishing features are as follows:

Acute inflammatory demyelinating polyneuropathy/Guillain–Barré syndrome	Transverse myelitis
Pain in the back or legs may be the initial presentation (sharp pain or tingling, itching paraesthesiae) followed by weakness	Weakness is usually the first presentation
	Weakness usually static after onset.
Progressive (typically ascending) weakness and areflexia	Reflexes brisk or depressed
Sphincter involvement less	Sphincter involvement common
Associated autonomic cardiac rhythm disturbances or blood pressure lability	Associated encephalopathy or visual impairment may occur

- Urgent neuraxis magentic resonance imaging will nevertheless be needed in a few children with probable Guillain–Barré syndrome when the clinical findings are uncertain
- A space-occupying lesion such as neuroblastoma may present with acute cord compression in infancy or childhood. Presentation is with acute-onset progressive weakness over hours to days and loss of weight-bearing. Examination may reveal a flaccid paraplegia, a distended bladder, and brisk lower limb reflexes with or without a palpable abdominal mass
- The symptoms and signs of acute cord compression should also raise the possibility of a spinal epidural abscess or haematoma. Presentation is with pain, sphincter disturbance, loss of weight bearing, and progressive weakness over hours to days (in association with fever in spinal epidural abscess).

SPINAL CORD TUMOURS
The signs and symptoms of the spectrum of spinal cord tumours may be non-specific and slowly progressive, often resulting in considerable delay in diagnosis (Wilne and Walker 2010). The symptoms may include progressive scoliosis, pain, altered sensation often ill-demarcated and poorly described including dysaesthesia (which in the young child may present as 'itchiness' only), slight weakness of one or more limbs, slow change in hand function or gait, which are often initially missed. Back pain is an unusual symptom in childhood and should be taken seriously. A bleed into a tumour may present as acute cord compression.

Examination reveals a slowly progressive spastic mono-, para-, or quadriparesis.

Cervico-medullary junction tumours may present with a stiff neck or torticollis, neck and shoulder pain and, sometimes, lower cranial nerve involvement. Tumours of the cauda equina cause flaccid weakness and atrophy of leg muscles and areflexia with sphincter disturbance and saddle anaesthesia.

RECOGNISING NON-ORGANIC MOTOR AND SENSORY SYMPTOMS

Non-organic presentations may mimic spinal cord disease and pose a diagnostic and therapeutic challenge. Discriminating elements in this clinical situation include the following:

• Age range usually in the second decade and rarely under 8 years old
• Inconsistent and fluctuating strength in limbs including a discrepancy between function on formal testing and function observed incidentally
• Bizarre and fluctuating postures and gait
• History suggestive of other medically unexplained symptoms
• A social history that puts the child in a vulnerable category for non-organic symptomatology
• 'Hoover's sign' (Hoover 1908) has been found in controlled studies to have good sensitivity and specificity (Ziv et al. 1998). It relies on the principle that flexion at one hip joint is accompanied by involuntary extension of the contralateral joint. The examiner cups the heel of the more affected leg and notes the strength of hip extension. They then note the strength of hip extension when the individual is asked to flex the contralateral hip. Discrepancy between voluntary hip extension (which is often weak) and involuntary hip extension (which should be normal) suggests functional paresis
• Inconsistent or patchy sensory loss not conforming to dermatomal distribution; circumferential distal sensory loss to all modalities is a common non-organic finding and is very unusual as a sign of organic pathology in children.
• It is important to recognize that careful imaging of the neuraxis is usually indicated at the time of presentation of medically unexplained neurological weakness or sensory symptoms. This is because (1) the symptoms may be the non-organic elaboration of a core organic pathology, for example in a child with underlying cord compression; (2) the child and family are likely to find a methodical organic approach before a definitive non-organic diagnosis, both reassuring in excluding organic pathology and engaging as a demonstration that the symptoms are being taken seriously; (3) medically unexplained neurological weakness or sensory symptoms may be a long-standing and fluctuating disorder, and an early diagnosis based purely on clinical judgement followed months later by a reversion to organic investigation is unlikely to inspire confidence in the child or family.

MYELOPATHY IN INTENSIVE CARE

It is important to remain vigilant about spinal injury in children in the paediatric intensive care unit. This may be due to spinal trauma unrecognized in the setting of major trauma elsewhere, after scoliosis repair, vascular events in severe meningitis, or embolism from deep veins owing to immobility, stasis, and indwelling vascular lines or demyelination from drugs such as methotrexate or as part of a disseminated encephalomyelitis (immune mediated or infective).

Although formal examination may be limited, careful observation may yield useful information:

- Observation may suggest a difference in colour, temperature, perspiration, and the skin may be cooler and dry below the level of the spinal cord lesion
- There may be a discrepancy between facial grimace to stimuli below and above a spinal level when assessing conscious level in a ventilated child
- Horner's syndrome (particularly miosis and ptosis) may suggest cervico-thoracic junction pathology but may also result from the placement of central lines in the neck.
- The back needs to be carefully examined (if it is deemed safe to move the child)
- Look for skeletal abnormalities secondary to pre-existing spinal cord dysfunction (congenital talipes, acquired bony deformities, dislocated hips, limb length discrepancy, scoliosis, and kyphosis)
- Fasciculation may be present in the acute stage of spinal injury at the level of the lesion
- As mechanical ventilation is withdrawn, observation of the breathing pattern to assess intercostal and diaphragmatic function may suggest cervical cord involvement. Lower cranial nerve signs may be a marker for an accompanying high cervical myelopathy
- When the urinary catheter is removed, the pattern of bladder function may indicate lesions above or below the bladder control level (S2–S4)
- Superficial and deep tendon reflexes are useful in localizing the lesion unless the child has been heavily sedated or paralysed.

Some important considerations for a child with suspected myelopathy on intensive care are the following:

- Blood pressure and heart rate measurements are important in individuals with spinal injury. Treatment with methylprednisolone or intravenous immunoglobulin may lead to high blood pressure. Autonomic involvement may lead to tachycardia or bradycardia, which may require cardiac monitoring including electrocardiogram monitoring for rhythm disturbances
- Respiratory function needs to be monitored and assessed (especially in suspected high cervical cord myelopathy) using appropriate techniques including pulse oximetry, end tidal CO_2 monitoring, transcutaneous CO_2 measurement, peak flow measurements plotted against height- and sex-normative data, cough impulse and sniff to assess crudely for diaphragmatic function. Involvement of the diaphragm either unilaterally or bilaterally may suggest the level of the spinal lesion (C3–C5)
- In an unconscious child with a suspected myelopathy, it is important to be aware of other systems being affected, in particular constipation and urinary retention and abdominal or chest trauma not immediately apparent, because of the confounding effects of neurogenic sensory and autonomic disturbance. During recovery there is a risk of embolism from deep veins which may be prevented by anticoagulation and/or compression bandages
- Neurogenic pain may need active therapeutic intervention

- Long-term immobilization and impaired autonomic and sensory function predisposes to skin breakdown and needs addressing with turning, meticulous skin care, and mattresses to relieve pressure points.

SPINAL CORD IN NON-ACCIDENTAL INJURY

The spinal cord may be involved in non-accidental trauma due to impact or shaking. This may result in contusion, diffuse axonal injury, and/or cord compression from haematomas, or ischaemic cord lesions from damage to the vascular supply. It should be considered in the differential diagnosis of any child who presents with an unexplained acute onset of weakness, sphincter disturbance, and encephalopathy, or where the history appears inconsistent with the clinical findings, but particularly in infants in the first year of life.

   Some important considerations are the following:

- Meticulous history of the preceding events taken in the presence of another professional and recorded contemporaneously
- A careful social history
- Detailed examination of the scalp, skin, mouth, ears, back, anus, and genitalia for evidence of trauma or of a bleeding diathesis
- Meticulous neurological examination including a formal retinal examination for retinal haemorrhage
- The pattern of weakness may range from a complete quadriplegia with abnormal breathing pattern to a mild upper limb weakness only
- It is highly likely in an infant that there will be an accompanying brain injury and consequent encephalopathy with or without seizures; this may be severe and obscure the accompanying myelopathy
- Sphincter dysfunction should be evaluated
- Spinal cord injury must be looked for when imaging for non-accidental head injury and must be considered even in the absence of radiological features (spinal cord injury without radiographic abnormality [SCIWORA])
- Full skeletal survey and detailed clotting studies are essential
- Other blunt abdominal or chest trauma may have occurred and should be evaluated.

Summary
- The identification and localization of cord pathology is dependent on a familiarity with cord anatomy and physiology.
- Spinal cord pathology and its clinical presentation is age dependent.
- The combination of motor, sensory, and sphincter disturbance is strongly suggestive of a cord lesion.
- Detailed history and examination including opportunistic observation will guide management.
- Detailed assessment of bladder and bowel symptoms with a high index of suspicion is required to identify sphincter disturbance in children.

- Great care must be taken to look for spinal cord involvement in the unconscious child and in the intensive care setting.
- Pain is an under-recognized symptom of spinal cord disease and its recognition and correct interpretation will allow for more rapid and appropriate investigation and treatment.
- Functional motor and sensory symptoms may coexist with organic cord pathology.
- The use of standardized examination scales guides the monitoring of recovery.

REFERENCES

Hoover CF. A new sign for the detection of malingering and functional paresis of the lower extremities. *JAMA* 1908; **51**: 746–747.

Maher CO, Smith E, Proctor M, Scott RM. In Kim DH, Betz RR, Huhn SL, Newton PL, editors. Surgery of the Paediatric Spine. New York, NY: Thieme, 2008: 337–343.

Ruggieri M, Smárason AK, Pike M. Spinal cord insults in the prenatal, perinatal, and neonatal periods. *Dev Med Child Neurol* 1999; **41**: 311–317.

Song D, Garton H, Fahim D, Maher CO. Spinal cord vascular malformations in children. *Neurosurg Clin N Am* 2010; **21**: 503–510.

Wilne S, Walker D. Spine and spinal cord tumours in children: a diagnostic and therapeutic challenge to healthcare systems. *Arch Dis Child Educ Pract Ed* 2010; **95**: 47–54.

Ziv I, Djaldetti R, Zoldan Y, Avraham M, Melamed E. Diagnosis of 'non-organic' limb paresis by a novel objective motor assessment: the quantitative Hoover's test. *J Neurol* 1998; **245**: 797–802.

2
IMAGING THE CORD

Gerardine Quaghebeur

Imaging of the spinal cord is a subsection of paediatric neuroradiology; the latter emerged as the first formal subspecialty of paediatric radiology during the late 1960s. It is now an effective combination of an age-related and specific-organ-directed clinical subspecialty that does require understanding of a wide spectrum of central nervous system (CNS) diseases. It also requires considerable technical adaptation and innovation within the diagnostic and therapeutic modalities that are used. The adaptation of techniques and equipment to accommodate and safely image patients of all sizes from fetus to young adults is necessary. Derek Harwood-Nash, considered by many to be the founder of paediatric neuroradiology, stated, 'there is a growing need for education and instruction in paediatric neuroradiological techniques and paediatric neuroradiological diseases within the neuroradiological fraternity as a whole' (Harwood-Nash and Fitz 1973). He went on to state, 'the child is not simply a small adult' and this can be further expanded to state that the infant is not a small child, the neonate is not a small infant and the fetus is not a small neonate.

Market forces have dictated that most imaging equipment will continue to be designed for (ever larger) adults. Thus creative thinking is needed to adapt, optimize, and use safely these technological advances in the paediatric population. The highest quality images are required to make a diagnosis, particularly for the spinal cord; this remains an imaging challenge even in adults.

The most important factor in obtaining high-quality imaging is lack of movement, which is particularly applicable to magnetic resonance imaging (MRI) and vascular imaging (Barkovich 2005, pp1–15).

The challenges include the following:

- The size of the individual patient, which may range from fetus to larger or heavier than adult patients
- Movement, which may be a result of fear, curiosity or inability to cooperate, pain, behavioural or developmental difficulties
- Comprehension/communication. There may be a difficulty with explanation to and/or engagement with the child
- The possible bio-effects of the imaging techniques used must be adequately managed to avoid excessive radiation exposure by means of paediatric computed tomography (CT)

protocols with increased speeds and reduced fields of view. In MRI it is similarly important to adapt scan protocols and not simply rely on adult protocols as these may be
non-diagnostic.

The solutions include the following:

• Creating a child- and parent-friendly environment
• This is easier if one is imaging in a dedicated children's hospital, but as most children
  will present to a mixed hospital, it may be appropriate to adapt one room within the
  neuradiology department
• Bright colours, visual stimulation, toys, murals, light and audiovisual displays are all
  helpful in helping children to collaborate with the investigation (Figs 2.1 and 2.2)
• Other solutions involve the need for the use of sedation or general anaesthesia.

There are different guidelines and policies about the use of sedation and anaesthesia
within radiology environments. Within the UK a document was produced by the Royal
College of Radiologists (2003) that highlights the importance of safe sedation and anaesthesia within the paediatric population in radiology departments. Adequate monitoring must
be available in all sedated infants and children and ideally MR-compatible monitors, though
expensive, should be available in all units. It is emphasized that children undergoing radiological examinations require a deeper level of sedation than adults, such that children are
not expected to be able to respond to verbal stimuli. This implies that sedation or anaesthesia
must be administered by anaesthetic staff skilled in paediatric airway management and life
support. There should be close collaboration between a radiology department and the local
paediatric anaesthetic department when designing protocols. It is recommended that most

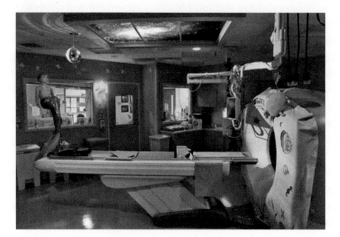

Fig. 2.1. An example of a child-focused computed tomography (CT) scanning suite with appropriate
modifications, including 'disguise' of the gantry and a ceiling-mounted fixture of the galaxy (Google
Images). A colour version of this figure is available in the plate section at the end of the book. Reproduced with permission from the Children's Hospital Pittsburgh.

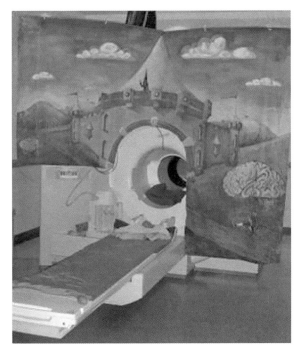

Fig. 2.2. A child-focused magnetic resonance imaging (MRI) scanner with brightly coloured mural and display: canvas overlay used to make MRI environment more friendly for young children, created by Scott Klein of the University of Oregon Brain Development Laboratory. A colour version of this figure is available in the plate section at the end of the book.

procedures on young children will be performed under general anaesthesia, conscious sedation is not encouraged within the UK (Royal College of Radiologists 2003), and there is particular emphasis on the importance of parental consent and information (Royal College of Radiologists 2003).

Neonates can often be scanned without sedation if they are kept warm and transferred as seamlessly as possible from their ward to the MR scanner and then fed immediately before the study. The use of dedicated neonatal MR-compatible incubators may be helpful in this population of patients. Preterm infants present additional problems of small size and inability to maintain body temperature; a decision to move these infants off the ward to an imaging environment must be made after careful consultation, taking into account the risk/benefit ratio. Control of body temperature is essential and an MR-compatible incubator is ideal.

In general, many children will be able to undergo CT with modern helical CT scanners without the need for sedation or general anaesthesia. Younger children may be gently restrained and older children will hold still long enough for a good CT examination to be obtained if the radiographer is able to initiate scanning while the patient is not moving. In some cases, however, sedation or anaesthesia will be required.

MRI scans can usually be obtained without sedation or general anaesthesia in most children over the age of 6 years provided the child has no other difficulties such as learning or behavioural problems. It is certainly worth trying to obtain the imaging without the use of sedation in these children. The use of a play specialist and familiarization with the room

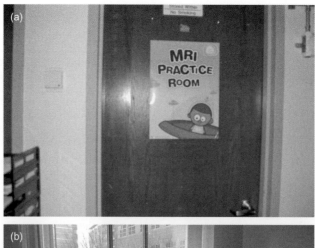

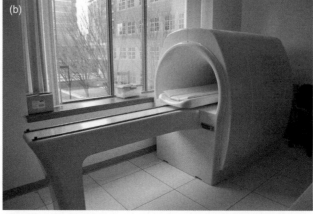

Fig. 2.3. (a, b) Personal images taken by the author of the MRI practice room and practice scanner located within the Department of Radiology, Children's Hospital of Philadelphia (March 2008).

and the equipment is often very helpful. Most children over the age of 6 will hold still for an MR study if they are distracted by music or a movie in those units fortunate enough to have audiovisual display. Those facilities fortunate enough to have a practice scanner available (Fig. 2.3) will find this especially helpful, particularly for those children who require repeated investigations, for example as part of tumour follow-up or radiotherapy staging. Fast MR techniques can also be used but most children under the age of 6 will require general anaesthesia for diagnostic MRI.

Imaging techniques
MRI is the method of choice for imaging the paediatric spine, particularly the cord. CT is a complementary technique and is useful particularly in the setting of acute trauma, and for evaluating bony or disc-based pathology, for instance scoliosis or potential infection. It

is not the method of choice (Barkovich 2005, pp1–15; Tortori-Donati 2005) when the initial presentation is with acute or progressive neurological dysfunction.

Ultrasound can be used in neonates and very young infants to exclude major developmental spine pathology but as the child grows older it becomes less useful, because ossification of the posterior elements of the spinal column limits the acoustic window from 3 to 4 months of age. It also remains debatable whether ultrasound will detect a fatty filum if the conus medullaris is at a normal level. If ultrasound does pick up an abnormality, then MRI is still required as it has been shown to pick up additional pathology in about 20% of cases (Rohrschneider et al. 1996).

Computed radiography/digital radiography of the spine is rarely used in either the adult or paediatric populations other than in evaluating congenital scoliosis (Musson et al. 2010) and assessing instability in cases of trauma or after surgical fusion and stabilization procedures.

Other techniques for evaluating the spinal cord include CT myelography in those patients where MRI is not possible; this would be unlikely in the paediatric age group. The vascular anatomy can be evaluated by non-invasive methods including magnetic resonance angiography and CT angiography; occasionally spinal catheter contrast angiography is still required for full evaluation and possible endovascular therapy of pathologies such as arteriovenous malformations.

Other techniques that are used for spinal imaging include nuclear medicine/isotope examinations, but these would rarely be used in evaluating the spinal cord as they are more suited for the vertebral marrow and other bone or disc-based pathologies.

It is extremely important that any imaging is closely correlated with history and clinical examination. Spinal cord dysfunction may present acutely, subacutely, or with chronic symptoms, and the symptoms may be very similar in many causes. Both compressive (surgical) and medical diseases can give rise to myelopathy, and clinical examination is extremely important to try to determine the site of the cord pathology. For instance, it is relevant to the radiologist whether the posterior columns are involved or spared when evaluating signal change within the cord. Knowledge of any abnormal cerebrospinal fluid (CSF) or serum results is helpful in decision making about which imaging sequences to use and whether contrast administration is likely to be helpful.

Spinal ultrasound

Ultrasound of the neonatal spine is a sensitive, readily available screening tool that is useful in evaluating the neonatal spine and cord (Aetna 2010). The recent advances in ultrasound mean that image quality is of similar diagnostic value to that of MRI in neonates. The main advantages of the technique are that it is readily available, can be performed either in the ultrasound department or on the neonatal unit with a portable machine and that sedation is not necessary.

Furthermore, this technique can then be used to decide whether any potential lesion requires urgent intervention or whether further diagnostic evaluation with MRI can be delayed until the patient is older and more magnetic resonance compatible, and when therapeutic intervention is likely to follow (Lowe et al. 2007a).

The examination is performed using a linear probe to obtain images in both the sagittal and axial plane along the spine. Different authors recommend different probe frequencies (7.5–10MHz [Dick et al. 2002] or 5–12Mhz [Lowe et al. 2007a]). The vertebral level is best determined by identifying the 12th rib and then counting from the lumbosacral junction or the tip of the coccyx. In cases of spinal dysraphism or complex vertebral body or rib abnormalities, it may be difficult to establish precisely the vertebral level and in that case correlation with radiographs may be helpful. On occasion, colour or Doppler ultrasound can be used to try to characterize any soft-tissue masses.

Neonatal ultrasound is generally possible up to the age of approximately 3 to 4 months as by that stage the posterior spinal elements will ossify from their original cartilaginous state and the acoustic window will therefore disappear.

The neonate is generally imaged prone, lying on a pillow, but imaging with the patient in a decubitus position is also possible.

The normal cord is identified as a tubular hypo-echoic structure with hyper-echoic walls. The central canal can be recognized as being hyper-echoic and the subarachnoid space surrounding the cord is hypo-echoic. The vertebral bodies are seen as echogenic structures lying anterior to the spinal cord. The important imaging features to note during the investigation include (1) the position of the conus medullaris, (2) the position of the cord within the spinal canal, (3) the presence of normal pulsatile movement of the cord and nerve roots, and (4) the thickness of the filum terminale (Dick et al. 2002).

It is essential for the ultrasonographer to appreciate that there are many normal variants that may simulate disorders so as to avoid misinterpretation and over-diagnosis, which could lead to referrals for inappropriate further imaging, possibly with the use of sedation or anaesthesia (Lowe et al. 2007b). The most common normal variants that may be confused with pathology include the following:

- Ventriculus terminalis
- Prominent filum terminale which should be recognized by the fact that the thickness is within normal limits and it has a normal midline course
- Pseudomass. This may result from clumping of nerve roots of the cauda equina and is a positional factor that may occur if the infant is scanned in the decubitus position. If an apparent mass is seen, turning the infant prone should resolve the appearances
- Unusual appearance of the coccyx. The coccyx can vary significantly in size and shape and on occasion may give rise to an apparent mass that could be palpated.

A competent and experienced sonographer will be familiar with these normal variants

Indications for spinal ultrasound in neonates include the following:

- Neonates with other congenital anomalies
- Complicated sacral dimple (located above the gluteal crease, where the bottom of the pit is not seen, where there is possible drainage of the dimple and where there are skin stigmata)

- A soft-tissue mass
- Where there has been inability to or failed lumbar puncture, which may suggest the presence of a subdural mass or collection (Lowe et al. 2007).

Low-risk lesions are simple midline dimples, without associated stigmata. High-risk lesions include atypical dimples, haemangiomas, hairy patches and skin tags, and lesions that are associated with CSF leakage. MRI remains the study of choice when surgical therapy is likely to be required, for example with open spinal dysraphism or where there is obvious CSF drainage from a skin dimple or sinus tract.

The obvious advantage of spinal ultrasound is that it allows screening and characterization of potential spinal abnormalities during the first days of life and is more readily available than MRI. It may also benefit the patient in that future imaging may be delayed till the child is older and therapeutic intervention is likely to be required; in many cases it will obviate the need for further imaging but in those patients who are likely to require surgical exploration and treatment, it is not likely to be the definitive diagnostic tool and spinal MRI will need to be used as a complementary method (Fig. 2.4).

Spinal MRI

MRI is the imaging method of choice for most conditions presenting with spinal cord dysfunction in children. The ultimate choice of scanning sequences and parameters may well be determined by a combination of the equipment available to the neuroradiologist, the clinical presentation and suspected pathology, and the clinical status of the individual patient. In some cases only a very rapid limited examination may be appropriate to avoid the use of anaesthesia; in others, long examinations such as those for the investigation of scoliosis are performed under anaesthesia and the examination should then be tailored to address fully all potential underlying abnormalities and answer all clinical questions.

There is a vast array of basic magnetic resonance pulse sequences available when designing protocols for imaging the spine and the optimal magnetic resonance technique may vary considerably depending on the type of scanner used, the region of interest, and the pathological process being studied. Some sequences take considerably longer than others and may only be appropriate if the child is able to keep still or is anaesthetized; differing sequences are susceptible to the presence of artefact, particularly chemical shift effect or susceptibility artefact due to the presence of any metal, possibly in the postoperative spine where there has been surgical implantation of stabilization devices.

Spin echo has high signal:noise and contrast:noise ratios but takes longer to acquire than gradient echo or fast spin-echo techniques. In most modern imaging protocols, fast spin-echo sequences are used as these can be obtained more quickly and they are generally applied in the sagittal and coronal plane. Gradient echo sequences have a shorter acquisition time but are more sensitive to chemical shift effect and any field inhomogeneity, so they are less useful in evaluating the postoperative spine. They are, however, good at evaluating cord signal change and are thus useful in evaluating myelopathy. Volume sequences (two- or three-dimensional) are useful in the axial plane to evaluate the exit foramena and nerve roots but are less sensitive at evaluating cord signal change.

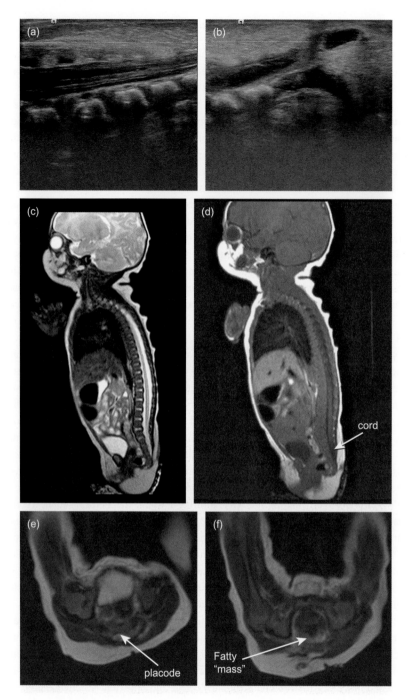

Fig. 2.4. (a, b) The ultrasound findings of a low-lying tethered cord and associated lipomyelomeningocoele. (c, d) Sagittal T_2- and T_1-weighted MRI scans obtained a few days later showing the low-lying tethered cord and lipomyelomengicolele. (e, f) Axial T_2-weighted MRI scans showing the neural placode extending into the fatty mass (arrows).

In summary, there is no single prescription for spinal cord imaging and the choice of imaging sequences will depend on the scanner, the patient, the clinical indication, and the supervising neuroradiologist.

In essence, it is important to obtain the highest resolution imaging possible for full evaluation of the spinal cord and thus ultra-thin sequences are suggested to cover the cord adequately, with less emphasis on the peripheral bony structures. The use of gradient moment nulling or flow compensation is extremely important in children, because they have very pulsatile CSF flow which causes significant artefact and loss of image quality. These artefacts (Fig. 2.5) may, on occasion, be misinterpreted as pathology. Gradient moment nulling or flow compensation is an option available on most commercial scanners and must be used routinely on long repetition time sequences (T_2, fluid-attenuated inversion recovery [FLAIR], and inversion recovery sequences).

When evaluating the cord, it is necessary to ensure that both the craniocervical junction and the cord termination are adequately demonstrated on the study. This means that the entire spinal column, including the sacral segments, should be included such that accurate localization of cord termination can be ascertained. If a surgical lesion is identified, it is essential that a method is provided whereby accurate localization can be determined. This

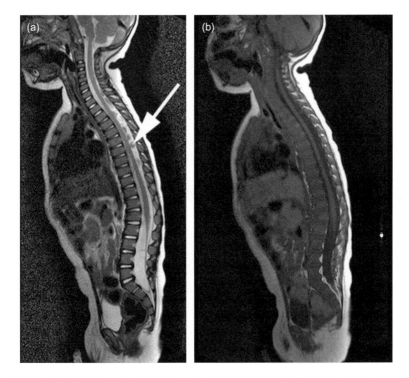

Fig. 2.5. (a) Sagittal T_2-weighted MRI scan showing apparent mass lesion posterior to the cord in the thoracic region as a result of turbulent CSF flow. White arrowhead indicates flow artefact. (b) Equivalent sagittal T_1-weighted scan which is not as susceptible to flow artefact, showing that the apparent lesions are not real. Flow nulling techniques should be used to avoid any potential misdiagnosis.

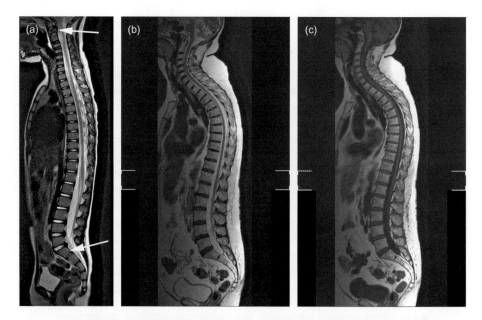

Fig. 2.6. (a) Sagittal T_2-weighted MRI scan demonstrating all the vertebral bodies such that accurate localization of any lesion level can be obtained. In a young child, this is often possible using a large field of view, but in larger children or adults the entire spine may not be demonstrated on a single sequence. Overlap and a method of identifying the level of any pathology is essential. Arrows demonstrate the C1 and S1 vertebral bodies. (b, c) The Philips Mobiview solution to allow a full image of the spinal canal to be obtained, even if the acquisitions are obtained in two separate scans (c, sagittal T_1-weighted scan).

means that a counting scan on which all vertebral segments are present is provided, typically in a single large field of view; alternatively there must be overlap of smaller fields of view by using an oil capsule to allow localization, or with modern software it may be possible to provide a full image of the spinal canal, even if the data are obtained in separate acquisitions (Fig. 2.6).

The choice of coil is important as it will significantly affect image quality. The choice will again be individual and may depend on the hardware available, and the size and age of the child. In the absence of dedicated paediatric coils, neonates are often imaged using the adult head coil; young infants can be imaged using either an adult extremity coil or in some cases an adult head and neck combined neurovascular coil. The advantage of extremity coils is that they generally are transmit/receive coils as opposed to simply receivers of radio frequency energy and as such increase field homogeneity and signal:noise ratio. If such a solution is possible, it may be practical to improve spatial resolution while being able to reduce imaging time and thus movement artefact.

In summary, when imaging the spinal cord, different techniques will be used or useful depending on both the clinical situation and the availability of scanner hardware and software. In the following section, examples are given of differing suggested imaging techniques for varying clinical situations.

IMAGING A CHILD WITH SUSPECTED OR CONFIRMED SPINAL DYSRAPHISM

In most cases, sagittal, axial, and coronal images will be required to demonstrate any potential malformation accurately. It is essential that the entire spinal column is imaged, and the sacrum must be included on the examinations to allow precise localization of cord termination. This is extremely relevant in cases of caudal regression syndrome. T_1-weighted sequences in the sagittal plane using 3mm slice thickness are often the most useful initial investigation. Axial images can then be obtained through any area of abnormality or suspected abnormality. Both axial T_1- and T_2-weighted sequences are useful, and high-resolution fast spin-echo T_2-weighted images are very useful when looking for dermoids or complications of cord tethering such as hydromyelia. The advantage of the T_1-weighted images is that they do not show the flow artefacts that are common on the T_2-weighted images and they are very useful at demonstrating any lipomas or abnormal fatty tissue. High-resolution T_2-weighted images are better at demonstrating the nerve roots of the cauda equina, any adhesions, and any possible bony or fibrous spurs. Diastematomyelia is the most challenging condition to diagnose on MRI as it is not always possible to identify the bony spur or the fibrous band. High-resolution three-dimensional CT is a useful adjunct in this case (Tortori-Donati et al. 2000, Tortori-Donati 2005, pp1551–1606) (Figs 2.7 and 2.8).

IMAGING THE CHILD WITH SUSPECTED CORD TRAUMA

The initial evaluation of spinal column or spinal cord trauma will be by plain radiographs or more likely helical CT. This allows accurate evaluation of the bony structures but does not allow evaluation of the cartilage, ligaments or spinal cord. Sagittal fast spin-echo T_1- and T_2-weighted images should be obtained using thin-section 3mm slices, to allow evaluation of the cord for the presence of contusion, oedema, or potential ischaemia. Supplementary axial planes are used if there is any evidence of spinal cord compression. The use of sagittal short-inversion recovery time (STIR) sequences (fat-suppressed fast spin-echo T_2-weighted images) is useful for evaluating vertebral body oedema and any associated ligamentous injury. Ligamentous lesions will be visualized as hyperintense signal on the STIR sequences, involving predominantly the posterior longitudinal ligament and the interspinous and super-spinous ligaments. This may be the only sign that an injury is potentially unstable (Figs 2.9 and 2.10).

MRI may also be required in evaluating the child after previous spinal cord trauma for late complications such as cord atrophy or the development of post-traumatic syringomyelia, or the development of a progressive neurogenic scoliosis.

The main indication for MRI of the cord potentially affected by trauma is in those cases where there are spinal cord symptoms and/or signs with negative radiological evaluation by means of routine radiographs: the so-called spinal cord injury without radiological abnormality (SCIWORA) syndrome.

IMAGING THE CHILD WITH SCOLIOSIS

These patients often present an imaging challenge and require long investigations, usually under general anaesthesia. It is extremely important to liaise closely with the referring clinician and in particular the spinal surgeon as corrective surgery may also require bony

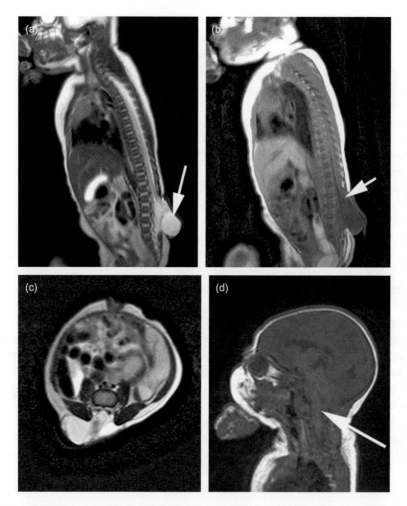

Fig. 2.7. (a) Sagittal T$_2$-weighted MRI sequence of a 1-day-old neonate showing open lumbosacral myelomeningocele (white arrow). These images were obtained after a feed with the infant wrapped in a blanket and imaged in the adult head coil. (b) Sagittal T$_1$-weighted sequence of 1-day-old neonate showing open lumbosacral myelomeningocele. On the T$_1$-weighted sequence the neural placode is more clearly identified within the sac (white arrow). (c) Axial T$_2$-weighted image at the level of the open myelomeningocele demonstrating the sac extending through the posterior fusion defect into the subcutaneous tissues and to the overlying skin. (d) Sagittal T$_1$-weighted sequence of the same child demonstrating associated Chiari II malformation with the cerebellar tonsils through the level of the foramen magnum (arrow).

imaging with high-resolution three-dimensional CT and multiplanar reformats. It is often useful to obtain both investigations under the same anaesthesia if the two scanning suites are co-located.

Initially, coronal T$_1$- or T$_2$-weighted images are best obtained to allow assessment of vertebral anomalies and planning of subsequent sagittal sequences. In many cases, several

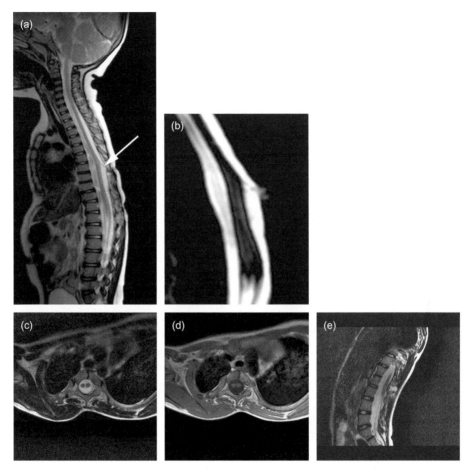

Fig. 2.8. (a) Sagittal T_2-weighted MRI sequence in a 7-year-old child who presented with a leaking lesion in mid-thoracic region. The conventional T_2-weighted sequence shows minor posterior displacement of the spinal cord with a dorsal dermal sinus track extending through the subarachnoid space into the overlying soft tissues (white arrow). (b) Sagittal reformat from high-resolution three-dimensional volume T_2-weighted acquisition demonstrating more detail of the spinal cord and the intraspinal tract. (c–e) Images demonstrating diastomatemyelia on MRI. Note the importance of acquiring at least two scan planes as the sagittal T_2-weighted sequence may be interpreted as normal.

oblique sagittal and axial planes will be required to give optimum information about the cord and to provide thorough imaging of its entirety. The study must include the craniocervical junction and the cord termination; ideally, the sacrum should also be visualized. If any abnormality is identified, axial sequences (both T_1 and T_2 weighted) should be placed to allow full evaluation of the abnormality: it should be possible to distinguish between the split cord and a central dilated canal or syringohydromyelia. The use of axial gradient echo sequences may be helpful for evaluating the presence of a fibrous band or bony spur in

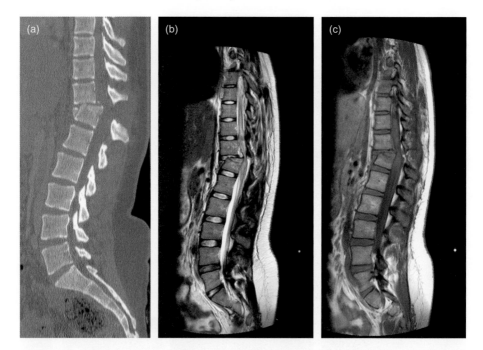

Fig. 2.9. (a–c) Sagittal CT reformat and sagittal T_2- and T_1-weighted MRI scans demonstrating a burst fracture at T12 with retropulsion of the bone causing canal compromise and cord compression, with oedema within the cord.

cases of diastematomyelia; however, as indicated in the section on imaging a child with suspected or confirmed spinal dysraphism, the use of CT is a useful adjunct for this.

Several authors have advocated the use of three-dimensional volume sequences, which may be helpful in evaluating these abnormalities (Figs 2.11 and 2.12) (Barkovich 2005, Musson et al. 2010, Kim et al. 1999, 2010).

IMAGING THE CHILD WITH SUSPECTED CRANIOCERVICAL JUNCTION PATHOLOGY
The craniocervical junction consists of the occiput, atlas, and axis. It effectively lies between the skull base and the cervical spine. It is an area that may be missed or ignored in conventional imaging unless the clinician guides the referring radiologist to disease likely to occur at this level.

There are several syndromes associated with craniocervical junction pathology. Examples include Down syndrome, Klippel–Feil syndrome, achondroplasia, osteogenesis imperfecta, and the mucopolysaccharidoses. In many of these syndromes, the pathology is considered to be due to softening of the skull base resulting in an acquired basilar invagination. In addition, congenital abnormalities such as the Chiari malformations may result in pathology at the craniocervical junction with identical or similar clinical presentation.

The clinical presentation varies and may be relatively insidious and progress slowly. The symptoms are usually attributable to compression of the neural structures at the

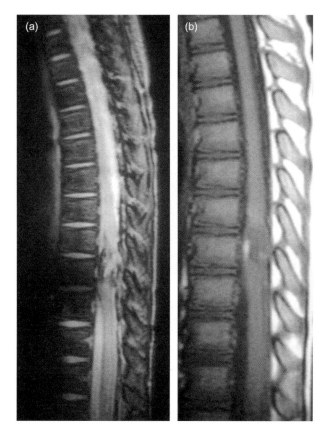

Fig. 2.10. (a, b) Sagittal T_2- and T_1-weighted MRI scans showing thoracic cord transection after hyperflexion injury without bony changes.

craniocervical junction and as such may relate to brainstem, cervical cord, cerebellum, lower cranial nerves, or cervical nerve roots.

The best method of imaging the craniocervical junction is MRI as it allows full evaluation of the soft tissues, the neural structures, and the ligaments. It will also allow contemporaneous imaging of the cranial cavity, which is a requirement in many of these patients as there may be associated congenital abnormalities or associated obstruction to intracranial CSF flow. In many, if not all, cases, there will also be the requirement of helical CT to allow full evaluation of the bony anatomy, particularly with sagittal and coronal reformats (Smoker and Khanna 2008).

One added benefit of CT is the availability or possibility of using CT angiography for preoperative planning to allow assessment of the position of the major vessels (Barker et al. 2009).

If a child presents with symptoms or signs possibly due to compression of the craniocervical junction, then MRI is the first imaging modality. Thin 3mm sagittal T_2- and

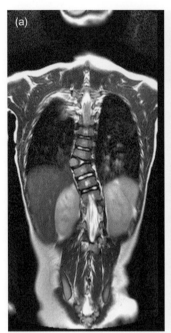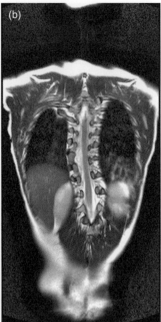

Fig. 2.11. (a, b) Sagittal and coronal T_2-weighted MRI sequences in evaluating scoliosis.

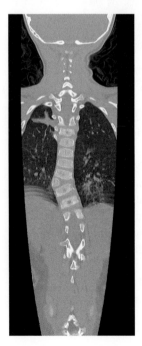

Fig. 2.12. Coronal CT reformat of the same child demonstrating bony abnormalities.

T_1-weighted sequences should be obtained to demonstrate the lower brainstem, craniocervical junction and upper cervical cord in the first instance. Depending on the imaging findings, other sequences will be tailored appropriately, and other imaging modalities such as CT examination can be prescribed.

If a cavity or syrinx is identified within the cord, confirmation that it is a cavity should be obtained by means of the T_1-weighted sequences and axial T_1- or T_2-weighted sequences should be obtained through the cavity to allow its localization within the cord. If the cavity extends into the medulla, the diagnosis of syringobulbia is made. If the cavity remains within the cord, the diagnosis of syringohydromyelia will be made. If a syrinx cavity is identified, then the search must be made for the possible cause. First, the foramen magnum must be evaluated with careful assessment of the position of the cerebellar tonsils. It is important to look for other causes of narrowing or stenosis of the foramen magnum, such as achondroplasia and other causes of basilar invagination, or mass lesions. If no abnormality is found at the craniocervical junction, then the cord termination must be carefully scrutinized for possible cord tethering. If no cause for the cavity can be made, then intravenous contrast should be administered to look for an underlying small obstructing lesion such as a tumour. A history of previous trauma, and/or infection which may have given rise to arachnoiditis, may indicate the cause of an identified syrinx cavity.

Some authors advocate the use of techniques that allow assessment of CSF flow within the ventricles and at the foramen magnum by the use of phase-contrast MRI. These techniques should allow flow dynamics of the CSF through the foramen magnum or past an obstructive lesion to be evaluated and they may be useful in the postoperative state (Brugieres et al. 2000).

It is important to recognize that not all dilatation of the central canal of the spinal cord is pathological. Petit-Lacour et al. (2000) found that in up to 1.5% of patients scanned there can be enlargement of the central canal without any associated pathology. These cavities are usually in the lower cervical or at mid-thoracic level, and they do not require follow-up. In practice, a single follow-up examination with contrast at 12 months is often considered to ensure that it is not the earliest phase of a cord neoplasm or syrinx, and any cause of cavities should obviously be excluded at the time of the examination (Fig. 2.13).

If MRI does not demonstrate classical features of syringohydromyelia/syringohydrobulbia with associated Chiari malformation, then the use of CT for evaluating the bony structures is generally recommended. In this case, one is looking for other causes of craniocervical junction compression and most of these will be related to the bony structure. Obtaining high-resolution bony imaging is important for consideration of any surgical planning or treatment. High-resolution CT with reformats in coronal and sagittal planes are typically obtained (Fig. 2.14).

The question of instability may arise in several of these patients, particularly those with Down syndrome where atlanto-axial subluxation is a recognized entity. If the child is cooperative, then flexion extension plain film examination is the method of choice; alternatively, supervised flexion extension CT of the craniocervical junction can be obtained but this does incur an increased radiation dose and requires close anaesthetic monitoring.

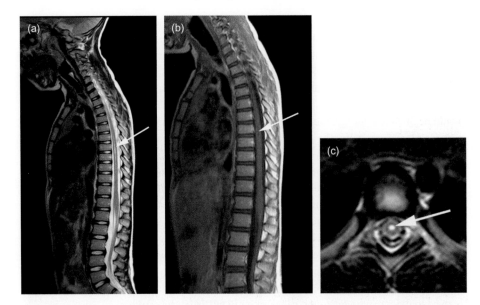

Fig. 2.13. (a) Sagittal T$_2$-weighted MRI sequence in a 7-year-old child who presented with non-specific back pain; the scan was obtained for 'reassurance'. The arrow indicates a normal mildly dilated central canal of the cord, a finding of no clinical significance. (b) Sagittal T$_1$-weighted sequence of the same child showing the linear hypointensity at the junction of the anterior and middle two-thirds of the cord and the typical distribution of the central canal (arrow). (c) Axial T$_2$-weighted scan showing the prominent but normal dilated canal of the cord (white arrow)

Achondroplasia can also lead to spinal problems at levels other than at the craniocervical junction. Many children will develop a thoracolumbar kyphosis, which may resolve spontaneously but up to 20% do not. Spinal stenosis tends to become symptomatic in later adolescence or adulthood rather than in childhood and may require imaging before consideration of surgical decompression (Barkovich 2005).

IMAGING THE CHILD WITH SUSPECTED ACQUIRED MYELOPATHY
There are a vast number of pathologies, both medical and surgical, that can give rise to symptoms of acquired myelopathy. A sagittal fast spin-echo T$_2$-weighted sequence is the best initial investigation as the subsequent examination can then be tailored on the basis of the initial imaging findings. It is important to appreciate that many pathologies can give rise to increased T$_2$ signal intensity of the cord and on imaging these may be indistinguishable. It is essential that there is a good clinical history available to the supervising neuro-radiologist so that the imaging sequences and ultimate report can be as accurate and relevant as possible. The duration of the history is essential and knowledge of any associated CSF findings is helpful in determining whether contrast administration should be considered.

It may be that the initial T$_2$-weighted sequence will be normal, which could be the result of the underlying pathology or the result of very early imaging. In those cases, the use of diffusion-weighted imaging should be considered as this may show pathology at an earlier

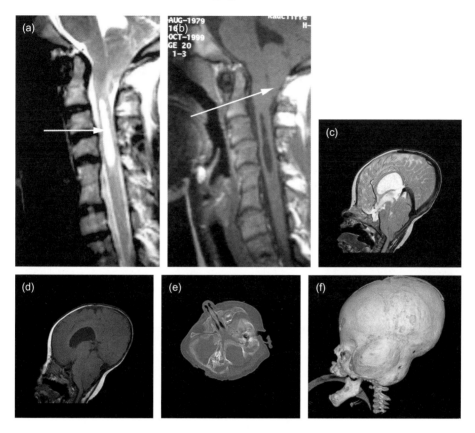

Fig. 2.14. (a) Sagittal T_2-weighted MRI scan demonstrating descent of cerebellar tonsils in keeping with Chiari I type malformation with associated syringohydromyelia. Arrow indicates syrinx cavity. (b) Sagittal T_1-weighted scan showing the same pathology with arrow indicating position of the cerebellar tonsils. (c–f) Sagittal T_2- and T_1-weighted sequences showing appearances at craniocervical junction in a child with craniosynostosis; note small posterior fossa and tonsillar descent. Axial CT and three-dimensional reformat demonstrates the bony anatomy.

stage than the conventional T_2-weighted sequence. If both these sequences are normal, then it is unlikely that the spinal cord is the cause of the clinical presentation and brain imaging should be considered. The following section will cover some of the commonest causes of acquired myelopathy, and suggested imaging techniques and findings.

Vascular disease
Ischaemic lesions of the cord do occur in children and may be arterial or venous in origin, arterial being the more likely. Children may present after minor trauma or sporting activity. The use of diffusion-weighted imaging should be considered in these patients as it may give a valuable clue to the diagnosis in the presence of normal appearing sagittal T_2-weighted sequences. Diffusion-weighted imaging has also been shown to be useful in other acute

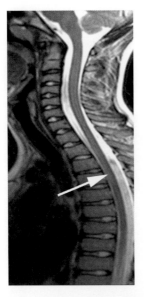

Fig. 2.15. Sagittal T$_2$-weighted MRI sequence in a 12-year-old child who presented with acute paraplegia after a baseball game. No definite abnormality is demonstrated on this examination although there is a suspicion of some increased T$_2$ signal intensity at the cervicothoracic level (see arrow).

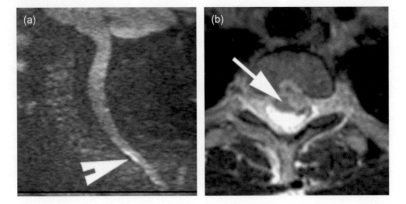

Fig. 2.16. (a) Sagittal T$_2$-weighted MRI scan of diffusion-weighted sequence in the same patient. This shows hyperintensity on the B1000 in the region of suspected abnormality in keeping with acute ischaemia (arrowhead). (b) Axial sequence demonstrating an apparent diffusion coefficient value within the cord at the level of suspected abnormality. There is hypointense signal demonstrated, in keeping with acute ischaemia (see arrow).

causes of myelopathy where the sagittal T$_2$-weighted scan has been negative (see Figs 2.15–2.17) (Marcel et al. 2010, Thurnher and Law 2009).

If spinal cord ischaemia is identified, the radiologist should also image for potential underlying causes such as neck artery dissections, particularly vertebral artery dissection.

Other vascular malformations are uncommon in the paediatric age group although intramedullary haematomas may occur as a result of arteriovenous malformations or

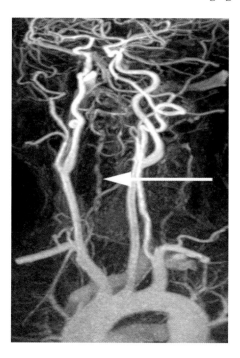

Fig. 2.17. Magnetic resonance contrast angiography demonstrating dissected right vertebral artery in a patient with spinal cord infarction (arrow).

cavernomas; dural arteriovenous fistulas are rare but are recognized in children, including those under the age of 1 year (Zuccaro 2010).

Presentation with spinal cord haemorrhage can occur as a result of intramedullary vascular malformations (Fig. 2.18). Evaluation of the spinal cord for an underlying vascular malformation by catheter angiography may be required, although in many cases no cause will be found in the acute stage. Follow-up spinal cord imaging is suggested to look for underlying vascular tumours such as haemangioblastoma or spinal cord cavernoma.

Mass lesions
In the case of a compressive aetiology, sagittal T_1 and/or STIR sequences with axial T_1- and T_2-weighted scans through the region of interest are recommended to allow full evaluation of the lesion and its extent. Contrast may be indicated although it is not always essential if the lesion is well demarcated, as in the case of a metastasis or primary bony tumour.

If an intramedullary mass lesion is identified, imaging must be tailored to demonstrate the precise extent, location, and internal structure of the mass, to try to narrow the differential diagnosis and guide future surgery and treatment. The MRI technique should include sagittal T_1- and T_2-weighted scans, with sagittal T_1-weighted scans after contrast enhancement and axial T_1- and/or T_2-weighted scans through the area of interest. The entire spinal canal should be imaged to evaluate the possibility of multifocal disease. Contrast-enhanced cranial imaging is also recommended to exclude associated intracranial pathology/dissemination. The use of gradient echo sequences should be considered if there is any possibility

41

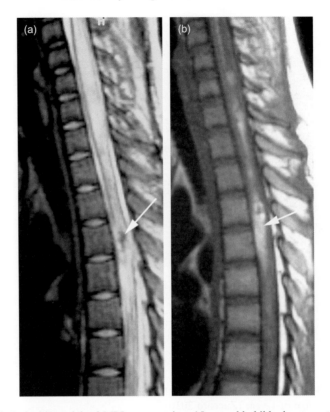

Fig. 2.18. (a) Sagittal T_2-weighted MRI sequence in a 15-year-old child who presented with acute paraplegia after a bicycle ride. This image shows oedema within the cord, which is swollen with a central hypointense area in keeping with acute haemorrhage (arrows). (b) Sagittal T_1-weighted scan in the same patient showing hyperintensity within the cord in keeping with acute to subacute haemorrhage (see arrow). Subsequent spinal angiography revealed no cause and nor did follow-up imaging. Presumed diagnosis is of cryptic intramedullary arteriovenous malformation.

of blood or blood breakdown products as this may again narrow the differential diagnosis (see Figs 2.19–2.21) (Do-Dai et al. 2010).

If a mass lesion is identified, the aim of the examination should be to allow precise localization of the mass. The report should state whether the lesion is intra- or extradural, and, if intradural, whether it is intra- or extra-medullary. The relationship to the cord and adjacent bony and soft-tissue structures should be described. The presence of any cord compression or intrinsic cord signal change should be documented. The precise level of the lesion should also be documented, ensuring that a counting scan is available to allow accurate surgical localization.

It is not possible to state accurately whether there is a plane of cleavage in many of these lesions; radiology has not shown high predictive value for this. It is, however, essential to identify the site of any contrast enhancement or solid portions of a tumour as these may guide surgical resection and biopsy. In the case of craniocervical or cervicomedullary

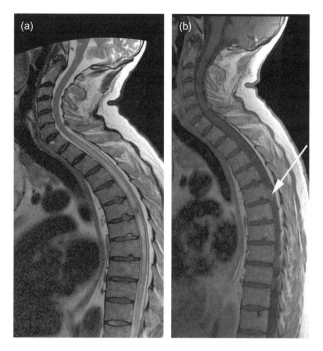

Fig. 2.19. (a) Sagittal T_2-weighted MRI scan showing the effects of an intramedullary metastasis with extensive associated oedema, distal and caudal to the lesion. (b) Sagittal T_1-weighted scan after contrast administration showing the enhancing lesion at the level of T5 (arrow).

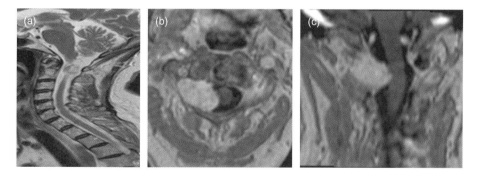

Fig. 2.20. (a) Sagittal T_2-weighted MRI scan showing lesion at the level of the craniocervical junction. On this sagittal sequence it is difficult to decide whether the lesion is intra or extra medullary. (b) Axial T_1-weighted sequence after contrast administration showing that the lesion is intradural but extramedullary, extending through a widened exit foramen in keeping with schwannoma. (c) Coronal T_1-weighted scan after contrast administration showing position of the extramedullary intradural mass lesion on the right.

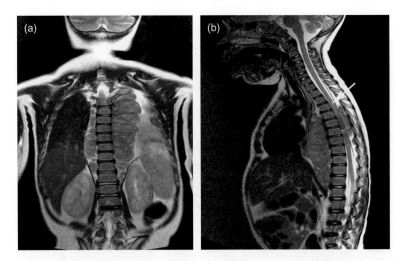

Fig. 2.21. (a) Coronal T_1-weighted MRI sequence showing extensive mediastinal involvement of intradural extramedullary gangliocytoma. This shows the benefit of coronal imaging in all spinal pathologies. (b) Sagittal T_2-weighted scan of childhood gangliocytoma showing the mediastinal component and the associated intraspinal component leading to cord compression. Note the high signal within the cord in keeping with oedema (arrow).

tumours, it is essential to obtain high-quality imaging to assess for any exophytic component as this may indicate a site of surgical biopsy or resection.

There are other pathologies that can give rise to mass lesions or compressive myelopathy. Trauma and infection may present with intraspinal mass lesions, and haemorrhage should be recognized by the imaging characteristics in the context of an appropriate history. Infection is usually associated with bone or disc-based changes, which should be identified on sagittal STIR sequences and will be delineated when using intravenous contrast on T_1-weighted sequences.

Inflammatory lesions
Most inflammatory causes of myelopathy will present with increased signal on the T_2-weighted sequence. The entire spinal cord should be evaluated for the presence of multiple lesions, and any lesion identified should be carefully evaluated to assess its precise extent. The extent of the signal change should be evaluated and the position on the axial scans should be reported. In classic inflammatory demyelination (multiple sclerosis), lesions are typically short, approximately 1.5 vertebral bodies in maximum length. They tend to be located posteriorly within the cord involving the posterior columns. They are often eccentrically located within the cord. They may be multiple. Acute lesions are often associated with mild cord swelling and, if contrast is administered, there may be pathological enhancement. Chronic lesions may be associated with cord atrophy.

In children, most acute inflammatory demyelination will be as a result of acute disseminated encephalomyelitis or as a result of neuromyelitis optica. The imaging findings

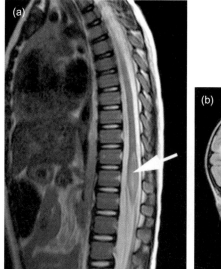
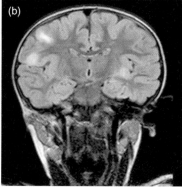

Fig. 2.22. (a) Sagittal T$_2$-weighted MRI scan of the thoracic cord demonstrating hyperintense signal on T$_2$-weighting signal with swelling at the level of the conus (arrow). This was the presentation in a child with acute disseminated encephalomyelitis. (b) Coronal fluid-attenuated inversion recovery (FLAIR) sequence of the brain in the same patient showing evidence of signal alteration in the cortex and subcortical white matter in keeping with acute disseminated encephalomyelitis.

may be very similar with extensive lesions within the cord up to seven to eight vertebral bodies in length. The lesions of neuromyelitis optica are typically central within the cord and may be associated with T$_1$ hypointensity. In the acute stages, the cord is often swollen and there may be contrast enhancement. The lesions of acute disseminated encephalomyelitis may be similarly longitudinally extensive and both conditions fall into the category now recognized as longitudinally extensive transverse myelitis. Contrast enhancement may be recognized in acute disseminated encephalomyelitis, and the T$_1$ hypointensity is less classical (Downer et al. 2012). On imaging findings alone, it may not be possible to distinguish between the two conditions; the full clinical picture and the use of adjunctive tests, including myelin oligodendrocyte glycoprotein and aquaporin-4 antibody evaluation, are necessary.

There are many other causes of an inflammatory demyelination that may also occur in the paediatric age group, although they are less common. Sarcoidosis and infective agents can give rise to identical imaging findings.

Sagittal T$_1$-weighted sequences should be obtained to look for hypointensity and to confirm that the T$_2$ signal change is not due to cystic change or cavitation as a result of hydromyelia. Contrast administration may be helpful in some cases, particularly if there is suspicion of an infectious aetiology or where the CSF is abnormal either in cytology or protein content (Figs 2.22–2.24).

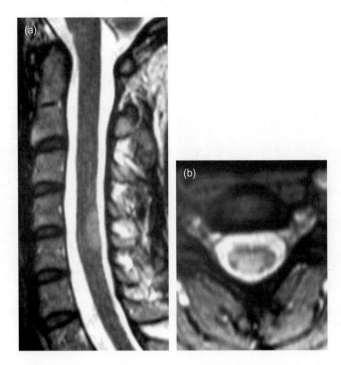

Fig. 2.23. (a) Sagittal T_2-weighted MRI scan showing typical lesion in multiple sclerosis. The lesion is less than 1.5 vertebral bodies in length, it occupies predominantly the posterior part of the cord, and there is minimal cord swelling. (b) Axial T_2-weighted scan of a patient with multiple sclerosis showing typical lesion affecting the posterior columns of the cord.

IMAGING THE FETAL SPINE

Fetal MRI has become established clinical practice in many parts of the world as complementary to antenatal ultrasound. Ultrasound of the fetal spine is a good imaging modality and is often more accurate than MRI in the precise localization of the defect and particularly the level. Although MRI of the spine and spinal cord does not necessarily offer significant advantage over the ultrasonography findings, the advantage of fetal MRI is that it does allow better evaluation of the brain and any associated posterior fossa or hindbrain abnormalities such as Chiari II malformation and cerebellar tonsillar ectopia. In the UK, fetal MRI after 20 weeks' gestation is generally obtained without any maternal sedation or fasting. The mother is scanned lying either supine or semi-recumbent, using a dedicated phased-array pelvis coil. Images are generally obtained using single-shot fast spin-echo T_2-weighted sequences, in the sagittal, coronal, and axial planes (Fig. 2.25) (Jokhi and Whitby 2011).

IMAGING THE BRAIN IN THE ASSESSMENT OF SPINAL CORD PATHOLOGY

In many cases, where the clinical presentation and symptomatology is a result of spinal cord disease, it may be appropriate to obtain tailored brain imaging at the time of the spinal investigation.

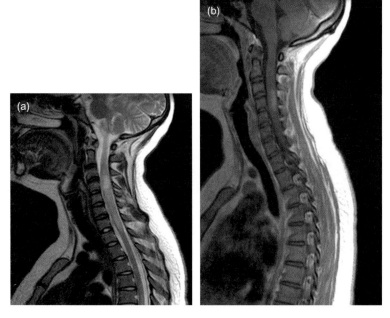

Fig. 2.24. (a) Sagittal T_2-weighted MRI scan showing a linearly extensive transverse myelitis in the cervical cord. The differential diagnosis lies between atypical multiple sclerosis, neuromyelitis optica, and acute disseminated encephalomyelitis. (b) Sagittal T_1-weighted scan after contrast administration showing enhancement of portion of the hyperintense lesion; this indicates acute pathology although it does not differentiate between the various differential diagnoses.

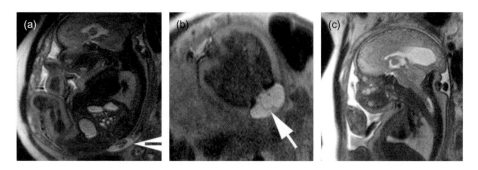

Fig. 2.25. (a) Sagittal T_2-weighted single-shot MRI sequence of the fetus showing a myelomeningocele (arrow). Detail of the spinal canal is not as good as might be obtained with ultrasound imaging, but the advantage of this technique is that it allows more careful evaluation of the craniocervical junction. (b) Axial sequence at the level of the myelomeningocele showing the large posterior fusion defect and meningocele sac (arrow). (c) Sagittal T_2-weighted sequence of the same fetus showing the Chiari II type malformation with relative absence of the fourth ventricle and the descent of the cerebellar tonsils leading to crowding at the craniocervical junction.

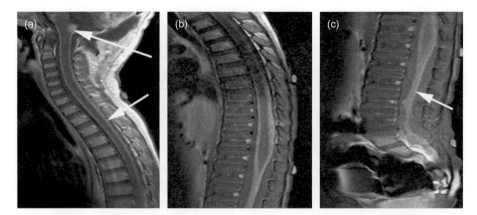

Fig. 2.26. (a) Sagittal T₁-weighted MRI scan of cervical and upper thoracic region in a 12-year-old child who presented with progressive quadriparesis. This shows extensive pathological enhancement within the subarachnoid space, in keeping with subarachnoid seeding or deposit. Notice the focal abnormality within the floor of the fourth ventricle, which was the site of the primary medulloblastoma (see arrows). (b) Sagittal T₁-weighted scan with contrast administration at the thoraco-lumbar region. Again there is pathological enhancement of the subarachnoid space with coating of the nerve roots of the cauda equina. (c) Sagittal T₁-weighted scan after contrast administration of lumbar and sacral region showing intensive enhancement within the cauda equina and dural space (arrow).

If a congenital spinal abnormality is demonstrated, then imaging of the entire neuraxis is suggested as there is association of cranial and spinal developmental abnormalities. It is also important to assess the ventricles, particularly for craniocervical junction abnormality or spinal cord disease where surgical intervention is proposed. It is thus suggested that in all patients who present with spinal dysraphism or who are being evaluated for a complex scoliosis with progressive neurology, full brain and spinal canal imaging is obtained.

In those children who present with apparent spinal cord disease, for instance gait disturbance or difficulties, then unless a cause for the symptomatology is demonstrated on spinal imaging, views of the brain should also be obtained. This is particularly relevant in patients who present with a progressive gait disorder.

The brain should be imaged in patients who are diagnosed with spinal tumours and spinal infection. Both pathologies can affect the entire neuraxis, and staging of spinal tumours is essential at the time of diagnosis. One should also remember that spinal cord dissemination may be a result of an intracranial primary tumour (classically, posterior fossa tumours) although the clinical presentation may be spine based. If leptomeningeal enhancement is demonstrated, then an intracranial cause of spinal seeding or dissemination must be excluded at the time of imaging (Fig. 2.26).

The question of whether to image the brain in cases of inflammatory demyelination is more difficult. If there are neurological manifestations in keeping with intracranial disease, then it is mandatory to obtain brain imaging, irrespective of what the spinal imaging shows. If the presentation is with a pure spinal (clinically isolated) syndrome, then the radiologist should be guided by the referring paediatric neurologist as to whether it is appropriate to obtain brain imaging at the time of the initial acute episode; however, a low threshold for such imaging is prudent given that silent brain demyelination may be present with significant diagnostic implications. If there are repeated episodes of inflammatory demyelination, then it is recommended that brain imaging should be obtained to look for dissemination in space as well as in time, to aid in the potential diagnosis of multiple sclerosis or other inflammatory demyelinating pathologies.

Summary

Imaging of the cord in children should be tailored according to the age, clinical presentation, and degree of cooperation of the child. Close relationships between imagers and their referrers are the most useful method of ensuring that any imaging examination effectively addresses the clinical question it is designed to answer.

REFERENCES

Aetna. Clinical policy bulletin: spinal ultrasound, number 0628. [Internet]. Hartford, CT: Aetna; 2010. Available from: http://www.aetna.com/cpb/medical/data/600_699/0628.html.

Barker R, Fareedi S, Thompson D. The use of CT angiography in the preoperative planning of cervical surgery in children. *Childs Nerv Syst* 2009; **25**: 955–959.

Barkovich J. Pediatric Neuroimaging (4th edition). Philadelphia, PA: Lippincott Williams & Wilkins, 2005.

Brugieres P, Idy-Perettia I, Iffeneckera C, et al. CSF flow measurements in syringomyelia. *Am J Neuroradiol* 2000; **21**: 1785–1792.

Dick E, Patal K, Owens C, de Bruyn R. Spinal ultrasound in infants. *Br J Radiol* 2002; **75**: 384–392.

Do-Dai DD, Brookes NK, et al. Magnetic resonance imaging of intramedullary spinal cord lesions: a pictorial review. *Curr Probl Diagn Radiol* 2010; **39**: 160–185.

Downer JJ, Leite MI, Carter R, et al. Diagnosis of neuromyelitis optica (NMO) spectrum disorders: is MRI obsolete? *Neuroradiology* 2012; **54**: 279–285.

Harwood-Nash DC, Fitz CR. Neuroradiology in Infants and Children. St Louis, MO: CV Mosby, 1973.

Jokhi RP, Whitby EH. Magnetic resonance imaging of the foetus. *Dev Med Child Neurol* 2011; **53**: 18–28.

Kim FM, Poussaint TY, Barnes PD. Neuroimaging of scoliosis in childhood. *Neuroimaging Clin N Am* 1999; **9**: 195–221.

Kim H, Kim HS, Moon ES, Yoon CS. Scoliosis imaging: what radiologists should know. *Radiographics* 2010; **30**: 1823–1842.

Lowe L, Johanek A, Moore C. Sonography of the neonatal spine: part 1, normal anatomy, imaging pitfalls, and variations that may simulate disorders. *AJR Am J Roentgenol* 2007a; **188**: 733–738.

Lowe L, Johanek A, Moore C. Sonography of the neonatal spine: part 2, spinal disorders. *AJR Am J Roentgenol* 2007b; **188**: 739–744.

Marcel C, Kramer S, Jeantroux J, et al. Diffusion weighted imaging and non-compressive myelopathies: a 33 patient prospective study. *J Neurol* 2010; **257**: 1438–1445.

Musson RE, Warren DJ, Bickle I, Connolly DJ, Griffiths PD. Imaging in childhood scoliosis: a pictorial review. *Postgrad Med J* 2010; **86**: 419–427.

Petit-Lacour MC, Lasjaunias P, Iffenecker C, et al. Visibility of the central canal on MRI. *Neuroradiology* 2000; **42**: 756–761.

Rohrschneider WK, Forsting M, Darge K, Tröger J. Diagnostic value of spinal ultrasound: comparative study with MR imaging in paediatric patients. *Radiology* 1996; **200**: 383–388.

Royal College of Radiologists. Publications and Guidance, Reference number BFCR(03)4, Safe Sedation, Analgesia and Anaesthesia within the Radiology Department. London: Royal College of Radiologists, 2003.

Smoker WRK, Khanna G. Imaging the craniocervical junction. *Childs Nerv Syst* 2008; **24**: 1123–1145.

Thurner MM, Law M. Diffusion weighted imaging, diffusion tensor imaging and fibre tractography of the spinal cord. *Magn Reson Imaging Clin N Am* 2009; **17**: 225–244.

Tortori-Donati P, Rossi A, Camma A. Spinal dysraphism: a review of neuroradiological features with embryological correlations and proposal for a new classification. *Neuroradiology* 2000; **42**: 471–491.

Tortori-Donati P, editor. Pediatric Neuroradiology, vol 2, Head, Neck and Spine. Berlin and Heidelberg: Springer, 2005.

Zuccaro G. Neurosurgical vascular malformations in children under one year of age. *Childs Nerv Syst* 2010; **26**: 1381–1394.

3
CLINICAL NEUROPHYSIOLOGY OF THE SPINAL CORD

Ravi Knight

Introduction

Neurophysiological assessment of the paediatric spinal cord is part of the clinical neurological evaluation of spinal cord dysfunction, and the clinical neurophysiologist participates in the diagnosis as well as in decisions that involve treatment. Conduction in the nervous system is essentially an electrical process, and current electrophysiological methods extend the clinical evaluation of sensory and motor dysfunction by refining the localization of neuropathology, by assessing severity, and by complementing neuroimaging techniques. Although magnetic resonance imaging (MRI) is now very sensitive at identifying anatomical lesions, clinical neurophysiological methods are useful in evaluating disordered function at a subclinical level, as part of the diagnostic process, as well as in monitoring spinal cord function, for instance in elective or emergency surgery.

The infant and child pose a special challenge to the clinical neurophysiologist, not only by virtue of size, and physical and emotional vulnerability, but also because of the effect of evolving and developing physiological processes such as neuronal maturation and myelination. Techniques used in adults are mostly transferrable to children with a few modifications, however. The child's cooperation is probably the single most important determinant of a successful study. It may not be possible to perform an extensive evaluation, and compromise will be needed between the completion of a comprehensive recording on the one hand and obtaining the key clinically relevant data from a more limited record on the other. Experienced technologists who enjoy working with children are essential to the success of the team. Clinical neurophysiologists should be aware of the finely judged balance involved in performing and interpreting a clinically relevant paediatric study.

Although the spinal cord comprises several ascending and descending pathways linking the peripheral with the central nervous system, for electrophysiological evaluation it is useful to envisage the spinal cord as comprising essentially two domains: the somatosensory (or posterior) and the motor (or anterior). The former includes the pre-ganglionic sensory roots (i.e. proximal to the dorsal root ganglia); the latter, the motor roots. An overview of the techniques involved in evaluating each of these domains, and their clinical applications, are discussed in the subsequent paragraphs. It is useful at the outset to review the fundamental aspects of physiology and spinal cord development relevant to the electrophysiologist.

Neuronal tissue is characterized by excitability, polarity, and spatial compartmentalization of cell function (Kandell 2000). The polarity of the nerve cell membrane is due to the ionic imbalance between sodium, calcium, and chloride on the outside of the cell, and potassium within the cell, that is maintained by selectively permeable ion channels. The equilibrium potential across a cell membrane depends upon the transmembrane concentration gradient as well as the electrical potential of the various ions, and is governed by the Nernst equation. The Goldman equation takes into consideration the relative contribution of different ions to the resting membrane potential. Polarity across the neuronal cell membrane and concentration of the extracellular ions is maintained by an energy-dependent sodium/potassium (Na/K) pump by the hydrolysis of adenosine triphosphate (ATP).

Ion channels, which are transmembrane proteins forming a hydrophilic pore, maintain membrane polarity by passively allowing ions in and out of cells, and are activated by the interaction between the electrochemical ionic gradient and the physicochemical properties of the pore. These include voltage-gated channels that respond to changes in membrane potential, ligand-gated channels that undergo configurational change in response to binding with a neurotransmitter and chemically (ATP)-gated channels (Hodgkin and Huxley 1952a, b).

Action potentials are generated by ionic flow through voltage-gated channels, and allow rapid transmission of information in the nervous system. At rest, the membrane potential is near the equilibrium potential of potassium. At threshold potential, there is a rapid influx of sodium ions through voltage-gated sodium channels when the membrane potential reaches a threshold of approximately 60mV, making the interior of the cell more positive, followed by the opening of potassium channels and the efflux of potassium. Inward sodium conductance is brief but of the order of 10^3, whereas that of potassium egress increases only to about 30-fold, but persists for longer. Sodium channels display transitions between the three states of rest, activation, and inactivation during an action potential, depending upon the duration of depolarization. The resting state is reached after brief depolarization while the channel is inactive if depolarization is maintained. Potassium channels are also inactive for some time, and contribute to the refractory period after an action potential.

Propagation of the action potential helps in the transmission of information along the nervous system. There is flow of ionic current from the area of depolarized membrane, with inward movement of sodium (positive) ions, and lateral movement towards the undepolarized parts of the membrane. This electrotonic potential generates an action potential in the adjacent membrane, which spreads further. The velocity of propagation varies directly with the diameter of the axon, and with the extent of myelination. Myelinated axons are denuded of myelin at the nodes of Ranvier, and transmembrane current flow across the sodium channels occurs at the node. These then depolarize the adjacent nodes to threshold, and propagate the action potential by saltatory conduction.

Synaptic transmission across nerve cell membranes may be electrical or chemical; the latter occur at specialized membrane junctions that allow only unidirectional flow across the synapse. Chemical synapses are characterized by a significant if brief delay for the flow of neurotransmitter, and spatio-temporal summation. The postsynaptic potentials may be excitatory or inhibitory. (An excellent animation of the action potential, produced by Harvard University, may be found at http://outreach.mcb.harvard.edu/animations/actionpotential.swf.)

In general, surface-recorded cortical activity represents the summated extracellular current flow from many neurons. The concepts of near-field and far-field volume conduction are both important in neurophysiological evaluation of the spinal cord. Near-field signals are those recorded in close proximity to, but not directly from, the source of the electrical signal, for example scalp electroencephalography (EEG) and needle electromyography (EMG). Far-field potentials are those recorded from some considerable distance from the source, and are important in the evaluation of somatosensory evoked potentials (SEPs) (Blum and Rutkove 2007).

EFFECTS OF MATURATION AND MYELINATION

In the peripheral nervous system, myelination starts in the sensory roots at 24 weeks post-conceptional age, continues into very early infancy, and is completed by 6 months after term (Minkowski et al. 1967). Posterior column tracts are discernible in the human fetus by 8 to 9 weeks post-conceptional age (Hughes 1976), with myelination starting in the medial longitudinal fasciculus at 20 weeks, and at 23 to 24 weeks elsewhere in the spinal cord. Mature degrees of myelination are observed by immunocytochemical techniques by 36 weeks in the cuneate fasciculus. At this stage, corticospinal and solitary tracts are still immature by comparison, and maturation continues into early childhood (Tanaka et al. 1995).

By contrast the presence of the motoneuron is detected at 4 weeks post-conceptional age (Sadler and Langman 2009).

Evaluation of sensory function

The neurophysiological evaluation of somatosensory dysfunction often includes routine nerve conduction studies as sensory disturbance in a child may be difficult to localize, and there may well be an underlying large fibre polyneuropathy responsible for the clinical features. In the clinical setting, summated responses from supra-maximal stimulation of a sensory nerve (sensory nerve action potential) and motor nerve (compound muscle action potential) are respectively recorded over the cutaneous course of the sensory nerve, and from the belly of the muscle, using surface electrodes applied to the skin. Needle EMG records electrical activity from within muscle, and describes the integrity of the motor unit—which comprises a single alpha-motoneuron and all of the muscle fibres it innervates.

Clinical neurophysiology exploits the electrical characteristics that are special to the neuron. In most neurons, electrical impulses are propagated over extensive distances through axons onto other neurons or target organs. Dendrites are fine processes that ramify from the cell body of the neuron and receive electrochemical input from other neurons. Together, the axons and dendrites contribute to over 90% of the neuronal cell volume.

The large diameter sensory neurons are located adjacent to the spinal cord in the dorsal root ganglion. These pseudounipolar (functionally bipolar neurons that have fused axons and dendritic processes) neurons branch into the peripheral component, which receives all non-noxious and non-thermal sensory input from the peripheral structures (muscles, skin, tendon), and the central component, which enters the spinal cord through the dorsal horn. Some of these form synapses with the corresponding anterior horn cells, whereas others ascend along the dorsal column in a laminar configuration (layers I–VI of Rexed (1952).

Cutaneous sensory input is mediated by laminae I to IV, whereas laminae V and VI are involved with proprioceptive sensory afferents as well as corticospinal projections from the sensory cortex. The fasciculus gracilis of the dorsal column receives sensory input from the most caudal body regions, whereas the lateral cuneate fasciculus starts at the mid-thoracic level. The cells of the dorsal column nuclei in the medulla oblongata display very high specificity for both the type and spatial location of the sensory impulse (Wall 1970).

Several neurotransmitter molecules have been described in the dorsal fibres, some still putative. These include substance P, vasoactive intestinal polypeptide, cholecystokinin, and angiotensin.

Pain, temperature, and coarse touch are mediated by unmyelinated and small myelinated nerve endings that project to the spinothalamic tracts. Second-order axons from pain and temperature fibres decussate in the ventral white commissure within one segment of their origin. Distinct lateral and ventral spinothalamic tracts serve pain and temperature, and coarse touch and pressure modalities, respectively. Axons from the ventral tract join the medial lemniscus in the lower brainstem, whereas the spinal lemniscus carries lateral tract axons to the thalamus. Somatotopic organization of the fibres is maintained throughout the tracts (Standring and Gray 2008).

During routine nerve conduction studies, stimulation of a peripheral nerve generates action potentials in individual motor and sensory nerve fibres that are summated to produce compound responses or potentials. These analogue triphasic signals are recorded by surface electrodes and undergo appropriate amplification, filtration, and digitization. Parameters such as amplitude, duration, latencies, and conduction velocities are analysed efficiently by computer software integral to modern neurophysiological equipment. Normative data for a range of nerves and muscles, and different age groups, enable quantification of any deviation from the norm. Conventional nerve conduction studies typically assess conduction and axonal integrity (deduced from the amplitude of the compound action potential) in the large fast conducting nerve fibres, principally the A beta fibres that mediate fine touch, with velocities in the range 40 to 60m/s in older children and 25 to 40m/s in infants. Pain and temperature sensation, mediated by slower conducting small myelinated A-III (conduction velocity 12–30m/s) and unmyelinated C fibres (conduction velocities 0.3–1.6m/s), cannot be assessed with standard nerve conduction tests. Evaluation of small fibre function requires specialized techniques accessible in a few neuroscience centres. These typically involve psychophysical methods, whereby the response time (clicking a hand-held switch) to a hot or cold thermal stimulus at a predetermined temperature over a defined, focal cutaneous area (e.g. dorsum of the foot, palm of the hand) is measured and compared with

normative data for age- and sex-matched comparisons. This assumes a degree of compre-
hension, cooperation, and manual dexterity that precludes their use in young children. Skin
biopsy to evaluate epidermal nerve fibre morphology and density is an alternative more
invasive option.

SEPs are particularly useful in evaluating pre-ganglionic sensory function, proximal to
the dorsal root ganglia. These are safe and non-invasive, and generally well tolerated by
infants and children. Although in theory any limb dermatome is amenable for study, in
practice only the median nerve SEPs, and to a lesser extent the tibial nerve SEPs, are studied
in children. Recording techniques and normative data are rather more robust for the median
nerve SEPs, which have been studied more extensively (Duckworth et al. 1976).

SEPs are evoked from cortical and sub-cortical generators in response to exogenous
stimulation of a peripheral nerve, and are electrical signals recorded from the head and
other parts of the body. Evoked potential activity can be assumed to represent the arrival
of sensory nerve activity at successive points along the peripheral and central sensory
pathways.

Typically, peripheral, and central sensory evoked potentials (SEPs) to median nerve
stimulation are recorded from the supra-clavicular area (Erb's point), the upper neck (C2
spine), and the somatosensory cortex (Fig 3.1).

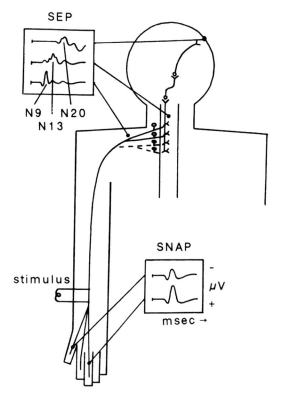

Fig. 3.1. The source of sensory evoked
potential signal generators. From Smith
and Knight (2011), with kind permission of Springer Science+Business
Media

SEPs resemble electroencephalograms in that they represent the summated electrical activity from underlying neural structures: they do not precisely represent the localization of the electrical signal and have relatively poor spatial resolution of the underlying sensory processes. The temporal resolution is superior, and is able to identify conduction delays of as little as 1 to 2ms.

Low-intensity current stimulation of a mixed peripheral nerve (median nerve at the wrist, tibial nerve at the ankle) produces potentials that are carried by the first-order axons with the fastest conducting myelinated fibres to the dorsal ganglia, and proceed to the median (gracile) or lateral (cuneate) nucleus in the medulla. Second-order axons carry the impulse to the ventrolateral nucleus of the thalamus, and third-order axons to the somato-sensory cortex.

The exact source of the generators of SEPs is not known. Clinically plausible, generally accepted generators are as follows:
Sources of generators of the median nerve SEPs (Jones 1977)
    N9: brachial plexus
    N11: dorsal roots/dorsal columns
    N13: dorsal horn (C6/7) plus passage through the foramen magnum ('P14' on scalp)
    N14: medial lemniscus ('P15' on scalp)
    N20: sensory cortex
Tibial nerve SEPs
    Lumbar N20: dorsal horn
    P40: sensory cortex

The evoked responses are of biphasic or triphasic morphology. The relative polarity, namely the negativity or positivity of the waveform, is referred to by the initials 'N' or 'P', and the numbers adjacent to these letters represent typical peak latencies. For example, the principal cortical N20 response to median nerve stimulation at the wrist occurs 20ms after the stimulus. Electrical stimulation with a square wave pulse is generally used, but other sensory modalities such as vibration may be tested in special circumstances. Cortical responses are recorded from the scalp using a modified EEG montage (Cracco et al. 1982). SEPs are generally small in amplitude, of the order of microvolts, and require averaging of several hundred responses to reduce background noise. Acquisition and analysis of the digitized signals are expedited by modern computer software technology. Standardization of technique according to published guidelines (Cruccu et al. 2008) enables consistency and facilitates comparison between patient groups, as well as the charting of the temporal evolution of disease in a patient.

SEPs amplitudes are less useful than latency measurements, with wide variability and a non-normal distribution in disease-free comparisons. A complete absence of response is clearly abnormal, however, and relative inter-side differences of greater than 50% are significant.

Inter-peak latency measurements are undertaken at multiple levels: Erb's point, second cervical vertebra, and the scalp. The peripheral N9 latency varies with arm length, and is determined by conduction along the median nerve and the brachial plexus. The central

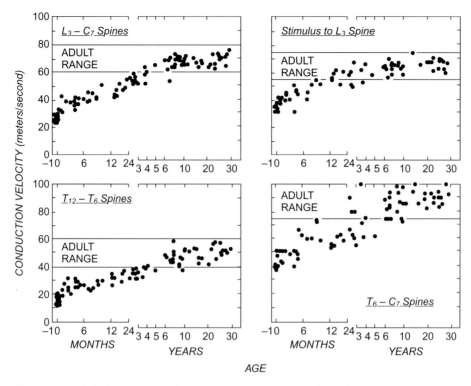

Fig. 3.2. The relation between age and conduction velocity of the spinal cord (L3–C7 spines), segmental velocity from thoracic spine (T12–T6 spines), and rostral (T6–C7) spines, to stimulation of the peroneal nerve. The most rapid increases in velocity are noted from the peroneal nerve and cauda equina, maximal in the first year of life. Redrawn from Cracco et al. (1979) with permission from Elsevier.

conduction time (measured by subtracting the peripheral N13 peak latency from that of the central N20) is a more robust indicator of a clinical lesion. The median nerve N20 decreases in infancy and early childhood until about 3 years of age, and increases through childhood to reach adult values by 14 to 18 years, in parallel with increasing arm length (Cracco et al. 1979) (Fig. 3.2).

Cortical somatosensory responses tend to be very variable in newborn infants, particularly in preterm infants, probably reflecting the variability in the extent of myelination of the thalamocortical and other long tracts (Gilles et al. 1983).

Clinical use of SEPs
SEPs are used in the study of a range of paediatric disorders, intrinsic as well as extrinsic, that involve the dorsal spinal cord.

Intrinsic cord diseases include hereditary neurodegenerative conditions such as Friedreich ataxia, ataxia telangiectasia, and the spinocerebellar ataxias (Scarpini et al. 1996, Velazquez et al. 2000, Velazquez Perez et al. 2007). Abnormalities of SEPs are frequent, mainly in the form of increased latencies with a dispersed/absent cortical response. Jones et al. (1980) described delayed and dispersed cortical responses in Freidreich's ataxia, in keeping with delayed conduction in the somatosensory pathways.

Thus SEPs provide objective evidence for dorsal column involvement, particularly when cerebellar features predominate.

The importance of SEPs in the setting of ataxia was highlighted by Fagan et al. (1987a, b). Abnormal SEPs in the context of childhood cerebellar ataxia point to a neuro-degenerative aetiology, and help refine the differential diagnosis. For instance, the presence of abnormal SEPs in a child with radiologically demonstrable cerebellar atrophy clearly indicates multisystem involvement, with evidence for dysfunction of the posterior column tracts.

SEPs have been extensively studied in leukodystrophies such as adrenomyeloneuropa-thy (Restuccia et al. 1997, Schmidt et al. 2001, Zgorzalewicz-Stachowiak et al. 2006, Matsumoto et al. 2010). Nearly all of 83 patients with elevated levels of very long chain fatty acids had prolonged or absent median and/or tibial SEPs (Kaplan et al. 1997). In comparison, definite EP abnormalities were detectable in 50% of clinically normal carriers of AML. SEPs have also been used to monitor response to treatment in adrenomyeloneu-ropathy (Korenke et al. 1995). Treatment with Lorenzo's oil remains controversial, with reports of clinical and neurophysiological improvement (Inagaki et al. 1995, Korenke et al. 1995), conflicting with other studies that show no improvement (Aubourg et al. 1993, Van Geel et al. 1999). Other leukodystrophies in which SEPs can be used to advantage include Alexander disease (Ichiyama et al. 1993), metachromatic leukodystrophy, Pelizaeus–Merzbacher disease, and Canavan disease where demyelination of the large fibre somatosensory pathways from the arms and legs can be deduced from prolongation or absence of the cortical responses (De Meirleir et al. 1988).

Evoked potentials have in the past had an important role in the diagnosis of multiple sclerosis (Turano et al. 1991). Despite the inroads made by MRI, the diagnosis of multiple sclerosis in childhood, although rare, remains challenging as it may not be possible to demonstrate dissemination of lesions in space. SEPs to tibial and median nerve stimulation were evaluated as part of a multimodality evoked potential study of 85 children with multiple sclerosis; the frequency of abnormal SEPs in relation to sensory symptoms at onset was 57% overall in this retrospective review of children who met McDonald or Poser criteria for multiple sclerosis as the 'criterion standard'. Children who had multimodal evoked potentials before the second clinical episode were selected for study. The diagnostic yield increased with the addition of visual evoked potentials, emphasizing the multimodal approach to assessment of somatosensory and visual function in these patients. Spatial dissemination was identified in 46% before the second clinical episode, highlighting the value of evoked potentials in childhood multiple sclerosis (Pohl et al. 2006).

Extrinsic cord compression in the child may occur as a result of congenital bony deformity from achondroplasia, as well from inherited disorders such as the mucopolysachhari-doses. SEPs are useful in the identification of subclinical somatosensory dysfunction in these cases. Abnormal SEPs indicate compressive cervical myelopathy in mucopolysaccharidoses. There is an increased risk of sudden death from myelopathy at the craniocervical junction in achondroplasia. SEPs, in particular subcortical SEPs, have been found to be very sensitive (78–92%) and specific (98–100%) compared with MRI as the 'criterion standard', in identifying cord compression and myelomalacia in a series of 30 children, with achondroplasia only seven of whom had clinical neurological abnormalities (Boor et al. 1999, Li et al. 2008). The authors of this study make a case for the use of SEPs to detect preclinical abnormality in early cervical myelopathy. Irretrievable spinal cord damage may be prevented by timely surgical decompression. These can also help in the evaluation of postoperative recovery of neurological function, as was demonstrated in the study by Boor et al. (1999) in which SEPs were used to document recovery of function objectively; improvement in the SEPs were seen in two of the three children who underwent surgical decompression.

Non-specific abnormalities of upper limb SEPs have been described in children with Down syndrome (Straumanis et al. 1973, Brandt and Rosen 1995, Chen and Fang 2005). Very few studies relate to the particular problem of the atlanto-axial instability that is seen in children with this condition. A cross-sectional study of 404 children with Down syndrome estimates the prevalence of radiological atlanto-axial instability at 4.6% (Pueschel and Scola 1987). A study by the same group compared radiologically confirmed atlanto-axial dislocation in asymptomatic and symptomatic patients with Down syndrome against those patients with Down syndrome but without radiologically evident dislocation; no significant differences were noted in conduction times between these groups, although subgroup analyses showed a correlation between the degree of prolongation of cortical latencies and the atlanto-dens interval measurements (Pueschel et al. 1987). The authors concluded that SEPs are useful as part of a multimodality (clinical, neurophysiological, and radiological) approach to asymptomatic atlanto-axial instability in this condition.

Lower limb (tibial nerve) SEPs have proven use in anatomical lesions such as the tethered cord syndrome, and demonstrate high correlation with clinical severity and degree of cord displacement (Roy et al. 1986). The presence of normal posterior tibial SEPs in patients with lower limb sensory symptoms correlated well with an absence of myelographic abnormality. Lower limb SEPs were used to determine the level of the conus medullaris and the degree of spinal cord displacement in this study.

Dissociated sensory loss is a clue to the diagnosis of syringomyelia; a clear correlation was found between abnormal pain and temperature sensibility and an abnormal cervical somatosensory response (Restuccia and Mauguiere 1991). SEPs have also been used successfully to distinguish between hydromyelia and syringomyelia (Roser et al. 2010), where abnormal somatosensory evaluation as well as the presence of central canal widening of more than 6 mm on MRI were used as exclusion criteria for hydromyelia.

SEPs are sensitive to the effects of nutritional deficiencies, and their treatment on the dorsal column, identifying abnormalities that are sometimes not apparent on neuroimaging. SEPs have been used in the diagnosis of neuromyelopathy from a range of micronutrient deficiency disorders including vitamin B_{12} (Jones et al. 1987, Misra et al. 2003, Puri et al. 2005, Misra and Kalita 2007), copper (Kumar et al. 2004), and vitamin E (Kaplan et al. 1988). These may produce combined degeneration of the somatosensory and corticospinal pathways and may be evaluated by a combination of SEP and motor evoked potential studies (see below).

In the operating theatre, intra-operative spinal cord monitoring with tibial and ulnar or median SEPs is undertaken routinely in extrinsic (e.g. scoliosis) as well as intrinsic surgery such as tumour removal (Master et al. 2008), although combined sensory and motor tract assessment appears more useful (Hyun et al. 2009). Sudden, or in some cases more gradual, waning of the amplitude of the cortical SSEP or MEP alerts the surgeon to cord compression and ischaemia; relief of pressure by surgical manipulation usually restores cord function which can be measured and documented.

Hirayama disease or juvenile distal upper extremity muscular atrophy bears special consideration in this section. There is pathological evidence for an underlying ischaemic cervical myelopathy (Hirayama 2000). Dynamic changes of the cervical dural sac and spinal cord induced by neck flexion are thought to play a role (Kwon et al. 2004).

A reduction in the subcortical N13 amplitude in response to neck flexion was reported as a unique finding in patients with Hirayama disease, as opposed to healthy controls and patients with other motoneuron disease (Restuccia et al. 2003). However, as a diagnostic test this is controversial and has been refuted by more recent studies that combined MRI with somatosensory evaluation (Misra et al. 2006, Ammendola et al. 2008). Clinical assessment, combined with needle EMG studies to confirm denervation in the C7 to T1 myotomes will help establish the diagnosis. This would indeed suggest that dynamic cord compression from neck flexion would not sufficiently explain the myelopathy associated with Hirayama disease.

Neurophysiological evaluation of spinal motor function: the anterior horn cell
Needle EMG is used by clinical neurophysiologists to assess the integrity of the motor unit. The motor unit as an anatomical entity comprises the anterior horn cell, and all the motor axons and muscle fibres that are innervated by the motoneuron. Needle EMG involves intramuscular insertion of a monopolar or concentric needle, with amplification and filtering of the digitized signal. Concentric needles are more widely used. Needle EMG therefore reflects the activity at the distal aspect of the motor unit and is very sensitive to dysfunction of any component of the motor unit (i.e. from the level of the anterior horn cell to the level of the motor and the muscle fibre). Overall, routine EMG for neurogenic change has been shown to have 100% agreement with clinical diagnosis and muscle biopsy in a series of childhood neuromuscular disorders. The range of neuromuscular diagnoses includes congenital myopathies, congenital myasthenia gravis, hereditary sensory and motoneuropathies, non-specific myopathies, and arthrogryposis congenita. A combined clinico-pathological criterion standard of diagnosis was eventually achieved on retrospective review of patient data, and EMG was shown to have a sensitivity of 100% for neurogenic disorders, in contradistinction to muscle biopsy with a sensitivity of 75%. For myopathic disease, the sensitivity of muscle biopsy was higher at 78%, whereas EMG had a sensitivity of 56% (Kang et al. 2003, Rabie et al. 2007).

However, it cannot differentiate between dysfunction (denervation) at the level of the motor axon, nerve, nerve root (radicle) or the motoneuron. It must also be remembered that muscle fibre atrophy and muscle splitting that characterize a primary myopathic process are also associated with 'denervation', namely loss of functional continuity with the motor axon supplying the muscle fibre. Thus fibrillations are also seen in muscle disorders as a result of muscle membrane instability. Chronic muscle disease may be associated with muscle fibre hypertrophy, and this may sometimes produce the impression of an apparently enlarged motor unit on EMG, mimicking neurogenic abnormality. It is the overall clinical interpretation that enables this distinction to be made.

ILLUSTRATIVE CASE

A 14-year-old male developed right foot drop and leg pain subacutely over 3 to 4 weeks after a game of rugby, and was referred for evaluation of possible peroneal neuropathy. His nerve conduction studies were normal, and argued against a focal neuropathy of the peroneal or sciatic nerves. Needle EMG sampling demonstrated fibrillations and reduced recruitment in the ankle invertor (i.e. tibialis posterior) as well as the ankle evertor and dorsiflexor (peroneus longus and tibialis anterior respectively) and localized the pathology to the L5 myotome. The features were therefore those of an L5 radiculopathy. Lateral lumbar disc herniation at L5/S1 was subsequently confirmed by neuroimaging.

Anterior horn neurons vary in size, with larger diameter (>25µm) cells innervating the extrafusal skeletal muscle fibres (alpha motoneurons), and smaller (15–25µm) cells supplying the muscle spindles (gamma motoneurons). Motoneurons are organized longitudinally into groups within the spinal cord that extend across multiple segments. The medial group is distributed throughout the cord, innervating the axial extensors and flexors. The lateral group innervates the limb muscles, and the central group is limited to some cervical and lumbosacral segments. As with the sensory system, there is somatotopic organization of the anterior horn neurons in the spinal cord (Standring and Gray 2008).

Unlike the sensory neuron, the motoneuron receives input from the dendrites as well as the cell body. Sensory input from more than 100 sensory neurons are required for a motoneuron to fire. A single motoneuron innervates several muscle fibres, with innervation ratios of 1:50 fibres for facial and other fine muscles, 1:250 for medium sized muscles such as the biceps, and up to 1:2000 in large muscles such as the gastrocnemius (Gath and Stalberg 1981).

The muscle action potential is generated when the nerve action potential at the terminal motor axon causes activation of calcium channels at the synaptic membrane. This prompts the quantal release of acetylcholine from storage vesicles in the synaptic cleft. Binding of acetylcholine to its receptor at the postsynaptic folds produces an endplate potential through an increase in membrane (sodium) cation permeability. Acetylcholine is rapidly metabolized by acetylcholinesterase at the synaptic cleft. The end plate potential depolarizes the postsynaptic membrane and, at a critical threshold level, opens sodium channels that propagate muscle fibre action potentials (Vincent 2008).

These traverse the interior of the muscle fibre through the T tubule, producing a near-synchronous activation of the muscle fibres. Calcium release from the sarcoplasmic reticulum into the sarcoplasm produces excitation–contraction coupling that leads to muscle contraction.

The size of the motoneuron is directly correlated with the diameter of the motor axons, the thickness of the myelin sheath, and the type of muscle fibres that it innervates. Henneman's size principle (Henneman and Olson 1965, Henneman et al. 1965, McPhedran et al. 1965) thus determines the properties of the motor unit, with the largest motoneurons with the fastest conducting axons innervating the fast twitch type II muscle fibres. Needle EMG usually involves analysis of motor units recruited at low levels of contraction, and is therefore biased towards the smaller, slow twitch type I muscle fibres and motor units (Preston and Shapiro 2005). Henneman and Olson (1965) related the properties of the motor unit to the electromechanical properties of motor unit recruitment, whereby the frequency firing of different motoneurons in a motor unit pool varies in proportion to the size of the motoneuron. The smallest motor units with lowest threshold are recruited initially, and units of successively increasing size are recruited with increasing force of muscle contraction. At a practical level this does not affect sampling, particularly in neurogenic disorders. Conditions that preferentially affect type II fibres (e.g. steroid myopathies) may be normal to needle EMG sampling.

The area of the recording surface varies with the size of the needle. The fine, Teflon®-coated 30-gauge facial needle with a recording area of $0.019\mu m^2$ is suitable for paediatric examinations. Dysfunction at the anterior horn cell manifests with abnormalities of the motor unit action potential and with spontaneous activity: fibrillations and fasciculations. Denervated muscle is characterized by spontaneous activity in the form of fibrillations. These represent spontaneously generated action potentials of individual muscle fibres that have lost their nerve supply (Daube 1991). They may be seen therefore in a range of pathologies that involve various components of the motor unit, including myopathies, motor axonopathies, and radiculopathies, as well as anterior horn cell disease. The amplitude of the fibrillation potential has been used as a marker of chronicity of denervation in the past, but has been shown to be unreliable in this regard (Dumitru and King 1998).

Fasciculations are summated, randomly firing action potentials of groups of muscle fibres from a single motor unit (Denny-Brown 1938). Consequently they assume the morphology of a single motor unit. In the appropriate clinical setting, these have high specificity for disorders of the anterior horn cell such as amyotrophic lateral sclerosis (Douglass et al. 2010), but can also be seen in other disorders involving the motor unit such as radiculopathy. More frequently they are seen in healthy children and adults, and are then termed benign fasciculations.

Typical needle EMG findings in spinal muscular atrophy include the presence of fibrillations, and reduced recruitment pattern of motor unit action potentials that have prolonged duration and increased amplitude. The actual electromyographic abnormality is similar in any disorder of the anterior spinal motoneurons. It is the pattern of weakness and the distribution of the EMG abnormality that helps make the distinction between the various forms of spinal muscular atrophy. Typically, spinal muscular atrophy shows diffuse or a proximal to distal gradient of severity, whereas this pattern of abnormality is reversed in the distal spinal muscular atrophies. Rather surprisingly, needle EMG-recorded fasciculations are reported to be unusual in survival motoneuron (SMN) protein-associated spinal muscular atrophy, to the extent of pointing away from this disorder (Hausmanowa-Petrusewicz and Karwanska 1986, Hausmanowa-Petrusewicz 1988). This may in fact relate to the relatively small recording surface area. Ultrasonography of muscle is sensitive to fasciculations and is a useful adjunct to neurophysiological evalution (Pillen et al. 2008).

The concept of the motor unit and its development owes much to the pioneering work of Adrian and Bronk (1928, 1929), as well as Sherrington and Denny-Brown (Sherrington 1925, Denny-Brown 1949).

The motor unit action potential generated by volitional muscle contraction is recorded by the intramuscular needle electrode and is analysed for duration, number of phases, and amplitude.

The summated action potential of all the muscle fibres in the motor unit contributes to the overall motor unit action potential. The amplitude of the motor unit action potential depends upon physiological variables such as age, temperature, distance from the recording electrode, and the type of muscle (proximal vs distal) (Buchthal et al. 1954). The motor unit action potential in young children and infants is relatively lower in amplitude and simpler in configuration than the mature form (Sacco et al. 1962).

Anterior horn cell disease enlarges the size of the motor unit, as the progressive drop-out of motoneurons causes the remaining motoneurons to re-innervate muscle fibres that have lost their 'parent' anterior horn cell (Denny-Brown 1950). This is reflected in the increased duration of the motor unit action potentials. Reinnervating muscle fibres and instability at the neuromuscular junction caused by nascent motor axonal connexions also increase the number of phases of the waveform, producing a wide and polyphasic potential.

Recruitment, the orderly addition of motor units and increase in the firing rate with increasing muscle contraction, is governed by Henneman's size principle, with the smaller motoneurons discharging first (Henneman et al. 1965, McPhedran et al. 1965, Olson et al. 1968). Motor neuronopathy, for example spinal muscular atrophy, is characterized by reduced recruitment, as fewer motor units fire at high frequencies to maintain a level of muscle contraction. A range of paediatric disorders involve the anterior horn cell, and the pattern of neurogenic change is described in Table 3.1.

SMN gene deletions account for over 93% of infants and children with spinal muscular atrophy (Chen et al. 2007). Genetic studies are rightly the investigation of choice in suspected spinal muscular atrophy. However, genetic diagnosis will prove difficult in a small but significant proportion with the typical phenotype. Clinical EMG is useful in this situation to confirm neurogenic muscle wasting, and would help to distinguish between a neuropathy that may involve sensory and motor axons, and a motoneuronopathy.

Electromyographic evaluation for anterior horn cell disease is particularly useful in clinical lower motoneuronal syndromes that are focal or regional in distribution. Hirayama disease, a relatively self-limited, asymmetrical disorder of the distal upper limb affecting mainly male adolescents (Hirayama 2000), is one such condition. In the era of global polio eradication and extensive coverage with polio vaccination, non-poliovirus infection of the spinal cord must still be considered in the setting of acute limb weakness.

TABLE 3.1

Neurogenic changes in paediatric disorders involving the anterior horn cell

Aetiology	Distribution of neurogenic abnormalities on needle electromyography	Examples
Inherited/familial	Diffuse, proximal > distal	Survival motoneuron (SMN) protein-associated spinal muscular atrophy
		Hexosaminidase deficicency
	Distal	Distal spinal muscular atrophy, glycyl-tRNA synthetase gene mutations (GARS)
	Focal, bulbospinal	Fazio–Londe disease
		Brown–Vialetto–Van Laere disease
		Kennedy disease (X-linked)
Acquired		
Infective	Patchy/regional	Poliomyelitis
		West Nile encephalomyelitis
		Human immunodeficiency virus
Compressive	Patchy/regional	Extrinsic compression (e.g. tumour)
	Focal	Intrinsic: syringomyelia
		?Hirayama disease
Nutritional	Regional/diffuse	Neurolathyrism (caused by ingestion of *Lathyrus sativus*, a legume that contains the neurotoxin β-oxalyl-amino-alanine (BOAA)
Traumatic	Segmental (cervical)	Birth trauma (Vialle et al. 2007, Goetz 2010)

ILLUSTRATIVE CASE

A five-year-old male with four-limb cerebral palsy was referred with flaccid weakness of the right leg after an acute febrile illness. He had been previously immunized with oral polio vaccine. Spinal neuroimaging and limb scans revealed no abnormality to account for the weakness. The diagnosis of a poliomyelitis-like anterior horn cell disease was suggested by neurophysiological assessment, which showed normal sensory and motor nerve action potentials, and fibrillations in a patchy distribution involving the lumbosacral segment of the right side, with a very reduced recruitment pattern on EMG. Evidence of acute Coxsackie A virus infection was obtained on serology.

Electromyography is also of particular value in the diagnostic evaluation of congenital arthrogryposis where clinical and genetic evaluation are unrevealing, particularly when combined with muscle biopsy (Kang et al. 2003). The frequency of neuromuscular disease as a cause of arthrogryposis multiplex congenita varies between 31% and 65% in the paediatric literature (Strehl et al. 1985, Banker 1986, Quinn et al. 1991). Recent studies have highlighted the importance of anterior horn cell disease as a frequent cause (Ambegaonkar et al. 2011). Needle EMG correctly identified all eight with 'neurogenic' arthrogryposis in a reported case series of 38 children from the Boston Children's Hospital (Kang et al. 2003). Two of these had motoneuronopathy with pontocerebellar hypoplasia. Concordant needle EMG and muscle biopsy findings had higher diagnostic use than either of these used on its own.

The compound muscle action potential, recorded in response to electrical stimulation of a peripheral nerve from its dependent muscle typically using surface electrodes, represents the summated action potential of all the muscle fibres of a given muscle generated in response to stimulation of the motor nerve. Although non-invasive, this has less clinical use than motor unit action potential in the evaluation of anterior horn cell disease, particularly in the acute or subacute setting. It is estimated that a reduction in the motor unit pool of the order of 50% would be required to produce a detectable reduction in the amplitude of the compound muscle action potential. However, as a proxy measure of the number of motor units supplying a muscle, it can be useful in the assessment of disease progression (Visser et al. 2008). Ulnar compound muscle action potential amplitude and area shows promise as a useful biomarker of response of spinal muscular atrophy to treatment with valproate (Lewelt et al. 2010).

Although the number of motor units innervating a muscle can be assessed semi-quantitatively during routine needle EMG by observing the recruitment pattern, it is also possible to quantify the number of motor units in a muscle by non-invasive means. Motor unit number estimation, using surface electrodes, provides an estimate of the number of motor units by dividing the amplitude of the supramaximal compound muscle action potential by the average amplitudes of the single motor unit potentials recorded by the electrode (Daube et al. 2000).

Various techniques using this principle have been described. It is neither necessary nor is it always feasible to perform these in young children to establish a diagnosis, but motor unit number estimation has a role in the research setting and has been used to establish the rate of anterior horn cell loss in spinal muscular atrophy (Bromberg and Swoboda 2002) and in evaluating the effect of treatment (Swoboda et al. 2009). Other more invasive, quantitative techniques such as multiple motor unit action potential analyis (Bischoff et al. 1994) may not be practicable in children. Automated techniques such as Willison's turns–amplitude interference pattern analysis (Smyth and Willison 1982), although beyond the scope of this book, may be useful in some situations.

F waves are generated by spinal anterior horn cells in response to supramaximal antidromic (i.e. conduction away from the terminal motor axons towards towards the soma of the anterior horn cells) activation along the peripheral nerve and are recorded by surface EMG electrodes. These are a measure of nerve conduction in the more proximal segments, where the peripheral nerve joins with its parent nerve roots at the level of the vertebral column. Their clinical use in disorders of the spinal cord is limited (Mesrati and Vecchierini 2004). There is normally some variability of the F-wave latency and amplitude, in keeping with the variability of the motoneuronal pool that is depolarized with each successive stimulation of the motor nerve. Minimum F latencies are useful in the computation of central motor conduction time.

Disorders of spinal interneurons, typified by tetanus which affects the Renshaw inhibitory cells (Benecke et al. 1977), pose no difficulty to the experienced clinician. Stiff person syndrome, usually caused by autoimmune dysfunction of the spinal interneuronal circuits, is well recognized in adults but its rarity in children may render its diagnosis challenging (Markandeyulu et al. 2001). Demonstration of abnormal exteroceptive motor reflexes to electrical nerve stimulation (absence of habituation, co-contraction of antagonist muscles) (Martinelli and Montagna 1985), and the presence of continuous motor unit activity on needle EMG, facilitate diagnosis (Meinck and Thompson 2002).

Evaluation of corticospinal motor pathways: motor evoked potentials and central motor conduction time

Magnetic stimulation of the head induces intracranial electrical currents that excite the central motor pathways (Barker et al. 1985, 1987, Hess et al. 1987). By the application of an induced field through a suitable magnetic coil over an appropriate area of the scalp, a compound muscle action potential is generated in a peripheral muscle after a period known as the cortical latency. The central conduction time is determined by subtracting the peripheral conducting time from the cortical latency. Peripheral conduction time from the level of the alpha motoneuron down the motor nerve to the muscle is conveniently calculated from the minimal F latency using the formula $(F + M - 1)/2$, where F is the minimum F latency and M the distal latency of the compound muscle action potential.

In paediatrics, motor evoked potentials are useful in monitoring anterior spinal cord function during spinal surgery (Deletis and Sala 2008). These are typically obtained by regular transcranial electrical stimulation of the motor cortex in the anaesthetized child, and recorded by using intramuscular electrodes from, for example, the tibialis anterior in the lower limb. The surgeon thus obtains continuous feedback about the integrity of the corticospinal pathways, and can respond in a timely fashion should monitoring indicate compromised anterior cord function. In the past the rather dramatic 'wake-up' test (which involved waking the child up during surgery and getting them to move their feet) was the only means available to assess motor dysfunction. Monitoring of MEPs is regarded as more sensitive than SEP monitoring in detecting preventable spinal cord damage.

Otherwise the role of motor evoked potentials in the diagnosis of spinal cord disease is somewhat limited; although generally safe and well tolerated, they are difficult to record in very young children, although Eyre et al. (2001) reported recording motor evoked potentials from active target muscles even in neonates. Widely replicated normative data are not available.

Transcranial magnetic stimulation has been used to document involvement of the anterior spinal pathways in transverse myelitis, although imaging is by far the more sensitive diagnostic modality (Noguchi et al. 2000). Abnormalities of motor evoked potentials (absence or prolongation of central motor conduction time) were more frequent than abnormalities of SEPs in an adult series (Kalita and Misra 2000).

Although they are not as sensitive as clinical evaluation of the corticospinal pathways, they may be of value in distinguishing subtypes of inherited spastic paraplegia. These may be used to distinguish between different genetic forms of hereditary spastic paraplegia, where, for example, abnormalities of intracortical inhibition have been reported in spastin- but not paraplegin-related mutations. Differences in central motor conduction times have been described in pedigrees showing different mutations within the spastin gene (Bonsch

66

et al. 2003, Nardone and Tezzon 2003). Magnetic evoked potentials have also been used to assess response to treatment with bone marrow transplant in adrenoleukodystrophy (Hitomi et al. 2003) and with d-penicillamine in Wilson disease (Meyer et al. 1991).

In the routine clinical setting, MEPs are of especial value in excluding spinal cord pathology in suspected psychogenic severe limb weakness and paraparesis (Meyer et al. 1992). Routine needle EMG may reveal an absence of spontaneous activity such as fibrillations and positive sharp waves that are expected in denervation, but in the absence of volitional contraction of the muscle it may not be possible to comment on any abnormality of the motor unit per se. However, the presence of normal motor evoked potentials to transcranial stimulation would provide some reassurance about the integrity of the corticospinal pathways.

Summary

The spinal cord in the human not only serves as a conduit for the transmission of sensory and motor signals between the brain and receptors in the skin, muscle, and internal viscera, but also as a modulator of these signals. Maturational changes in infancy and childhood add to its physiological complexity. A range of neurophysiological techniques are available that can be modified to study different age groups in infancy and childhood.

SEPs evaluate posterior spinal column function, whereas EMG and transcranial magnetic stimulation techniques help with appraising the anterior horn cell and the motor pathways. The clinical neurophysiologist can assist with the diagnosis of spinal cord dysfunction by determining the likely level of the anatomical lesion, and by excluding other pathology such as peripheral neuropathy or a disorder of the neuromuscular junction. In addition, response to any available treatment of a spinal cord disorder, be it surgical (e.g. foramen magnum decompression) or medical (e.g. Lorenzo's oil for adrenomyeloneuropathy) may be assessed more objectively by neurophysiological techniques. Spinal cord monitoring of sensory and motor function is rapidly becoming a routine part of the surgical management of compressive spinal pathology, and helps in early identification and prevention of iatropathic cord injury.

Clinical neurophysiology fulfils a useful role in the diagnosis and management of spinal cord disorders; close interdisciplinary interaction involving the paediatric neurologist, neurosurgeon, and radiologist, along with the neurophysiologist, will help optimize the care of children with these challenging conditions.

REFERENCES

Adrian ED, Bronk DW. The discharge of impulses in motor nerve fibres: part I. Impulses in single fibres of the phrenic nerve. *J Physiol* 1928; **66:** 81–101.

Adrian ED, Bronk DW. The discharge of impulses in motor nerve fibres: part II. The frequency of discharge in reflex and voluntary contractions. *J Physiol* 1929; **67:** i3–151.

Ambegaonkar G, Manzur AY, Robb SA, Kinali M, Muntoni F. The multiple phenotypes of Arthrogryposis multiplex congenita with reference to the neurogenic variant. *Eur J Paediatr Neurol* 2011; **15:** 316–319.

Ammendola A, Gallo A, Iannaccone T, Tedeschi G. Hirayama disease: three cases assessed by F wave somatosensory and motor evoked potentials and magnetic resonance imaging not supporting flexion myelopathy. *Neurol Sci* 2008; **29:** 303–311.

Aubourg P, Adamsbaum C, Lavallard-Rousseau MC, et al. A two-year trial of oleic and erucic acids ("Lorenzo's oil") as treatment for adrenomyeloneuropathy. *N Engl J Med* 1993; **329:** 745–752.

Banker BQ. Arthrogryposis multiplex congenita: spectrum of pathologic changes. *Hum Pathol* 1986; **17:** 656–672.

Barker AT, Freeston IL, Jalinous R, Jarratt JA. Magnetic stimulation of the human brain and peripheral nervous system: an introduction and the results of an initial clinical evaluation. *Neurosurgery* 1987; **20:** 100–109.

Barker AT, Jalinous R, Freeston IL. Non-invasive magnetic stimulation of human motor cortex. *Lancet* 1985; **i:** 1106–1107.

Benecke R, Takano K, Schmidt J, Henatsch HD. Tetanus toxin induced actions on spinal Renshaw cells and Ia-inhibitory interneurones during development of local tetanus in the cat. *Exp Brain Res* 1977; **27:** 271–286.

Bischoff C, Stalberg E, Falck B, Eeg-Olofsson KE. Reference values of motor unit action potentials obtained with multi-MUAP analysis. *Muscle Nerve* 1994; **17:** 842–851.

Blum AS, Rutkove SB. The Clinical Neurophysiology Primer. Totowa, NJ: Humana, 2007.

Bonsch D, Schwindt A, Navratil P, et al. Motor system abnormalities in hereditary spastic paraparesis type 4 (SPG4) depend on the type of mutation in the spastin gene. *J Neurol Neurosurg Psychiatry* 2003; **74:** 1109–1112.

Boor R, Fricke G, Bruhl K, Spranger J. Abnormal subcortical somatosensory evoked potentials indicate high cervical myelopathy in achondroplasia. *Eur J Pediatr* 1999; **158:** 662–667.

Brandt BR, Rosen I. Impaired peripheral somatosensory function in children with Down syndrome. *Neuropediatrics* 1995; **26:** 310–312.

Bromberg MB, Swoboda KJ. Motor unit number estimation in infants and children with spinal muscular atrophy. *Muscle Nerve* 2002; **25:** 445–447.

Buchthal F, Pinell P, Rosenfalck P. Action potential parameters in normal human muscle and their physiological determinants. *Acta Physiol Scand* 1954; **32:** 219–229.

Chen WJ, Wu ZY, Lin MT, et al. Molecular analysis and prenatal prediction of spinal muscular atrophy in Chinese patients by the combination of restriction fragment length polymorphism analysis, denaturing high-performance liquid chromatography, and linkage analysis. *Arch Neurol* 2007; **64:** 225–231.

Chen YJ, Fang PC. Sensory evoked potentials in infants with Down syndrome. *Acta Paediatr* 2005; **94:** 1615–1618.

Cracco JB, Cracco RQ, Stolove R. Spinal evoked potential in man: a maturational study. *Electroencephalogr Clin Neurophysiol* 1979; **46:** 58–64.

Cracco RQ, Anziska BJ, Cracco JB, Vas GA, Rossini PM, Maccabee PJ. Short-latency somatosensory evoked potentials to median and peroneal nerve stimulation: studies in normal subjects and patients with neurologic disease. *Ann N Y Acad Sci* 1982; **388:** 412–425.

Cruccu G, Aminoff MJ, Curio G, et al. Recommendations for the clinical use of somatosensory-evoked potentials *Clin Neurophysiol* 2008; **119:** 1705–1719.

Daube JR. AAEM minimonograph #11: needle examination in clinical electromyography. *Muscle Nerve* 1991; **14:** 685–700.

Daube JR, Gooch C, Shefner J, Olney R, Felice K, Bromberg M. Motor unit number estimation (MUNE) with nerve conduction studies. *Suppl Clin Neurophysiol* 2000; **53:** 112–115.

De Meirleir LJ, Taylor MJ, Logan WJ. Multimodal evoked potential studies in leukodystrophies of children. *Can J Neurol Sci* 1988; **15:** 26–31.

Deletis V, Sala F. Intraoperative neurophysiological monitoring of the spinal cord during spinal cord and spine surgery: a review focus on the corticospinal tracts. *Clin Neurophysiol* 2008; **119:** 248–264.

Denny-Brown D. Interpretation of the electromyogram. *Arch Neurol Psychiatry* 1949; **61:** 99–128.

Denny-Brown D. Effect of poliomyelitis on the function of the motor neuron. *Arch Neurol Psychiatry* 1950; **64:** 141–145.

Denny-Brown D. Fibrillation and fasciculation in voluntary muscle. *Brain* 1938; **61:** 311–334.

Douglass CP, Kandler RH, Shaw PJ, McDermott CJ. An evaluation of neurophysiological criteria used in the diagnosis of motor neuron disease. *J Neurol Neurosurg Psychiatry* 2010; **81:** 646–649.

Duckworth T, Yamashita T, Franks CI, Brown BH. Somatosensory evoked cortical responses in children with spina bifida. *Dev Med Child Neurol* 1976; **18**: 19–24.

Dumitru D, King JC. Fibrillation potential amplitude after denervation. *Am J Phys Med Rehabil* 1998; **77**: 483–489.

Eyre JA, Taylor JP, Villagra F, Smith M, Miller S. Evidence of activity-dependent withdrawal of corticospinal projections during human development. *Neurology* 2001; **57**: 1543–1554.

Fagan ER, Taylor MJ, Logan WJ. Somatosensory evoked potentials: part I. A review of neural generators and special considerations in pediatrics. *Pediatr Neurol* 1987a; **3**: 189–196.

Fagan ER, Taylor MJ, Logan WJ. Somatosensory evoked potentials: part II. A review of the clinical applications in pediatric neurology. *Pediatr Neurol* 1987b; **3**: 249–255.

Gath I, Stalberg E. In situ measurement of the innervation ratio of motor units in human muscles. *Exp Brain Res* 1981; **43**: 377–382.

Gilles FH, Leviton A, Dooling EC, editors. The Developing Human Brain: Growth and Epidemiologic Neuropathology. Boston, MA: J Wright-PSG, 1983.

Goetz E. Neonatal spinal cord injury after an uncomplicated vaginal delivery. *Pediatr Neurol* 2010; **42**: 69–71.

Hausmanowa-Petrusewicz I. Electrophysiological findings in childhood spinal muscular atrophies. *Rev Neurol (Paris)* 1988; **144**: 716–720.

Hausmanowa-Petrusewicz I, Karwanska A. Electromyographic findings in different forms of infantile and juvenile proximal spinal muscular atrophy. *Muscle Nerve* 1986; **9**: 37–46.

Henneman E, Olson CB. Relations between structure and function in the design of skeletal muscles. *J Neurophysiol* 1965; **28**: 581–598.

Henneman E, Somjen G, Carpenter DO. Excitability and inhibitability of motoneurons of different sizes. *J Neurophysiol* 1965; **28**: 599–620.

Hess CW, Mills KR, Murray NM. Responses in small hand muscles from magnetic stimulation of the human brain. *J Physiol* 1987; **388**: 397–419.

Hirayama K. Juvenile muscular atrophy of distal upper extremity (Hirayama disease): focal cervical ischemic poliomyelopathy. *Neuropathology* 2000; **20** (Suppl): S91–S94.

Hitomi T, Mezaki T, Tsujii T, et al. Improvement of central motor conduction after bone marrow transplantation in adrenoleukodystrophy *J Neurol Neurosurg Psychiatry* 2003; **74**: 373–375.

Hodgkin AL, Huxley AF. Propagation of electrical signals along giant nerve fibers. *Proc R Soc Lond B Biol Sci* 1952a; **140**: 177–183.

Hodgkin AL, Huxley AF. A quantitative description of membrane current and its application to conduction and excitation in nerve. *J Physiol* 1952b; **117**: 500–544.

Hughes A. The development of the dorsal funiculus in the human spinal cord. *J Anat* 1976; **122**: 169–175.

Hyun SJ, Rhim SC, Kang JK, Hong SH, Park BR. Combined motor- and somatosensory-evoked potential monitoring for spine and spinal cord surgery: correlation of clinical and neurophysiological data in 85 consecutive procedures. *Spinal Cord* 2009; **47**: 616–622.

Ichiyama T, Hayashi T, Ukita T. Two possible cases of Alexander disease. Multimodal evoked potentials and MRI. *Brain Dev* 1993; **15**: 153–156.

Inagaki M, Maegaki Y, Ohtani K, Asano J, Suzuki Y. Reappearance of visual and somatosensory evoked potentials in a patient with childhood adrenoleukodystrophy after bone marrow transplantation and dietary erucic acid therapy *Acta Paediatr Jpn* 1995; **37**: 125–128.

Jones SJ. Short latency potentials recorded from the neck and scalp following median nerve stimulation in man. *Electroencephalogr Clin Neurophysiol* 1977; **43**: 853–863.

Jones SJ, Baraitser M, Halliday AM. Peripheral and central somatosensory nerve conduction defects in Friedreich's ataxia. *J Neurol Neurosurg Psychiatry* 1980; **43**: 495–503.

Jones SJ, Yu YL, Rudge P, et al. Central and peripheral SEP defects in neurologically symptomatic and asymptomatic subjects with low vitamin B12 levels. *J Neurol Sci* 1987; **82**: 55–65.

Kalita J, Misra UK. Neurophysiological studies in acute transverse myelitis. *J Neurol* 2000; **247**: 943–948.

Kandell E, Schwartz JH, Jessell TM, editors. Principles of Neural Science. New York, NY: McGraw Hill, 2000.

Kang PB, Lidov HG, David WS. et al. Diagnostic value of electromyography and muscle biopsy in arthrogryposis multiplex congenita. *Ann Neurol* 2003; **54**: 790–795.

Kaplan PW Rawal K, Erwin CW, D'Souza BJ, Spock A. Visual and somatosensory evoked potentials in vitamin E deficiency with cystic fibrosis. *Electroencephalogr Clin Neurophysiol* 1988; **71**: 266–272.

Kaplan PW, Tusa RJ, Rignani J, Moser HW. Somatosensory evoked potentials in adrenomyeloneuropathy. *Neurology* 1997; **48**: 1662–1667.

Korenke GC, Hunneman DH, Kohler J, Stockler S, Landmark K, Hanefeld F. Glyceroltrioleate/glyceroltri-erucate therapy in 16 patients with X-chromosomal adrenoleukodystrophy/adrenomyeloneuropathy: effect on clinical biochemical and neurophysiological parameters. *Eur J Pediatr* 1995; **154**: 64–70.

Kumar N, Gross JB Jr, Ahlskog JE. Copper deficiency myelopathy produces a clinical picture like subacute combined degeneration *Neurology* 2004; **63**: 33–39.

Kwon O, Kim M, Lee KWA. Korean case of juvenile muscular atrophy of distal upper extremity (Hirayama disease) with dynamic cervical cord compression. *J Korean Med Sci* 2004; **19**: 768–771.

Lewelt A, Krosschell KJ, Scott C, et al. Compound muscle action potential and motor function in children with spinal muscular atrophy. *Muscle Nerve* 2010; **42**: 703–708.

Li L, Muller-Forell W, Oberman B, Boor R. Subcortical somatosensory evoked potentials after median nerve and posterior tibial nerve stimulation in high cervical cord compression of achondroplasia. *Brain Dev* 2008; **30**: 499–503.

Markandeyulu V, Joseph TP, Solomon T, Jacob J, Kumar S, Gnanamuthu C. Stiff-man syndrome in childhood *J R Soc Med* 2001; **94**: 296–297.

Martinelli P, Montagna P. Exteroceptive reflexes abnormalities in stiff-man syndrome. *J Neurol Neurosurg Psychiatry* 1985; **48**: 92–93.

Master DL, Thompson GH, Poe-Kochert C, Biro C. Spinal cord monitoring for scoliosis surgery in Rett syndrome: can these patients be accurately monitored? *J Pediatr Orthop* 2008; **28**: 342–346.

Matsumoto H, Hanajima R, Terao Y, et al. Efferent and afferent evoked potentials in patients with adreno-myeloneuropathy. *Clin Neurol Neurosurg* 2010; **112**: 131–136.

McPhedran AM, Wuerker RB, Henneman E. Properties of motor units in a heterogeneous pale muscle (m gastrocnemius) of the cat. *J Neurophysiol* 1965; **28**: 85–99.

Meinck HM, Thompson PD. Stiff man syndrome and related conditions. *Mov Disord* 2002; **17**: 853–866.

Mesrati F, Vecchierini MF. F-waves: neurophysiology and clinical value. *Neurophysiol Clin* 2004; **34**: 217–243.

Meyer BU, Britton TC, Benecke R. Wilson's disease: normalisation of cortically evoked motor responses with treatment. *J Neurol* 1991; **238**: 327–330.

Meyer BU, Britton TC, Benecke R, Bischoff C, Machetanz J, Conrad B. Motor responses evoked by magnetic brain stimulation in psychogenic limb weakness: diagnostic value and limitations. *J Neurol* 1992; **239**: 251–255.

Minkowski A, Council for International Organizations of Medical Sciences France Délégation Générale à La Recherche Scientifique et Technique. Regional Development of the Brain in Early Life. Philadelphia, PA: FA Davis, 1967.

Misra UK, Kalita J. Comparison of clinical and electrodiagnostic features in B12 deficiency neurological syndromes with and without antiparietal cell antibodies. *Postgrad Med J* 2007; **83**: 124–127.

Misra UK, Kalita J, Das A. Vitamin B12 deficiency neurological syndromes: a clinical MRI and electrodi-agnostic study. *Electromyogr Clin Neurophysiol* 2003; **43**: 57–64.

Misra UK, Kalita J, Mishra VN, Phadke RV, Hadique A. Effect of neck flexion on F wave, somatosensory evoked potentials, and magnetic resonance imaging in Hirayama disease. *J Neurol Neurosurg Psychiatry* 2006; **77**: 695–698.

Nardone R, Tezzon F. Transcranial magnetic stimulation study in hereditary spastic paraparesis. *Eur Neurol* 2003; **49**: 234–237.

Noguchi Y, Okubo O, Fuchigami T, Fujita Y, Harada K. Motor-evoked potentials in a child recovering from transverse myelitis. *Pediatr Neurol* 2000; **23**: 436–438.

Olson CB, Carpenter DO, Henneman E. Orderly recruitment of muscle action potentials. *Arch Neurol* 1968; **19**: 591–597.

Pillen S, Arts IM, Zwarts MJ. Muscle ultrasound in neuromuscular disorders. *Muscle Nerve* 2008; **37**: 679–693.

Pohl D, Rostasy K, Treiber-Held S, Brockmann K Gartner J, Hanefeld F. Pediatric multiple sclerosis: detection of clinically silent lesions by multimodal evoked potentials *J Pediatr* 2006; **149**: 125–127.

Preston DC, Shapiro BE. Electromyography and Neuromuscular Disorders: Clinical-Electrophysiologic Correlations (2nd edition). Philadelphia, PA; Butterworth-Heinemann, 2005.

Pueschel SM, Findley TW, Furia J, Gallagher PL, Scola FH, Pezzullo JC. Atlantoaxial instability in Down syndrome: roentgenographic, neurologic, and somatosensory evoked potential studies. *J Pediatr* 1987; **110**: 515–521.

Pueschel SM, Scola FH. Atlantoaxial instability in individuals with Down syndrome: epidemiologic, radiographic, and clinical studies. *Pediatrics* 1987; **80**: 555–560.

Puri V, Chaudhry N, Goel S, Gulati P, Nehru R, Chowdhury D. Vitamin B12 deficiency: a clinical and electrophysiological profile. *Electromyogr Clin Neurophysiol* 2005; **45**: 273–284.

Quinn CM, Wigglesworth JS, Heckmatt J. Lethal arthrogryposis multiplex congenita: a pathological study of 21 cases. *Histopathology* 1991; **19**: 155–162.

Rabie M, Jossiphov J, Nevo Y. Electromyography (EMG) accuracy compared to muscle biopsy in childhood. *J Child Neurol* 2007; **22**: 803–808.

Restuccia D, Di Lazzaro V, Valeriani M, et al. Abnormalities of somatosensory and motor evoked potentials in adrenomyeloneuropathy: comparison with magnetic resonance imaging and clinical findings. *Muscle Nerve* 1997; **20**: 1249–1257.

Restuccia D, Mauguiere F. The contribution of median nerve SEPs in the functional assessment of the cervical spinal cord in syringomyelia. A study of 24 patients. *Brain* 1991; **114**: 361–379.

Restuccia D, Rubino M, Valeriani M, Mirabella M, Sabatelli M, Tonali P. Cervical cord dysfunction during neck flexion in Hirayama's disease. *Neurology* 2003; **60**: 1980–1983.

Rexed B. The cytoarchitectonic organization of the spinal cord in the cat. *J Comp Neurol* 1952; **96**: 414–495.

Roser F, Ebner FH, Sixt C, Hagen JM, Tatagiba MS. Defining the line between hydromyelia and syringomyelia A differentiation is possible based on electrophysiological and magnetic resonance imaging studies. *Acta Neurochir (Wien)* 2010; **152**: 213–9.

Roy MW, Gilmore R, Walsh JW. Evaluation of children and young adults with tethered spinal cord syndrome. Utility of spinal and scalp recorded somatosensory evoked potentials. *Surg Neurol* 1986; **26**: 241–248.

Sacco G, Buchthal F, Rosenfalck P. Motor unit potentials at different ages *Arch Neurol* 1962; **6**: 366–373.

Sadler TW, Langman J. Langman's Medical Embryology. Baltimore, MD: Lippincott Williams and Wilkins, 2009.

Scarpini C, Mondelli M, Guazzi GC, Federico A. Ataxia-telangiectasia: somatosensory, brainstem auditory and motor evoked potentials in six patients. *Dev Med Child Neurol* 1996; **38**: 65–73.

Schmidt S, Traber F, Block W, et al. Phenotype assignment in symptomatic female carriers of X-linked adrenoleukodystrophy. *J Neurol* 2001; **248**: 36–44.

Sherrington CS. Recruitment and some other features of reflex inhibition. *Proc R Soc Lond Ser B* 1925; **97**: 488–518.

Smith S, Knight R. In Birch R, editor. Surgical Disorders of the Peripheral Nerves. London: Springer, 2011: 197.

Smyth DP, Willison RG. Quantitative electromyography in babies and young children with no evidence of neuromuscular disease. *J Neurol Sci* 1982; **56**: 209–217.

Standring S, Gray HA. Gray's Anatomy: The Anatomical Basis of Clinical Practice. Edinburgh: Churchill Livingstone, 2008.

Straumanis JJ Jr, Shagass C, Overton DA. Somatosensory evoked responses in Down syndrome. *Arch Gen Psychiatry* 1973; **29**: 544–549.

Strehl E, Vanasse M, Brochu P. EMG and needle muscle biopsy studies in arthrogryposis multiplex congenita. *Neuropediatrics* 1985; **16**: 225–227.

Swoboda KJ, Scott CB, Reyna SP, et al. Phase II open label study of valproic acid in spinal muscular atrophy. *PLoS One* 2009; **4**: e5268.

Tanaka S, Mito T, Takashima S. Progress of myelination in the human fetal spinal nerve roots spinal cord and brainstem with myelin basic protein immunohistochemistry. *Early Hum Dev* 1995; **41**: 49–59.

Turano G, Jones SJ, Miller DH, Du Boulay GH, Kakigi R, McDonald WI. Correlation of SEP abnormalities with brain and cervical cord MRI in multiple sclerosis. *Brain* 1991; **114**: 663–681.

Van Geel BM, Assies J, Haverkort EB, et al. Progression of abnormalities in adrenomyeloneuropathy and neurologically asymptomatic X-linked adrenoleukodystrophy despite treatment with "Lorenzo's oil". *J Neurol Neurosurg Psychiatry* 1999; **67**: 290–299.

Velazquez L, Medina E, Alvarez A, et al. [Neurophysiological clinical study of 70 patients with type 2 spinocerebellar ataxia.] (In Spanish.) *Rev Neurol* 2000; **30**: 109–115.

Velazquez Perez L, Sanchez Cruz G, Canales Ochoa N, et al. Electrophysiological features in patients and presymptomatic relatives with spinocerebellar ataxia type 2. *J Neurol Sci* 2007; **263**: 158–164.

Vialle R, Pietin-Vialle C, Ilharreborde B, Dauger S, Vinchon M, Glorion C. Spinal cord injuries at birth: a multicenter review of nine cases. *J Matern Fetal Neonatal Med* 2007; **20**: 435–440.

Vincent A. Autoimmune disorders of the neuromuscular junction. *Neurol India* 2008; **56**: 305–313.

Visser J, De Visser M, Van Den Berg-Vos RM, et al. Interpretation of electrodiagnostic findings in sporadic progressive muscular atrophy. *J Neurol* 2008; **255**: 903–909.

Wall PD. The sensory and motor role of impulses travelling in the dorsal columns towards cerebral cortex. *Brain* 1970; **93**: 505–524.

Zgorzalewicz-Stachowiak M, Stradomska TJ, Bartkowiak Z, Galas-Zgorzalewicz B. Cerebral childhood and adolescent X-linked adrenoleukodystrophy. Clinical presentation neurophysiological neuroimaging and biochemical investigations. *Folia Neuropathol* 2006; **44**: 319–326.

4
SPINAL CORD MALFORMATIONS

Michel Zerah and Abhaya V Kulkarni

Malformations of the spinal cord are one of the most frequent malformations in the embryo. They have been described for as long as humans have walked on the planet and many anthropological excavations have uncovered spines with typical stigmata seen in children with spinal dysraphism, most of which were myelomeningocele (MMC) (Fig. 4.1). As there were no treatments for these malformations, we can assume that most did not survive. However, many ancient sculptures and drawings provide evidence of adults with such spinal deformities or lesions, which can be related to open or, more often, occult dysraphisms. These spinal dysraphisms belong to the family of malformations called neural tube defects (NTDs), which includes anencephaly, exencephaly, encephaloceles, and meningoceles.

Ancient medical care for these children was virtually non-existent and even Aristotle recommended infanticide in this situation (Bekker 1843, Singer 1993), starting an ongoing ethical debate about the antenatal diagnosis and management of the most severe cases of MMC. Early attempts at treatment included unsuccessful ligation of the sac and application of sclerosing solutions (Goodrich 2008). Only the past two centuries have seen progressive improvement in treatment including surgery for closure of the sac and the effective treatment of hydrocephalus.

Classifications
These malformations must be clearly divided into two different families.

OPEN DYSRAPHISM
This consists mostly of MMC. It is a frequent (prevalence approximately 0.5–1.0 per 1000 pregnancies [Shaer et al. 2007]), very severe malformation in which the spinal canal is open to the external surface with its external edge attached to the edges of a skin defect. The muscles are absent or pushed laterally and the posterior elements of the vertebral column are absent or open (spina bifida).

OCCULT DYSRAPHISM
This is a heterogeneous group of malformations including lipomas of the filum and the conus, diastematomyelias, neurenteric cysts, dermal sinuses, and more complex conditions, often associated with malformation syndromes, including anorectal malformations.

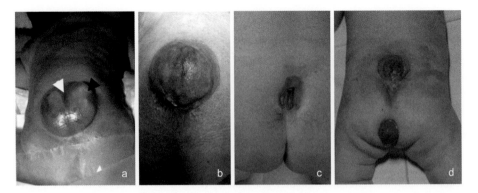

Fig. 4.1. Myelomeningocele (MMC). (a) Non-rupture MMC (white arrow, meningocele; black arrow, neural plate). (b) Partly epithelialized MMC. (c) Rachischisis (externalized neural plate, without meningocele). (d) Very severe form with anal prolapse.

Caudal regression syndrome is probably distinct from the previous malformations and will be treated separately

Embryology (Afonso and Catala 2003)

The term 'spina bifida' was suggested by Nicolas Tulp in 1641 (Tulpius 1641) in his first description of MMC. It was proposed solely to describe a duplication of the spinous process of the vertebra. This term, incorrect though it might be, is still used to describe any malformation occurring in the lower spine.

GASTRULATION

After fertilization and approximately five rounds of cell division, the human embryo comprises a spherical blastocele (the future placenta) and an eccentrically placed cluster of cells, the inner cell mass (the future embryo).

By the end of the first embryonic week, it will be composed of two layers, the epiblast and the hypoblast. This establishes a ventrodorsal axis.

During the second week, a rostrocaudal axis develops and the epiblast cells in the caudal region of the embryo migrate towards the midline to form the primitive streak. At the cranial end of the primitive streak lies the primitive knot or Hensen's node. Cells from the primitive streak and Hensen's node invaginate beneath the epiblast in a process known as gastrulation. This invagination creates a three-layered embryo (endoderm, mesoderm, and ectoderm). The ectodermal cells give rise to the surface ectoderm and the neuroectoderm or neuroepithelium. The regression of the primitive streak, the primitive pit, the notocordal canal, and the notocordal plate has been described in the avian embryo but is still debated in more evolved species (there is no evidence of a neurenteric canal in mammals for example). Some complex dysraphisms (MMC, split cord malformations) are related to this period of embryogenesis.

PRIMARY NEURULATION (CATALA ET AL. 1996)

During the third embryonic week, the ectoderm forms two morphologically distinct tissues: the centrally located neuroectoderm and the more peripherally located cutaneous ectoderm. The neuroectoderm is visible on embryonic day (D)16. Between D16 and D28, the neuroectoderm undergoes several morphologic changes referred to as neurulation to form the neural tube. A midline neural groove develops. Elevation, growing, and medial convergence of the neural folds bring the neuroectoderm together in the midline to form the neural tube. Fusion of the neural folds and separation from the overlying cutaneous ectoderm completes the process. This process starts at the middle part of the embryo and progresses rostrally to close at D24 to D26 at the level of the anterior neuropore (future commissural plate lamina terminalis) and caudally to close 2 days later (caudal neuropore) at the level of the second sacral segment where it joins the process of secondary neurulation.

The entire process of primary neurulation is finished at the end of the fourth week.

SECONDARY NEURULATION (CATALA 1999)

This involves a mechanism entirely different from primary neurulation. The most caudal part of the neural tube develops from a pluripotent group of cells. Secondary neurulation involves the independent formation and canalization of multiple secondary tubules from the caudal cell mass and subsequent fusion of adjacent tubules to form a secondary neural tube. It will eventually fuse with the primary neural tube.

SPINAL OCCLUSION

This begins at the time of anterior neuropore closure (D24) and ends a week later. It initiates the rapid growth of the neural tube and the dilatation of the ventricular system. Failure to maintain this spinal and spinal cord occlusion may produce MMC and the mesenchymal and brain anomalies referred to as the Chiari II malformation.

ASCENT OF THE CONUS MEDULLARIS

By approximately gestation day 45, the caudal end of the neural tube extends to the coccygeal spinal level. Thereafter, the caudal end of the neural tube begins to ascend to more cranial spinal levels. This involves two mechanisms: retrogressive differentiation and, more importantly, the differential growth between the spine and the spinal cord during embryonic and fetal life. By 1 or 2 months after birth, the conus medullaris lies at its final location, opposite the L1 to L2 disk space. Any problem during this relative ascent (e.g. in secondary neurulation) can lead to a low and tethered spinal cord.

EMBRYOLOGY OF MYELOMENINGOCELE (TILL 1969, LEMIRE 1983)

Many theories have been discussed (non-closure, reopening, overgrowth, over-distension). The non-closure theory has gained almost universal acceptance but there is no definitive evidence to refute the others. Numerous teratogenic agents and genetic disorders (e.g. trisomies 13 and 18, congenital hemidysplasia with ichthyosiform erythroderma and limb

defects [CHILD], Frazer, Waardenburg, and Meckel–Gruber syndromes) have been identified which act on specific parts of the neurulation sequence to produce NTDs. The role of
folate deficiency has also been identified as one of the main causes of open dysraphism
and can be largely prevented by folate supplementation before conception and during the
early stages of pregnancy (Czeizel and Dudas 1992). The exact mechanism by which folate
reduces the risk of open NTDs is unclear.

Embryology of the Occult Dysraphisms
Although the embryology of these disorders remains largely unknown in humans, it is
clearly a different mechanism from that causing MMC (Till 1969, Lemire 1983, Belzberg
et al. 1991, Catala 1998, 2002, Tortori-Donati et al. 2000, Li et al. 2001, Afonso and Catala
2003, Finn and Walker 2007, Muthukumar 2009).

Open dysraphism: MMC
Epidemiology
MMC (Fig. 4.1) is one of the most frequent human malformations. Its mean incidence is
one per 1000 live births, with a wide variation based on ethnicity, race, geography, and
temporal trends. In Europe, the highest rates are found in Ireland and Wales (five per 1000
live births) compared with southeast Europe (0.1–0.6 per 1000 live births) (Group 1991).
In Canada and the USA, a higher incidence has been reported along the East Coast. In
China, the incidence rates north of the YangTze River are six times those of the Southern
Province. Pockets of higher incidence have also been identified in India without any systematic geographical pattern (Frey and Hauser 2003).

Ethnicity also has an effect on the rates of MMC. In the USA, the Hispanic population
has the highest risk. This risk remains among Hispanics even after controlling for other
factors. When a low prevalence ethnic group migrates to a region of high incidence, they
tend to maintain their low rates or at least a rate lower than that of the native population.
When a high prevalence ethnic group migrates to a region of low incidence, they maintain
a higher rate than the native population, but there is always a significant reduction in risk.
These geographical and ethnic considerations have led to a search for environmental and
nutritional factors, specifically the folates (Canfield et al. 1996a,b, 2009).

Observations in the UK in the mid-1970s that lower red-cell folate level in women of
lower socio-economic status was associated with a higher prevalence of NTDs implicated
folate deficiency as an aetiological factor (Rosano et al. 1999). In the early 1980s, initial
randomized trials in the UK were strongly supportive of a role for folate supplementation
in the prevention of NTDs.

From 1988 to 1995 several case–control studies indicated a risk reduction of 30 to
75% in those receiving peri-conceptual folic acid supplements. The Medical Research
Council Vitamin Study Group (UK) in 1991 reported the results of a double-blind randomized controlled study (33 centres, seven countries) which showed that peri-conceptional
folic acid supplementation (4mg/d), in mothers with a previous history of NTD, was
associated with a risk reduction of 72% (Smithells et al. 1976, 1983, Laurence et al. 1980,
1981).

In 1991 the US Centres for Disease Control and Prevention therefore recommended 4mg/day supplementation for mothers with a high risk of MMC by virtue of a previously affected pregnancy (Pitkin 2007).

In 1992, a randomized study of 4156 low-risk Hungarian women found a statistically significant reduction of NTDs with folic acid supplementation (800µg/d). This led to the further recommendation by the Centres for Disease Control and Prevention that all repro-ductive-aged women should take 400µg folic acid daily in addition to a folate-rich diet (Czeizel et al. 1992, Czeizel and Dudas 1992, Dudas and Czeizel 1992).

PREVENTION

Because folic acid supplementation has been shown to reduce the risk of NTD, the mainstay of prevention is now aimed at increasing the intake of folic acid in the target population of women. This can be achieved in three ways, as follows.

Increasing folate-rich foods in the diet

Even if foods high in folate are numerous (broccoli, spinach, green salad), it is difficult to get enough folate from natural sources alone to reduce the risk of NTD. Therefore a recom-mendation to increase folate intake through food is not an adequate measure in isolation.

Folic acid supplementation

Since 1993, public health strategies in many countries have aimed to promote the taking of folic acid by women of childbearing age. The recommended dose is 400µg daily (McNulty et al. 2000). Women who have had a previous NTD-affected pregnancy or who are otherwise at high-risk (close relative with a NTD, type 1 diabetes mellitus, epilepsy treated with val-proic acid or carbamazepine) are recommended 4mg per day. This needs to be taken for at least 1 month before conception and continued throughout the first trimester of pregnancy.

However, these strategies have not been successful in substantially reducing the numbers of affected births. The likely reason for this is that up to 50% of all pregnancy are unplanned and folate must be taken before conception to have an effect.

Fortification of foods with folic acid

Because the above measures are often unsuccessful, food fortification policies (in the UK, Australia, Mongolia) have instead been used to provide a more widespread and reliable intake of folic acid. Since 1998, mandatory fortification of flour has been introduced in Canada, Indonesia, and some South American and Asian countries. Recent data have con-firmed that rates of NTDs have dropped in the USA and Canada by 26% and 46% compared with pre-fortification rates. In Chile, where fortification was introduced in 2000, there has been a 40% drop (Lopez-Camelo et al. 2000, 2005, Hertrampf and Cortes 2004, Llanos et al. 2007, Nazer et al. 2007). In France there has been a reluctance to follow such policies. The most recent results were published in 2009, after Brazil introduced fortification of flours made of corn and wheat in the state of Rio Grande do Norte in 2002 (M. Bezerra, personal communication). Only an insignificant decrease in the incidence of MMC was found, prob-ably related to a poor consumption of industrial flour in poor families.

ANTENATAL DIAGNOSIS AND MANAGEMENT

Until a few decades ago, the prenatal detection rate was relatively low and mostly occurred in developed countries. Serum screening (alpha-fetoprotein, acetylcholinesterase) (Wald and Cuckle 1980) was used in conjunction with ultrasound. Using this type of approach, detection rates as high as 80% were reached. Over the past 20 years, the detection rate has dramatically increased to almost 100%, following the recognition that indirect cerebral findings were present in the overwhelming majority of cases of MMC. These cerebral findings include ventriculomegaly, the lemon sign (frontal bossing), the banana sign (deformation of the cerebellum), and the obliteration of the cisterna magna (Fig. 4.2). Direct signs best detectable in the axial plane are a C or U shape of the affected vertebra, interruption of the skin contour with or without a meningocele, and splaying of the lateral processes (Fig. 4.2).

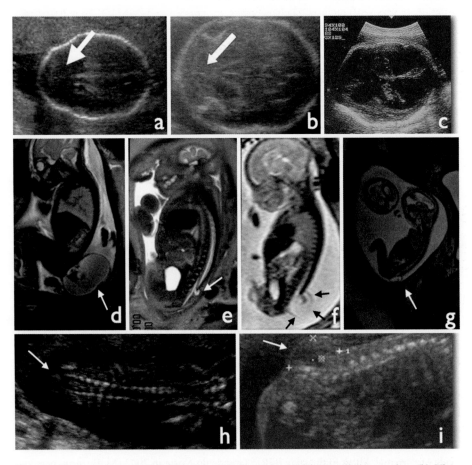

Fig. 4.2. Myelomeningocele (MMC). Antenatal diagnosis. (a) Ultrasound: lemon sign. (b) Ultrasound: banana sign. (c) Ultrasound: antenatal hydrocephalus. (d–g) Sagittal MRI: MMC (in a twin pregnancy in g). (h, i) Ultrasound: coronal and sagittal images of an MMC.

It has become possible to achieve a diagnosis progressively earlier in gestation (10th or 12th week in some cases, 18th–24th in most cases) (Nicolaides et al. 1986, Filly 1989a,b, Van Den Hof et al. 1990, Sebire et al. 1997, Monteagudo et al. 2000, Rossi et al. 2004a,b, Ghi et al. 2006).

Magnetic resonance imaging (MRI) and fetal karyotyping are not routinely recommended. These can, however, reveal chromosomal anomalies (8–16%) or other associated malformations.

Once the diagnosis has been made, the weight of the ethical and moral decisions falls squarely on the shoulders of the parents and physicians as they consider what course to follow. The termination of the fetus has always been at the centre of the moral debate about the right to life and hinges on the status of the fetus. In many countries, termination remains illegal even in cases of severe malformation. In most countries where termination is permitted, the period for legal termination is up to and no later than the 18th to 28th week of gestation. In very few countries, such as France, termination remains legal for lethal or very severe malformations such as MMC, until the last day of pregnancy. The termination rate is 23% in the USA and 78% in Europe (Czeizel et al. 1979, Dommergues et al. 1999, 2006, Koszutski et al. 2009).

In utero treatment of MMC has been proposed (Bruner et al. 2000, 2004, Walsh et al. 2001, Hirose et al. 2003, Tubbs et al. 2003, Tulipan et al. 2003, Hamdan et al. 2004, Tulipan 2004, Johnson et al. 2006, Sutton 2008, Hirose and Farmer 2009). It remains very controversial and is undertaken in very few centres in the world. Preliminary reports show no improvement in limb deficits or in sphincter dysfunction, but possibly a reduction in the rate of Chiari malformation and hydrocephalus (from 90 to 50%). A strictly controlled prospective clinical trial began in 2003 involving three major centres in the USA. The final results of this study, published in 2011 (Adzick et al. 2011), suggest that fetal surgery before 26 weeks' gestation may preserve neuromotor function, reverse Chiari malformation, reduce the need for ventriculo-peritoneal shunting, and possibly improve cognitive function. However, these data also demonstrate that fetal surgery is associated with maternal (uterine scarring and pulmonary oedema) and fetal (preterm birth) risks. Further research is necessary to define the optimal surgical technique (open or endoscopic), the ideal timing, and to evaluate the long-term outcome for mother and infant (Danzer et al. 2012).

Where the decision is taken to continue the pregnancy, early consultation should be organized with a paediatric neurosurgeon to explain to the future parents the initial postnatal care and the short- and long-term follow-up.

INITIAL MANAGEMENT AT BIRTH
Delivery by Caesarean section is recommended by many authors to minimize trauma to and possible infection of the MMC during transit through the birth canal, although this indication is still controversial and not evidence-based (Cochrane et al. 1991, Merrill et al. 1998, Lewis et al. 2004, Hamrick 2008).

Even if it remains impracticable in many countries for most children, early surgery is the criterion standard treatment for MMC. If surgery is not done during the first few days, most children will die from early infection or later (sometimes after several months) from chronic hydrocephalus.

In addition to supplies routinely needed in the delivery room, sterile gauze, warm saline, and non-permeable covers for the dressing should be provided. Infants with open dysraphism are at high risk of latex allergy. In a recent study, 48% of patients with MMC showed a biological (specific immunoglobulin E greater than 0.7kU/l) latex sensitization and 15% were allergic to latex with clinical manifestations. These results underline the importance of avoiding latex exposure from the beginning. All diagnostic and therapeutic procedures should therefore be conducted in a latex-free environment (Buck et al. 2000, Niggemann et al. 2000, Rendeli et al. 2006, Woodhouse 2008, Majed et al. 2009).

Careful neonatal paediatric and neurosurgical assessment is the first step before surgical procedure planning. Other than determining the lesion's level, this evaluation aims to identify the site, extent, and characteristics of the spinal malformation and to identify any related spinal deformity (scoliosis, severe kyphosis, split cord malformation) that may have an impact on surgery. Ascertaining the presence of or absence of hydrocephalus (rarely present at birth) is crucial in ensuring the correct surgical strategy, as is identifying any wider associated malformation syndrome not already prenatally identified.

Closure of MMC within 24 to 48 hours is customary. The role of the surgery is to place the spinal cord back within the spinal canal and to close dura, fascia, muscle, and skin in separate layers. In some large defects, plastic-surgery closure techniques can be useful.

Early postoperative mortality is near zero. However, the morbidity due to complications of the repair (wound-healing problems, cerebrospinal fluid leak, meningitis) can be significant. They may affect the patient's quality of life and are usually due to a largely avoidable faulty technique.

As many as 90% of infants with open dysraphism develop hydrocephalus before the end of the second week (Chakraborty et al. 2008). It can be detected by clinical examination and ultrasound, and treated by ventriculo-peritoneal shunt. Most infants with MMC exhibit some degree of Chiari II malformation, but the exact number of those who will develop clinical signs and need surgery remains controversial (5–30%); the need for surgery to a Chiari malformation during the first day of life is exceptional (Pollack et al. 1996).

Parents of infants with MMC may experience feelings of crisis, stress, anxiety, helplessness, denial, and lowered self-esteem. The initial approach of the paediatric team is extremely important. As during prenatal consultations, in the postnatal preoperative period, the paediatric neurosurgeon should spend sufficient time with the family explaining the diagnosis, treatment, complications, and potential outcome. Unduly optimistic or pessimist explanations should be avoided. The paediatric urology team should also be involved at the early neonatal stage (see below).

LATE COMPLICATIONS
Vertebral problems and deformities
Children with MMC have a high incidence of vertebral deformity (scoliosis, kyphosis, or lordosis). The deformities are either congenital or secondary to paralysis. They are often progressive and bracing can be ineffective, leading to surgical treatment in most cases.

Neuropathic bladder

This is the most frequent complication of MMC and needs to be closely followed from birth to minimize the risk of urological deterioration (chronic infections, urinary incontinence, vesicouretral reflux). All children with MMC should be assessed neonatally by the paediatric urology team and followed regularly with kidney and bladder ultrasound and urodynamic studies.

Chiari II malformation and syringomyelia (La Marca et al. 1997, Caldarelli et al. 1998)

The Chiari II malformation is specific to MMC (Fig. 4.3). It occurs in more than 90% of cases but is rarely symptomatic. The brainstem has abnormal disposition and angulation. The posterior fossa is smaller than normal. The fourth ventricle is caudally displaced and elongated. The foramen magnum is large, there is significant prolapse of the vermis, and the lower part of the tonsils are low or very low (lower cervical or even upper thoracic spine). It is very often associated with brain and ventricular malformations (dysgenesis or agenesis of the septum pellucidum, colpocephaly, enlarged massa intermedia, malformation of the floor of the third ventricle).

Clinical manifestations of the Chiari II malformation can be related to brainstem compression, usually seen during the first weeks of life (poor feeding, recurrent vomiting, high-pitched cry or stridor due to vocal cord paralysis, episodes of apnoea, pulmonary aspiration, nystagmus or bradycardia, torticollis, opisthotonus, lower cranial nerve dysfunction). The incidence of these symptoms is estimated to be 5 to 10%. The indications for

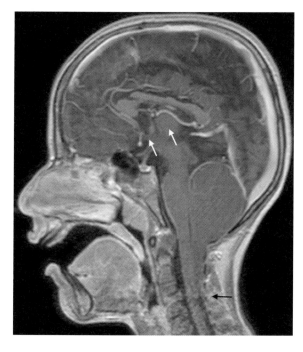

Fig. 4.3. Myelomeningoele. Chiari II malformation. The tip of the level is at the level of C4 (black arrow). The region of the third ventricle is typically abnormal with an enlarged mass intermedia and a verticalization of the floor of the third ventricle (white arrows).

early craniovertebral junction surgical decompression are controversial, but this can some-times be associated with good clinical results. Problems related to the hindbrain hernia can also be seen later in life, in childhood or in adulthood. Syringomyelia is very frequent but remains, in most cases, asymptomatic. However, it can worsen the neurological, orthopae-dic, or urological status of the child. In these situations, craniovertebral decompression is also controversial and must not be performed until cord re-tethering and, most importantly, shunt malfunction has been ruled out.

Tethered cord (Hoffman et al. 1976, Yamada et al. 1981, Pierz et al. 2000, Phuong et al. 2002, Hertzler et al. 2010, Mehta et al. 2010, 2011, Vandertop 2010)
This occurs in about 20% of initially operated MMC. The clinical diagnosis is difficult, but decline in lower extremity strength, a change in sphincter function, rapid worsening of scoliosis, gait change, spasticity, and the development of pain (usually back pain and less commonly, leg pain) are the more frequent symptoms. MRI, unfortunately, is of little help in making the diagnosis, which usually rests on careful serial clinical evaluation and indi-vidual judgement. The decision as to whether to untether surgically is based on the rate of progression of symptoms, the elimination of other possible causes (especially shunt dys-function), and a discussion between the paediatric neurosurgical team and the family and patient. In most cases, surgery is performed during the pre-adolescent period.

It is vital always to bear in mind that by far the most common cause of neurological change in MMC is shunt malfunction. This can mimic any of the symptoms of the above complications; therefore shunt function must always be checked before any surgical inter-vention such as cranio-vertebral junction decompression or cord untethering. Even in cases of severe shunt malfunction the ventricular size may remain small or unchanged, and so many neurosurgeons recommend a surgical shunt exploration in all cases of unclear clinical deterioration, regardless of imaging results. Although intracranial monitoring may be of value, pressures are not infrequently only mildly elevated.

Occult dysraphism
THE CUTANEOUS SYNDROME
Cutaneous anomalies are present in 90% of cases (Fig. 4.4). These skin anomalies have considerable diagnostic value and their absence in individual cases is often responsible for delayed diagnosis. These anomalies are often in the midline (72% in our series) but when lateral they were predominantly on the left side (75%, $p<0.01$). In all series the most common of these anomalies was a subcutaneous lump representing the subjacent presence of a lipoma or a meningocele. When the subcutaneous lipoma is caudally situated, the lump is associated with a gluteal fold deviation. The diagnostic value of these lumbosacral cuta-neous lesions in asymptomatic children as an indicator of an occult spinal dysraphism is variable. In a previous study we retrospectively reviewed 54 children referred to the Depart-ment of Paediatric Dermatology in our hospital (Guggisberg et al. 2004). Occult spinal dysraphism was detected in three out of 36 patients with an isolated midline lesion and in 11 out of 38 patients with the combination of two or more different skin lesions. These skin anomalies can be divided into three groups of varying risk: group 1 (high risk), two or more

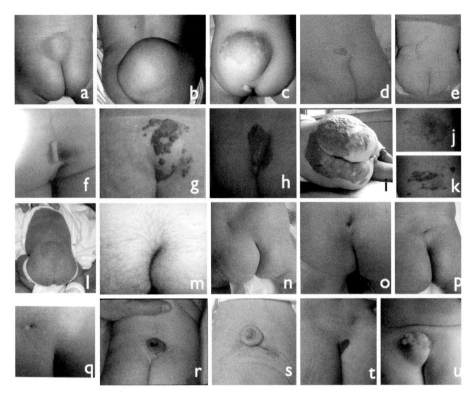

Fig. 4.4. Occult dysraphism. Skin anomalies. (a–c) Subcutaneous lipomas (a, median; b, lateralized; c, associated with an angioma and a lump). (d–f) Caudal appendix. (g–k) Angiomas. (l) Skin hamartoma. (m, n) Deviation of the gluteal furrow. (o–q) Dermal sinuses. (r–s) 'Meningocele manqué' (mostly seen in limited dorsal myeloschisis). (t) Naevus. (u) Complex form with lipoma, angioma, caudal appendix, and deviation of the gluteal furrow.

lesions (of any type), subcutaneous lipoma, tail, dermal sinus, 'queue de faune'; group 2 (low risk), atypical dimple, aplasia cutis, deviation of the gluteal furrow; group 3 (very low risk), hemangioma, port-wine stain, hypertrichosis, fibroma pendulum, pigmentary naevus, coccygeal dimple (Fig. 4.5).

LIPOMA

Congenital lumbosacral lipomas are the most common form of closed NTD. In most cases, they are now diagnosed prenatally or at birth. They may lead to progressive neuro-orthopaedic and sphincter deterioration. However, their natural history is poorly understood. Prophylactic surgery has been the criterion standard of treatment, but considering the deterioration after prophylactic de-tethering over time, especially in the case of lipoma of the conus, the performance of systematic prophylactic surgery has been questioned (Kulkarni 2004, Zerah 2008, Pang et al. 2010a).

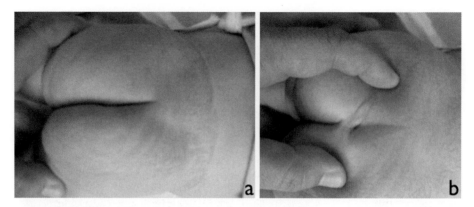

Fig. 4.5. Sacrococcygeal dimple. A benign coccygeal dimple must be hidden by the gluteal furrow, located at less than 2.5cm of the anal margin, and size less than 2.5cm in diameter. There is no relationship between the deepness of the groove and the risk of dysraphism.

General considerations (Pierre-Kahn et al. 1997)

Among more than 2500 cases reported in the literature, there is a significant female predominance (females:males 1.2:1, $p<0.001$). This contrasts with the equal sex ratio generally found in MMC and the male predominance in isolated osseous spina bifida occulta or neurenteric cyst.

The real incidence of this malformation is uncertain. In a previous paper, we attempted to approach the epidemiology of this malformation in two French regional registries. A minimum incidence of four to eight per 100 000 was found. Routine autopsy has provided a prevalence of incidental lipomas ranging from 0 to 6% (mean 0.003%). Recent MRI studies of adults investigated for suspected disc disease or lumbar stenosis have revealed an incidence of 1.5 to 5%. All of these studies, however, were of small size and restricted to the filum.

These lipomas are essentially mature teratomas (and not tumours). They typically consist of normal mature adipocytes separated into clusters by numerous collagen bands. In our series, 77% included, in addition, a wide variety of ectodermal, endodermal, or mesodermal tissues. The most frequent were from mesodermal origin (nerves and striated muscle fibres). The metabolic activity in the lipoma was similar to that observed in normal adipose tissue. Consequently, adipocytes from congenital lipomas are capable of growth or regression commensurate with increase or decrease in the rest of the body's fat, with consequent clinical deterioration or improvement.

Lipoma of the filum (Pierre-Kahn et al. 1997)

This is the simplest malformation. The fatty infiltration of the filum may involve the whole length of the filum or only a part of it (Fig. 4.6). The roots of the cauda equina are generally free and not malformed. In most cases, lipomas of the filum are asymptomatic at birth and only diagnosed because of the cutaneous stigmata. Ultrasound, if done early enough

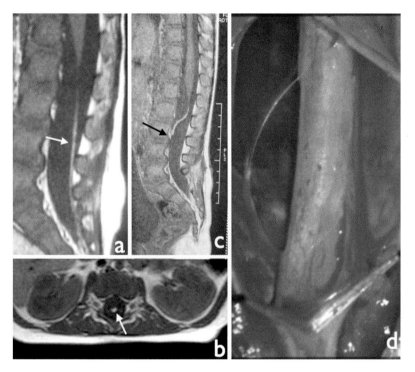

Fig. 4.6. Lipoma of the filum. (a, b) Axial, sagittal, and coronal T_1-weighted MRI of the filum (white arrows). (c) Sagittal T_1-weighted MRI after the section (black arrow). (d) Operative view.

(before the sixth week of life), is often sufficient to make the diagnosis. There is no need for MRI before the third month. A small filum lipoma is best appreciated on axial T_1-weighted images. Although systematic prophylactic surgery (division of the filum) is often proposed with excellent results, this is controversial (Kulkarni 2004, Zerah 2008, Pang et al. 2010a). If the diagnosis is not made at birth, it is possible that neurological or urological deterioration may occur later in life. Surgery is indicated if this occurs, but the expectation is of the stabilization of symptoms rather than improvement.

Lipoma of the conus (Pierre-Kahn et al. 1995, 1997, Lellouch-Tubiana et al. 1999,
Kulkarni et al. 2004, Zerah et al. 2008)
Different anatomical forms of lipoma of the conus have been described. All have in common an insertion on to the lumbar spinal cord and some relationship with the roots. It extends typically from L2 to S3, with a median rostrocaudal length of four vertebral levels. The zone of insertion on the cord is usually wide. Chapman classified lipomas into four types according to localization (dorsal, dorsolateral or lateral, caudal, and dorsocaudal). In our series, very complex forms were found in most patients (62.9%). In lipomyelomeningoceles, a subcutaneous meningocele is associated with an extra-spinal extension of the spinal

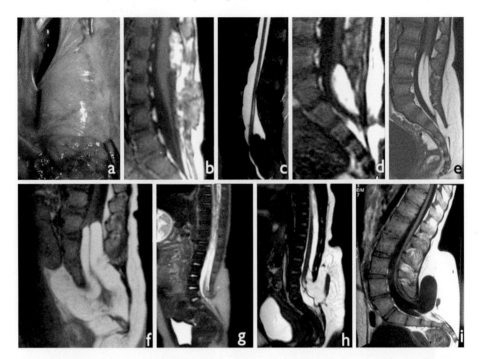

Fig. 4.7. Lipoma of the conus. (a) Operative view. (b–i) Sagittal MRI scans of (b) posterior lipoma, (c) posteroterminal lipoma, (d) terminal lipoma, (e) transitional lipoma, (f) complex chaotic form with anterior expansion, (g, h) lipomyelocele, (i) lipomyelocystocele.

cord. In lipomyeloceles, the spinal cord extends extra-spinally within the subcutaneous lipoma. In lipomyelocystoceles, which are rare, the spinal cord ends in a pseudocystic terminal hydromyelia closed superficially by the lipoma itself (Fig. 4.7).

The neurological syndrome associated with lipomas of the conus involves neurological deficits in the lower limbs, sphincter disturbance, and orthopaedic deformities. Sphincter disorders are the most common problem (60% of symptomatic cases), of which urinary difficulties are the most common, with incontinence associated in most cases with dysuria, urgency of micturition, and incomplete voiding. Bladder infection and pyelonephritis are also common and may be the first or only manifestation of the condition.

Neuro-orthopaedic syndrome is less common (32%), affecting the distal lower limbs. Paralysis or sensory deficits are usually associated with muscular atrophy and/or progressive foot deformity. The upper level of the deficit is almost never above L4.

Back and leg pain is also frequent, especially in adults (33%). Progressive deterioration has been well documented. It may start at any age including in adulthood and in the elderly. It usually occurs slowly and insidiously. The real incidence of deterioration is controversial. Fifteen years ago, we started a prospective study following a cohort of asymptomatic lipomas of the filum at birth. We have enrolled more than 150 children. Only one-third of

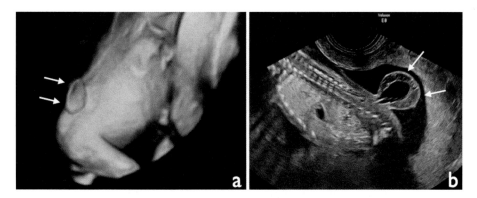

Fig. 4.8. Lipoma of the conus. Antenatal ultrasound at 15 weeks of gestation. (a) Three-dimensional image with the skin covered lump (white arrows). (b) Two-dimensional image. The normal thick skin allows differentiation of occult dysraphism from MMC (white arrows).

them have deteriorated so far, with a return to a completely normal status after surgery in half. With this protocol of conservative management 94% of children have a normal life at 15 years' follow-up (unpublished data).

Prenatal diagnosis is possible in some cases from week 15 of gestation on the basis of lumbosacral meningocele and overlying hyperechogenic skin (Fig. 4.8). Unlike MMC, no associated hydrocephalus or Chiari malformations are found. There is a low-lying terminal cord and, over time, the meningocele component diminishes and the lipoma becomes more prominent. In no case, in our experience, did prenatal MRI provide more information than ultrasound.

Ultrasound is the examination of choice in neonates and up to 6 weeks. Our preference is to recommend ultrasound as the first investigation, although MRI remains the main investigation before surgery (Fig. 4.9). Sagittal and axial views in T_1- and T_2-weighted images are necessary to analyse the lipoma and its relationship to the spinal cord, the roots, and the spine. There is a consensus opinion in favour of surgical de-tethering and subtotal removal of the lipoma in symptomatic patients (Zerah et al. 2008). For asymptomatic patients, based on our 15 year prospective study, we advocate conservative management.

DIASTEMATOMYELIA

(Sheptak and Susen 1967, McMaster 1984, Han et al. 1985, Szalay et al. 1987,
Maiuri et al. 1989, Kogler et al. 1991, Pang et al. 1992, Kim et al. 1994,
Dias and Pang 1995, Unsinn et al. 2000, Gan et al. 2007)

The word diastematomyelia was introduced by Ollivier in 1837. It came from the Greek διαστεμα (diastema, meaning slit or cleft) and μψελοσ (myelos, meaning cord). Ollivier clearly states that this definition applies to a division of the spinal cord in two halves. It must not be confused with diplomyelia, which is a supplementary, completely formed spinal cord situated anterior or posterior to the original one. Diplomyelia is an exceptionally rare malformation, described in mutated animals but only described in autopsy in humans. On

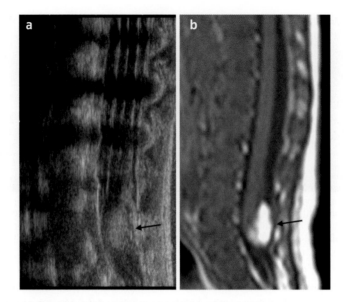

Fig. 4.9. Lipoma of the conus. Comparison between (a) ultrasound and (b) MRI.

the other hand, dimyelia is a true duplication of the spinal cord found only in conjoined twins.

Classification

Since 1991, most authors have followed the classification proposed by Pang. He proposed the term of split cord malformation and clearly differentiated two main types of diastematomyelia.

Type I is characterized by two hemicords, having their own dural envelope, separated by an osteocartilaginous septum or spur. In this type, spinal anomalies (hemi-, butterfly, or fused vertebra) are present in the large majority of cases.

Type II occurs where the two hemicords are contained in a single dural sac with or without a fibrous septum; in this type of diastematomyelia, spinal bony anomalies are rare.

The embryology of diastematomyelia continues to be the subject of debate. The classical explanation of the persistence of the neurenteric canal cannot be accepted in the absence of any evidence for the existence of this canal in primates. Disorders of neurulation or adherence between endoderm and mesoderm have also been proposed, but the most popular theory is based on abnormal gastrulation with an abnormally wide primitive stalk.

In most cases of diastematomyelia, the lower spine is affected. Fifty-five per cent of cases are in the lumbosacral region, 32% are thoracolumbar, and only 13% above. In 5 to 10% of cases, several clefts coexist at different levels so it is particularly important that the full length of the cord is imaged.

In diastematomyelia, hydromyelia may involve one or both the hemicords. A tight filum or a low cord is often present in a low diastematomyelia. Lipoma, dermal sinus, MMC, and hemimyelomeningocele have also been described in association with diastematomyelia of either type. On the other hand, Chiari malformation is a rare association.

Clinical symptoms and signs

Most cases are sporadic, with a female predominance reported in all series (1.2:1 to 1.5:1). It has been described in every part of the world but seems to be rarer in Asia (excluding the Indian sub-continent) and more frequent around the Mediterranean (especially in Turkey).

Diastematomyelia can be easily diagnosed before birth and, in our personal antenatal clinics, is the commonest cause of antenatally diagnosed dysraphism. For the past five years, two-thirds of our cases have been diagnosed before birth.

Postnatally, type II diastematomyelia is asymptomatic (and undiagnosed) in most cases. Type I diastematomyelia is usually diagnosed on the basis of skin stigmata, orthopaedic anomalies, or a spinal dysraphic neurological syndrome. Any of the skin markers described above can be associated with type 1 diastematomyelia, but the presence of a hairy patch ('queue de faune') is present in more than 90% of cases and is quasi-pathognomonic of type I diastematomyelia (Fig. 4.10a–c). The typical orthopaedic syndrome is characterized by a severe and progressive scoliosis (more rarely kyphosis) relating to spinal bony anomalies as well as the spinal cord malformation. In our experience, the scoliosis is twice as common where a hydromyelia is also present.

The neurological syndrome is related to the level of the malformation. Gait difficulties, asymmetric weakness and limb atrophy (on the side of the smaller cord), sensory deficit, pain, and sphincter dysfunction are the most frequent symptoms.

Radiological findings

Antenatal diagnosis is based on ultrasonography and confirmed by MRI (Fig. 4.11). This should separate an isolated diastematomyelia, which is of good prognosis, from more complex forms associated with other malformations of the CNS and other organ systems, which have a less favourable prognosis.

Postnatal diagnosis can also be achieved by ultrasonography during the first weeks of life. Computed tomography, MRI, and radiograph will help to secure the diagnosis and to decide on appropriate treatment (Fig. 4.10d–o).

Management

The treatment of diastematomyelia remains controversial. Some authors are in favour of prophylactic surgery, even in asymptomatic type II diastematomyelia. We do not support this approach. By contrast, in type I diastematomyelia, neurosurgery must be performed in all symptomatic children, before or in combination with spinal surgery. We are also in favour of prophylactic surgery in asymptomatic type I diastematomyelia because of the high risk of clinical deterioration with age, the difficulty of surgery in older children, and because postoperative improvement is rare in symptomatic patients. In the case of antenatally

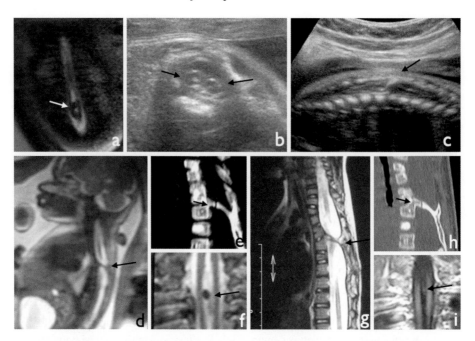

Fig. 4.10. Diastematomyelia. Antenatal diagnosis. (a–c) Coronal, axial, and sagittal ultrasound. (d–i) Pre- (d–f) and postnatal (g–i) images in the same child. (d, g) Sagittal T_2-weighted MRI, (e, h) CT, (f) coronal T_2-, and (i) T_1-weighted MRI.

diagnosed diastematomyelia, we prefer to perform the surgery between 6 months and one year of age because of the risk of haemorrhage in very young infants. The goal of surgery, is to remove the bony spur and to resect the intermedullary dura to avoid the late regrowth of the spur. Where there is an associated dysraphism (e.g. lipoma of the filum), this malformation is operated on during the same procedure (Pang and Parrish 1983).

DERMAL SINUS
(Kuharik et al. 1985, Gok et al. 1995, Bajpai et al. 1997, Hattori et al. 1999,
Jindal et al. 1999, Santiago Medina et al. 1999, Ackerman and Menezes 2003,
Emmez et al. 2004, Sen et al. 2005, Lode et al. 2008)
Dermal sinuses (Fig. 4.11o–q) must be differentiated from benign coccygeal pits (Fig. 4.5). They represent a true track going from a small hole in the skin to the spinal canal. In 60 to 70% of cases they reach the subarachnoid space, with half attaching to the filum or the conus. The track includes both dermal and epidermal elements. It can end in an intradural dermoid or epidermoid cyst or, rarely, a teratoma.

This entity must be diagnosed as soon as possible after birth. The diagnosis is usually made on the basis of the skin stigmata. It presents as a midline dimple, higher than the

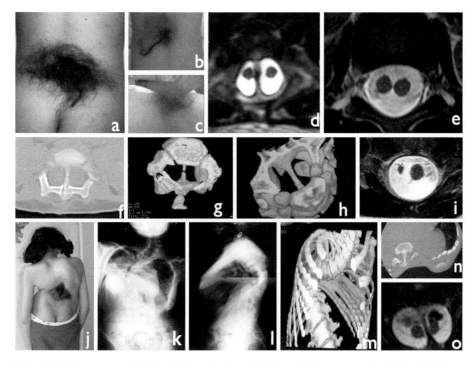

Fig. 4.11. Diastematomyelia. (a–c) 'Queue de faune'. (d) Type I diatematomyelia. (e) Type II diaste-matomyelia. (f–h) Bony spur on two- and three-dimensional computed tomography (CT) image. (i) Asymmetry of the spinal hemicord. (j–o) Diastematomyelia with severe kyphoscoliosis (j, qeue de faune; k, l, plain radiograph; m, three-dimensional CT image; n, axial CT; o, T_2-weighted MRI).

coccygeal pit. It may be associated with hairy tufts, hemangiomas, or telangiectasia, hypo-, or hyperpigmentation or any other skin marker.

The main complication of the dermal sinus is infection with resultant severe bacterial meningitis or intramedullary abscess. These infections may lead to permanent neurological deficits so there is a clinical urgency for neonatal diagnosis and surgery. The diagnosis may be by ultrasound, but the most detailed examination remains MRI. T_1-weighted sagittal and axial images with gadolinium injection and fat saturation is the criterion standard (Fig. 4.12). Although this usually demonstrates the sinus, it may fail to determine whether the track ends in the intra- or extradural space.

A distinctive form of dermal sinus has recently been described: the limited dorsal myeloschisis (Pang et al. 2010b), characterized by two constant features: 'a focal closed midline defect and a fibroneuronal stalk that links the skin lesion to the underlying cord' with both flat and saccular variants. In contrast to the dermal sinus, where there is a perme-able track to the surface, the fibroneuronal stalk of the limited dorsal myeloschisis does not usually provide access from the surface and in consequence has a low risk of secondary meningitis.

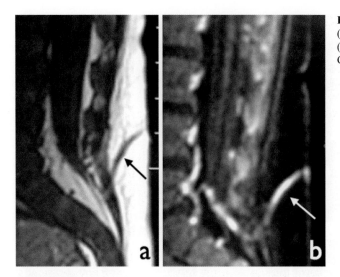

Fig. 4.12. Dermal sinus.
(a) Sagittal T_1-weighted and
(b) T_1-weighted FATSAT
GADO MRI.

NEURENTERIC CYST
(Mann et al. 1984, McMaster 1984, Pang et al. 1992, Catala and Poirier, 1996,
Muraszko and Youkilis 2000, Rauzzino et al. 2001, Rossi et al. 2004b,
de Oliveira et al. 2005, D'Andrea et al. 2008, Aouad et al. 2008, Cai et al. 2008,
Garg et al. 2008, Menezes 2008, Muzumdar et al. 2008, Rendle et al. 2008,
Yasuda et al. 2008, Aydin et al. 2009, Mittal et al. 2009, Gadodia et al. 2010,
Savage et al. 2010, Theret et al. 2010, Tucker et al. 2010, Zenmyo et al. 2010)
Neurenteric cysts are one of the rarer occult dysraphisms (0.3% of spinal tumours). We
reported the largest paediatric series to date, with 16 children operated on over a 14 year
period (De Oliveira et al. 2005). These cysts can occur at any level of the neuraxis from
the posterior clinoid to the coccyx. They are most often found in the cervical and upper
thoracic regions. They are generally located ventral to the spinal cord. It is generally
accepted that they result from the embryological remnants of the neurenteric canal. However,
although it has been well described in birds, there is no evidence in the literature of the
existence of a neurenteric canal during embryological life in mammals. Neurenteric cysts
are lesions consisting of an intradural cyst lined by mucin-producing non-ciliated epithelium that is simple or pseudostratified. The cyst can be ciliated or it can have a mixture of
gastrointestinal, pancreatic, respiratory, or squamous epithelium.

Clinical presentation
In the paediatric age group, there is a male predominance (60.4%) with a mean age of
presentation of 6 years 5 months. In 40% of the cases, the diagnosis follows the onset of
acute neurological symptoms (para- or teraparesis) or meningitis. Pain, myelopathy, and
spinal deformity are the most frequent signs in slow-growing forms. Occasionally, signs
may be absent even in the presence of severe compression of the spinal cord. In recurrent

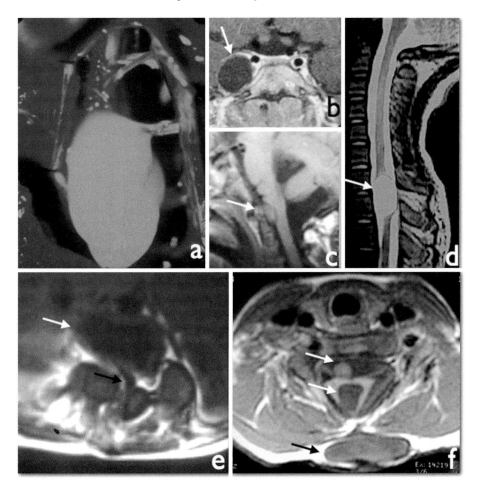

Fig. 4.13. Neurenteric cyst. (a) Operative view. (b) Neurenteric cyst within the cavernous sinus. (c) Retroclival form. (d) Premedullary cervicodorsal neurenteric cyst. (e) Prespinal form (white arrow) with a spinal body split and a tract between the cyst and the spinal cord (black arrow). (f) Cervical, prespinal, premedullary, and retrospinal cysts (arrows).

meningitis, neurenteric cyst must be considered and thoroughly searched for with full neuraxis MRI.

Radiology

Few antenatally diagnosed cases have been reported. Because of the association of the cyst with complex bony spinal malformations, plain spine radiography, CT and MRI must be performed. In some small cysts presenting with recurrent meningitis, the cyst can be missed, especially if located at the anterior craniovertebral junction, and repeat examinations may be required (Fig. 4.13).

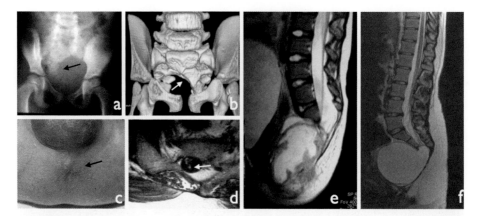

Fig. 4.14. Currarino syndrome. (a, b) Hemisacral agenesia (two- and three-dimensional CT image). (c) Anal imperforation. (d) Lipoma of the filum (T_1-weighted MRI). (e) Presacral teratoma (T_2-weighted MRI). (f) Anterior meningocele (T_2-weighted MRI).

Treatment

Complete excision is the aim of surgical treatment. If total removal is achieved, the prognosis is excellent. In the case of incomplete treatment, the risk of recurrence is high and often results in subsequent more complex surgery.

COMPLEX FORMS

(Currarino et al. 1981, Gudinchet et al. 1997, Ross et al. 1998, Riebel et al. 1999, Belloni et al. 2000, Hagan et al. 2000, Lynch et al. 2000, Kochling et al. 2001, Le Caignec et al. 2003, Horn et al. 2004, Martucciello et al. 2004, Urioste et al. 2004, Emans et al. 2005, Verlinsky et al. 2005, Cretolle et al. 2006, 2007, Garcia-Barcelo et al. 2006, Kilickesmez et al. 2006, Merello et al. 2006)

Currarino syndrome is an autosomal dominant congenital malformation characterized by three main clinical features: anterior sacral bone defect (sickle-shaped sacrum or sacral agenesis below S2), hindgut anomaly, and a pre-sacral mass (anterior meningocele, teratoma, rectal duplication, or a combination of these) (Fig. 4.14). Additional associated malformations have been described, namely renal or ureteric duplications, hydronephrosis, horseshoe kidney, bicornuate uterus, and NTD including tethered cord and lipoma of the filum, lipoma of the conus, dermal sinuses, and diastematomyelia.

More complex malformations may incorporate any of the neurological lesions described above, with or without visceral, spinal, or limb anomalies.

Caudal regression syndromes

This group is a heterogeneous collection of caudal malformations including agenesis of the caudal spinal column, imperforate anus, and genital anomalies. The lower extremities are usually dysplastic or atrophic. Fusion and atrophy result in the most severe case (sirenomelia). They can be part of syndromic complexes such as omphalocele, imperforate anus, exstrophic

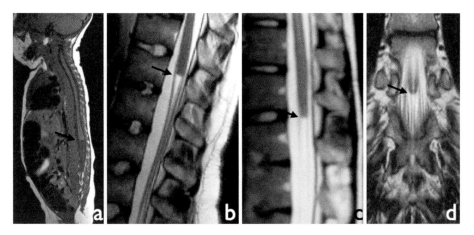

Fig. 4.15. Caudal regression. (a) The end of the spinal cord at T10. (b–d) T_2-weighted sagittal (b, c) and coronal (d) MRI. Typical spectrum of caudal regression with absence of the tip of the conus and horizontal clear cut spinal cord.

bladder, spinal defect (OIES) (Kallen et al. 2000, Keppler-Noreuil 2001, Kumar and Chandra 2002, Mittal et al. 2004, Kosaki et al. 2005, Ben-Neriah et al. 2007, Chen 2008, Morioka et al. 2008, Tokunaga et al. 2009) or vertebral anomalies, imperforate anus, tracheo-oesophageal fistula, renal abnormalities, and limb deformities (VACTERL) (Kuo et al. 2007).

In less severe forms, there is only a partial sacral agenesis, a short intergluteal fold and a short spinal cord ending above D12 (Fig. 4.15). Clinically, sphincter problems are frequent (bowel rather than bladder) and there is often a history of maternal diabetes.

Summary
Spinal dysraphysm must be differentiated into two completely different entities, as follows.

Open dysraphism (MMC) is the first entity, with emphasis on the importance of folic acid prophylaxis, antenatal diagnosis, and management (including the ethical and legal issues around the termination of pregnancy and, in the immediate future, the role of antenatal surgery) and, postnatally, the immediate management (surgery of the malformation, treatment of the hydrocephalus, urological evaluation) and the long-term management of the later complications (orthopaedic, urological, and re-tethering).

Occult dysraphism is a more diverse group of conditions. By far the most frequent are the spinal lipomas; where lipomas of the filum are a benign and usually easily managed group, lipomas of the conus are a significantly more severe entity, with possible immediate and/or late neurological and urological deficits. Because of the difficulty and the risk of the surgery, the management of asymptomatic forms remains controversial (prophylactic surgery or conservative approach).

The association of some occult dysraphisms with multi-organ malformation (especially anorectal, urological, and genital malformations) presents a particular multi-faceted management challenge.

REFERENCES

Ackerman LL, Menezes AH. Spinal congenital dermal sinuses: a 30-year experience. *Pediatrics* 2003; **112**: 641–647.

Adzick NS, Thom EA, Spong CY, et al. A randomized trial of prenatal versus postnatal repair of myelomeningocele. *N Engl J Med* 2011; **364**: 993–1004.

Afonso ND, Catala M. Neurosurgical embryology. Part 7: development of the spinal cord, the spine and the posterior fossa. *Neurochirurgie* 2003; **49**: 503–510.

Aouad RK, Dagher WI, Shikani AH. Neurenteric cyst of the clivus. Otolaryngol Head *Neck Surg* 2008; **139**: 863–864.

Aydin AL, Sasani M, Ucar B, Afsharian R, Ozer AF. Prenatal diagnosis of a large, cervical, intraspinal, neurenteric cyst and postnatal outcome. *J Pediatr Surg* 2009; **44**: 1835–1838.

Bajpai M, Kataria R, Gupta DK, Agarwala S. Occult spinal dysraphism. *Indian J Pediatr* 1997; **64**: 62–67.

Bekker I. Corpus Scriptorum Historiae Byzantinae. Bonn 1843; Politica vii: 16.

Belloni E, Martucciello G, Verderio D, et al. Involvement of the HLXB9 homeobox gene in Currarino syndrome. *Am J Hum Genet* 2000; **66**: 312–319.

Belzberg AJ, Myles ST, Trevenen CL. The human tail and spinal dysraphism. *J Pediatr Surg* 1991; **26**: 1243–1245.

Ben-Neriah Z, Withers S, Thomas M, et al. OEIS complex: prenatal ultrasound and autopsy findings. *Ultrasound Obstet Gynecol* 2007; **29**: 170–177.

Bruner JP, Tulipan N, Reed G, et al. Intrauterine repair of spina bifida: preoperative predictors of shunt-dependent hydrocephalus. *Am J Obstet Gynecol* 2004; **190**: 1305–1312.

Bruner JP, Tulipan NB, Richards WO, Walsh WF, Boehm FH, Vrabcak EK. In utero repair of myelomeningocele: a comparison of endoscopy and hysterotomy. *Fetal Diagn Ther* 2000; **15**: 83–88.

Buck D, Michael T, Wahn U, Niggemann B. Ventricular shunts and the prevalence of sensitization and clinically relevant allergy to latex in patients with spina bifida. *Pediatr Allergy Immunol* 2000; **11**: 111–115.

Cai C, Shen C, Yang W, Zhang Q, Hu X. 2008. Intraspinal neurenteric cysts in children. *Can J Neurol Sci* 2008; **35**: 609–615.

Caldarelli M, Di Rocco C, La Marca F. Treatment of hydromyelia in spina bifida. *Surg Neurol* 1998; **50**: 411–420.

Canfield MA, Annegers JF, Brender JD, Cooper SP, Greenberg F. Hispanic origin and neural tube defects in Houston/Harris County, Texas. I. Descriptive epidemiology. *Am J Epidemiol* 1996a; **143**: 1–11.

Canfield MA, Annegers JF, Brender JD, Cooper SP, Greenberg F. Hispanic origin and neural tube defects in Houston/Harris County, Texas. II. Risk factors. *Am J Epidemiol* 1996b; **143**: 12–24.

Canfield MA, Marengo L, Ramadhani TA, Suarez L, Brender JD, Scheuerle A. The prevalence and predictors of anencephaly and spina bifida in Texas. *Paediatr Perinat Epidemiol* 2009; **23**: 41–50.

Catala M. Embryonic and fetal development of structures associated with the cerebro-spinal fluid in man and other species. Part I: the ventricular system, meninges and choroid plexuses. *Arch Anat Cytol Pathol* 1998; **46**: 153–169.

Catala M. From conception to the child. *Childs Nerv Syst* 1999; **15**: 613–619.

Catala, M. Genetic control of caudal development. *Clin Genet* 2002; **61**: 89–96.

Catala M, Poirier J. Neurenteric cyst of anterior cranial fossa. *Br J Neurosurg* 1996; **10**: 526–527.

Catala M, Teillet MA, De Robertis EM, Le Douarin ML. A spinal cord fate map in the avian embryo: while regressing, Hensen's node lays down the notochord and floor plate thus joining the spinal cord lateral walls. *Development* 1996; **122**: 2599–2610.

Chakraborty A, Crimmins D, Hayward R, Thompson D. Toward reducing shunt placement rates in patients with myelomeningocele. *J Neurosurg Pediatr* 2008; **1**: 361–365.

Chen CP. Syndromes, disorders and maternal risk factors associated with neural tube defects (III). *Taiwan J Obstet Gynecol* 2008; **47**: 131–140.

Cochrane D, Aronyk K, Sawatzky B, Wilson D, Steinbok P. The effects of labor and delivery on spinal cord function and ambulation in patients with meningomyelocele. *Childs Nerv Syst* 1991; **7**: 312–315.

Cretolle C, Sarnacki S, Amiel J, et al. Currarino syndrome shown by prenatal onset ventriculomegaly and spinal dysraphism. *Am J Med Genet A* 2007; **143**: 871–874.

Cretolle C, Zerah M, Jaubert F, et al. 2006. New clinical and therapeutic perspectives in Currarino syndrome (study of 29 cases). *J Pediatr Surg* 2006; **41**: 126–131.

Currarino G, Coln D, Votteler T. Triad of anorectal, sacral, and presacral anomalies. *AJR Am J Roentgenol* 1981; **137**: 395–398.

Czeizel A, Kerekes L, Meretey K, et al. National programme for prevention of the recurrence of neural tube defects. *Acta Paediatr Acad Sci Hung* 1979; **20**: 315–319.

Czeizel AE, Dudas I. Prevention of the first occurrence of neural-tube defects by periconceptional vitamin supplementation. *N Engl J Med* 1992; **327**: 1832–1835.

Czeizel AE, Dudas I, Fritz G, Tecsoi A, Hanck A, Kunovits G. The effect of periconceptional multivitamin-mineral supplementation on vertigo, nausea and vomiting in the first trimester of pregnancy. *Arch Gynecol Obstet* 1992; **251**: 181–185.

D'Andrea G, Mencarani C, Necci V, Di Stefano D, Occhiogrosso G, Frati A. High cervical neurenteric cyst; acute post-traumatic rupture and respiratory failure: a case report. *Zentralbl Neurochir* 2008; **69**: 51–53.

Danzer E, Johnson MP, Adzick NS. Fetal surgery for myelomeningocele: progress and perspectives. *Dev Med Child Neurol* 2012; **54**: 8–14.

De Oliveira RS, Cinalli G, Roujeau T, Sainte-Rose C, Pierre-Kahn A, Zerah M. Neurenteric cysts in children: 16 consecutive cases and review of the literature. *J Neurosurg* 2005; **103**: 512–523.

Dias MS, Pang D. Split cord malformations. *Neurosurg Clin N Am* 1995; **6**: 339–358.

Dommergues M, Benachi A, Benifla JL, Des Noettes R, Dumez Y. The reasons for termination of pregnancy in the third trimester. *Br J Obstet Gynaecol* 1999; **106**: 297–303.

Dommergues M, Mandelbrot L, Mahieu-Caputo D, Boudjema N, Durand-Zaleski I. Termination of pregnancy following prenatal diagnosis in France: how severe are the foetal anomalies? *Prenat Diagn* 2006; **30**: 531–539.

Dudas I, Czeizel AE. Use of 6,000 IU vitamin A during early pregnancy without teratogenic effect. *Teratology* 1992; **45**: 335–336.

Emans PJ, Kootstra G, Marcelis CL, Beuls EA, Van Heurn LW. The Currarino triad: the variable expression. *J Pediatr Surg* 2005; **40**: 1238–1242.

Emmez H, Guven C, Kurt G, Kardes O, Dogulu F, Baykaner K. Terminal syringomyelia: is it as innocent as it seems? *Neurol Med Chir (Tokyo)* 2004; **44**: 558–561.

Filly RA. Radiology residency training in diagnostic sonography. *J Ultrasound Med* 1989a; **8**: 475.

Filly RA. Radiology residency training in diagnostic sonography: recommendations of the Society of Radiologists in Ultrasound. *Radiology* 1989b; **172**: 577.

Finn MA, Walker ML. Spinal lipomas: clinical spectrum, embryology, and treatment. *Neurosurg Focus* 2007; **23**: 1–12.

Frey L, Hauser WA. Epidemiology of neural tube defects. *Epilepsia* 2003; **44** (Suppl. 3): 4–13.

Gadodia A, Sharma R, Jeyaseelan N, Aggarwala S, Gupta P. Prenatal diagnosis of mediastinal neurentric cyst with an intraspinal component. *J Pediatr Surg* 2010; **45**: 1377–1379.

Gan YC, Sgouros S, Walsh AR, Hockley AD. Diastematomyelia in children: treatment outcome and natural history of associated syringomyelia. *Childs Nerv Syst* 2007; **23**: 515–519.

Garcia-Barcelo M, So MT, Lau DK, et al. Population differences in the polyalanine domain and 6 new mutations in HLXB9 in patients with Currarino syndrome. *Clin Chem* 2006; **52**: 46–52.

Garg N, Sampath S, Yasha TC, Chandramouli BA, Devi BI, Kovoor JM. Is total excision of spinal neurenteric cysts possible? *Br J Neurosurg* 2008; **22**: 241–251.

Ghi T, Pilu G, Falco P, et al. Prenatal diagnosis of open and closed spina bifida. *Ultrasound Obstet Gynecol* 2006; **28**: 899–903.

Gok A, Bayram M, Coskun Y, Ozsarac C. Unusual malformations in occult spinal dysraphism. *Turk J Pediatr* 1995; **37**: 391–397.

Goodrich JT. In: Ozek M, Cinalli G, Maixner W, editors. Spina Bifida. Management and Outcome. Springer, 2008: 3–18.

Group EW. Prevalence of neural tube defects in 20 regions of Europe and their impact on prenatal diagnosis, 1980–1986. *J Epidemiol Comm Health* 1991; **45**: 52–58.

Gudinchet F, Maeder P, Laurent T, Meyrat B, Schnyder P. Magnetic resonance detection of myelodysplasia in children with Currarino triad. *Pediatr Radiol* 1997; **27**: 903–907.

Guggisberg D, Hadj-Rabia S, Viney C, et al. Skin markers of occult spinal dysraphism in children: a review of 54 cases. *Arch Dermatol* 2004; **140**: 1109–1115.

Hagan DM, Ross AJ, Strachan T, et al. Mutation analysis and embryonic expression of the *HLXB9* Currarino syndrome gene. *Am J Hum Genet* 2000; **66**: 1504–1515.

Hamdan AH, Walsh W, Bruner JP, Tulipan N. Intrauterine myelomeningocele repair: effect on short-term complications of prematurity. *Fetal Diagn Ther* 2004; **19**: 83–86.

Hamrick SE. Cesarean delivery and its impact on the anomalous infant. *Clin Perinatol* 2008; **35**: 395–406.

Han JS, Benson JE, Kaufman B, et al. Demonstration of diastematomyelia and associated abnormalities with MR imaging. *Am J Neuroradiol* 1985; **6**: 215–219.

Hattori H, Higuchi Y, Tashiro Y. 1999. Dorsal dermal sinus and dermoid cysts in occult spinal dysraphism. *J Pediatr* **134**: 793.

Hertrampf E, Cortes F. Folic acid fortification of wheat flour: Chile. *Nutr Rev* 2004; **62**: S44–S48.

Hertzler DA 2nd, Depowell JJ, Stevenson CB, Mangano FT. Tethered cord syndrome: a review of the literature from embryology to adult presentation. *Neurosurg Focus* 2010; **29**: E1.

Hirose S, Farmer DL. Fetal surgery for myelomeningocele. *Clin Perinatol* 2009; **36**: 431–438.

Hirose S, Meuli-Simmen C, Meuli M. Fetal surgery for myelomeningocele: panacea or peril? *World J Surg* 2003; **27**: 87–94.

Hoffman HJ, Hendrick EB, Humphreys RP. The tethered spinal cord: its protean manifestations, diagnosis and surgical correction. *Childs Brain* 1976; **2**: 145–155.

Horn D, Tonnies H, Neitzel H, et al. Minimal clinical expression of the holoprosencephaly spectrum and of Currarino syndrome due to different cytogenetic rearrangements deleting the Sonic Hedgehog gene and the *HLXB9* gene at 7q36.3. *Am J Med Genet A* 2004; **128**: 85–92.

Jindal A, Mahapatra AK, Kamal R. Spinal dysraphism. *Indian J Pediatr* 1999; **66**: 697–705.

Johnson MP, Gerdes M, Rintoul N, et al. Maternal-fetal surgery for myelomeningocele: neurodevelopmental outcomes at 2 years of age. *Am J Obstet Gynecol* 2006; **194**: 1145–1150.

Kallen K, Castilla EE, Robert E, Mastroiacovo P, Kallen B. OEIS complex—a population study. *Am J Med Genet* 2000; **92**: 62–68.

Keppler-Noreuil KM. OEIS complex (omphalocele-exstrophy-imperforate anus-spinal defects): a review of 14 cases. *Am J Med Genet* 2001; **99**: 271–279.

Kilickesmez O, Gol IH, Uzun M, Oruk C. Complete familial Currarino triad in association with Hirschsprung's disease: magnetic resonance imaging features and the spectrum of anorectal malformations. *Acta Radiol* 2006; **47**: 422–426.

Kim SK, Chung YS, Wang KC, Cho BK, Choi KS, Han DH. Diastematomyelia—clinical manifestation and treatment outcome. *J Korean Med Sci* 1994; **9**: 135–144.

Kochling J, Karbasiyan M, Reis A. Spectrum of mutations and genotype-phenotype analysis in Currarino syndrome. *Eur J Hum Genet* 2001; **9**: 599–605.

Kogler A, Arsenic B, Marusic-Della Marina B, Kovac D, Sore B. Diastematomyelia—case report. *Neurol Croat* 1991; **41**: 57–64.

Kosaki R, Fukuhara Y, Kosuga M, et al. OEIS complex with del(3)(q12.2q13.2). *Am J Med Genet A* 2005; **135**: 224–226.

Koszutski T, Kawalski H, Kudela G, Wroblewska J, Byrka-Owczarek K, Bohosiewicz J. Babies with myelomeningocele in Poland: parents' attitudes on fetal surgery versus termination of pregnancy. *Childs Nerv Syst* 2009; **25**: 207–210.

Kuharik MA, Edwards MK, Grossman CB. Magnetic resonance evaluation of pediatric spinal dysraphism. *Pediatr Neurosci* 1985; **12**: 213–218.

Kulkarni AV, Pierre-Kahn A, Zerah M. Conservative management of asymptomatic spinal lipomas of the conus. *Neurosurgery* 2004; **54**: 868–873.

Kumar R, Chandra A. Terminal myelocystocele. *Indian J Pediatr* 2002; **69**: 1083–1086.

Kuo MF, Tsai Y, Hsu WM, Chen RS, Tu YK, Wang HS. Tethered spinal cord and VACTERL association. *J Neurosurg* 2007; **106**: 201–204.

La Marca F, Herman M, Grant JA, McLone DG. Presentation and management of hydromyelia in children with Chiari type-II malformation. *Pediatr Neurosurg* 1997; **26**: 57–67.

Laurence KM, James N, Miller M, Campbell H. Increased risk of recurrence of pregnancies complicated by fetal neural tube defects in mothers receiving poor diets, and possible benefit of dietary counselling. *Br Med J* 1980; **281**: 1592–1594.

Laurence KM, James N, Miller MH, Tennant GB, Campbell H. Double-blind randomised controlled trial of folate treatment before conception to prevent recurrence of neural-tube defects. *Br Med J (Clin Res Ed)* 1981; **282**: 1509–1511.

Le Caignec C, Winer N, Boceno M, et al. Prenatal diagnosis of sacrococcygeal teratoma with constitutional partial monosomy 7q/trisomy 2p. *Prenat Diagn* 2003; **23**: 981–984.

Lellouch-Tubiana A, Zerah M, Catala M, Brousse N, Kahn AP. Congenital intraspinal lipomas: histological analysis of 234 cases and review of the literature. *Pediatr Dev Pathol* 1999; **2**: 346–352.

Lemire RJ. Neural tube defects: clinical correlations. *Clin Neurosurg* 1983; **30**: 165–177.

Lewis D, Tolosa JE, Kaufmann M, Goodman M, Farrell C, Berghella V. Elective cesarean delivery and long-term motor function or ambulation status in infants with meningomyelocele. *Obstet Gynecol* 2004; **103**: 469–473.

Li YC, Shin SH, Cho BK, et al. Pathogenesis of lumbosacral lipoma: a test of the 'premature dysjunction' theory. *Pediatr Neurosurg* 2001; **34**: 124–130.

Llanos A, Hertrampf E, Cortes F, Pardo A, Grosse SD, Uauy R. Cost-effectiveness of a folic acid fortification program in Chile. *Health Policy* 2007; **83**: 295–303.

Lode HM, Deeg KH, Krauss J. Spinal sonography in infants with cutaneous birth markers in the lumbo-sacral region – an important sign of occult spinal dysrhaphism and tethered cord. *Ultraschall Med* 2008; **29** (Suppl. 5): 281–288.

Lopez-Camelo JS, Castilla EE, Orioli IM. Folic acid flour fortification: impact on the frequencies of 52 congenital anomaly types in three South American countries. *Am J Med Genet A* 2000; **152**: 2444–2458.

Lopez-Camelo JS, Orioli IM, Da Graca Dutra M, et al. Reduction of birth prevalence rates of neural tube defects after folic acid fortification in Chile. *Am J Med Genet A* 2005; **135**: 120–125.

Lynch SA, Wang Y, Strachan T, Burn J, Lindsay, S. Autosomal dominant sacral agenesis: Currarino syndrome. *J Med Genet* 2000; **37**: 561–566.

Maiuri F, Gambardella, A, Trinchillo, G. Congenital lumbosacral lesions with late onset in adult life. *Neurol Res* 1989; **11**: 238–244.

Majed M, Nejat F, Khashab ME, et al. Risk factors for latex sensitization in young children with myelomeningocele. *J Neurosurg Pediatr* 2009; **4**: 285–288.

Mann KS, Khosla VK, Gulati DR, Malik AK. Spinal neurenteric cyst. Association with vertebral anomalies, diastematomyelia, dorsal fistula, and lipoma. *Surg Neurol* 1984; **21**: 358–362.

Martucciello G, Torre M, Belloni E, et al. Currarino syndrome: proposal of a diagnostic and therapeutic protocol. *J Pediatr Surg* 2004; **39**: 1305–1311.

McMaster MJ. Occult intraspinal anomalies and congenital scoliosis. *J Bone Joint Surg Am* 1984; **66**: 588–601.

McNulty H, Cuskelly GJ, Ward M. Response of red blood cell folate to intervention: implications for folate recommendations for the prevention of neural tube defects. *Am J Clin Nutr* 2000; **71**: 1308S–1311S.

Mehta VA, Bettegowda C, Ahmadi SA, et al. Spinal cord tethering following myelomeningocele repair. *J Neurosurg Pediatr* 2010; **6**: 498–505.

Mehta VA, Bettegowda C, Amin A, El-Gassim M, Jallo G, Ahn ES. Impact of tethered cord release on symptoms of Chiari II malformation in children born with a myelomeningocele. 2011; *Childs Nerv Syst* 2011; **27**: 975–978.

Menezes AH. Surgical approaches: postoperative care and complications 'posterolateral-far lateral transcondylar approach to the ventral foramen magnum and upper cervical spinal canal'. *Childs Nerv Syst* 2008; **24**: 1203–1207.

Merello E, De Marco P, Mascelli S, et al. HLXB9 homeobox gene and caudal regression syndrome. *Birth Defects Res A Clin Mol Teratol* 2006; **76**: 205–209.

Merrill DC, Goodwin P, Burson JM, Sato Y, Williamson R, Weiner CP. The optimal route of delivery for fetal meningomyelocele. *Am J Obstet Gynecol* 1998; **179**: 235–240.

Mittal A, Airon, RK, Magu, S, Rattan, KN, Ratan SK. Associated anomalies with anorectal malformation (ARM). *Indian J Pediatr* 2004; **71**: 509–514.

Mittal S, Petrecca K, Sabbagh AJ, et al. Supratentorial neurenteric cysts–a fascinating entity of uncertain embryopathogenesis. *Clin Neurol Neurosurg* 2009; **112**: 89–97.

Monteagudo A, Timor-Tritsch IE, Mayberry P. Three-dimensional transvaginal neurosonography of the fetal brain: 'navigating' in the volume scan. *Ultrasound Obstet Gynecol* 2000; **16**: 307–313.

Morioka T, Hashiguchi K, Yoshida F, et al. Neurosurgical management of occult spinal dysraphism associated with OEIS complex. *Childs Nerv Syst* 2008; **24**: 723–729.

Muraszko K, Youkilis A. Intramedullary spinal tumors of disordered embryogenesis. *J Neurooncol* 2000; **47**: 271–281.

Muthukumar N. Congenital spinal lipomatous malformations: part I – classification. *Acta Neurochir (Wien)* 2009; **151**: 179–188.

Muzumdar D, Bhatt Y, Sheth J. Intramedullary cervical neurenteric cyst mimicking an abscess. *Pediatr Neurosurg* 2008; **44**: 55–61.

Nazer HJ, Cifuentes OL, Aguila RA, et al. 2007 Effects of folic acid fortification in the rates of malformations at birth in Chile. *Rev Med Chil* 2007; **135**: 198–204.

Nicolaides KH, Campbell S, Gabbe SG, Guidetti R. Ultrasound screening for spina bifida: cranial and cerebellar signs. *Lancet* 1986; **ii**: 72–74.

Niggemann B, Buck D, Michael T, Haberl H, Wahn U. Latex allergy in spina bifida: at the turning point? *J Allergy Clin Immunol* 2000; **106**: 1201.

Pang D, Parrish RG. Regrowth of diastematomyelic bone spur after extradural resection. *J Neurosurg* 1983; **59**: 887–890.

Pang D, Dias MS, Ahab-Barmada M. Split cord malformation: Part I: a unified theory of embryogenesis for double spinal cord malformations. *Neurosurgery* 1992; **31**: 451–480.

Pang D, Zovickian J, Oviedo A. Long term outcome of total and near total resection of spinal cord lipomas and radical reconstruction of the neural placode, part II: outcome analysis and preoperative profiling. *Neurosurgery* 2010a; **66**: 253–272.

Pang D, Zovickian J, Oviedo A, Moes GS. Limited dorsal myeloschisis: a distinctive clinicopathological entity. *Neurosurgery* 2010b; **67**: 1555–1579.

Phuong LK, Schoeberl KA, Raffel C. Natural history of tethered cord in patients with meningomyelocele. *Neurosurgery* 2002; **50**: 989–993.

Pierre-Kahn A, Zerah M, Renier D. Lipomes malformatifs intrarachidiens. *Neurochirurgie* 1995; **41** (Suppl. 1): 1–134.

Pierre-Kahn A, Zerah M, Renier D, et al. Congenital lumbosacral lipomas. *Childs Nerv Syst* 1997; **13**: 298–334.

Pierz K, Banta J, Thomson J, Gahm N, Hartford J. The effect of tethered cord release on scoliosis in myelomeningocele. *J Pediatr Orthop* 2000; **20**: 362–365.

Pitkin RM. Folate and neural tube defects. *Am J Clin Nutr* 2007; **85**: 285S–288S.

Pollack IF, Kinnunen D, Albright AL. The effect of early craniocervical decompression on functional outcome in neonates and young infants with myelodysplasia and symptomatic Chiari II malformations: results from a prospective series. *Neurosurgery* 1996; **38**: 703–710.

Rauzzino MJ, Tubbs RS, Alexander E 3rd, Grabb PA, Oakes WJ. Spinal neurenteric cysts and their relation to more common aspects of occult spinal dysraphism. *Neurosurg Focus* 2001; **10**: e2.

Rendeli C, Nucera E, Ausili E, et al. Latex sensitisation and allergy in children with myelomeningocele. *Childs Nerv Syst* 2006; **22**: 28–32.

Rendle DI, Durham AE, Bestbier M, Smith KC, Boswell JC. Neurenteric cyst with associated butterfly vertebrae in a seven-month-old colt. *Vet Rec* 2008; **162**: 558–561.

Riebel T, Maurer J, Teichgraber UK, Bassir C. The spectrum of imaging in Currarino triad. 1999; *Eur Radiol* **9**: 1348–1353.

Rosano A, Smithells D, Cacciani L, et al. Time trends in neural tube defects prevalence in relation to preventive strategies: an international study. *J Epidemiol Community Health* 1999; **53**: 630–635.

Ross AJ, Ruiz-Perez V, Wang Y, et al. A homeobox gene *HLXB9*: is the major locus for dominantly inherited sacral agenesis. *Nat Genet* 1998; **20**: 358–361.

Rossi A, Biancheri R, Cama A, Piatelli G, Ravegnani M, Tortori-Donati P. Imaging in spine and spinal cord malformations. *Eur J Radiol* 2004a; **50**: 177–200.

Rossi A, Cama A, Piatelli G, Ravegnani M, Biancheri R, Tortori-Donati P. Spinal dysraphism: MR imaging rationale. *J Neuroradiol* 2004b; **31**: 3–24.

Santiago Medina L, Al-Orfali M, Zurakowski D, Poussaint TY, Dicanzio J, Barnes PD. Occult lumbosacral dysraphism in children and young adults: diagnostic performance of fast screening and conventional MR imaging. *Radiology* 1999; **211**: 767–771.

Savage JJ, Casey JN, McNeill IT, Sherman, JH. Neurenteric cysts of the spine. *J Craniovertebr Junction Spine* 2010; **1**: 58–63.

Sebire NJ, Noble PL, Thorpe-Beeston JG, Snijders RJ, Nicolaides KH. Presence of the 'lemon' sign in fetuses with spina bifida at the 10–14-week scan. *Ultrasound Obstet Gynecol* 1997; **10**: 403–405.

Sen O, Kayaselcuk F, Yalcin O, et al. Lumbar meningeal hamartoma and epidermoid cyst associated with spinal dysraphism in an elderly patient. *Neurosurg Rev* 2005; **28**: 159–162.

Shaer CM, Chescheir N, Schulkin J. Myelomeningocele: a review of the epidemiology, genetics, risk factors for conception, prenatal diagnosis, and prognosis for affected individuals. *Obstet Gynecol Surv* 2007; **62**: 471–9PMID: 17572919.

Sheptak PE, Susen AF. Diastematomyelia. *Am J Dis Child* 1967; **113**: 210–213.

Singer P. Practical Ethics (2nd edition). Cambridge University Press, 1993: 83.

Smithells RW, Nevin NC, Seller MJ, et al. Further experience of vitamin supplementation for prevention of neural tube defect recurrences. *Lancet* 1983; **i**: 1027–1031.

Smithells RW, Sheppard S, Schorah CJ. Vitamin deficiencies and neural tube defects. *Arch Dis Child* 1976; **51**: 944–950.

Sutton LN. Fetal surgery for neural tube defects. *Best Pract Res Clin Obstet Gynaecol* 2008; **22**: 175–188.

Szalay EA, Roach JW, Smith H, Maravilla K, Partain CL. Magnetic resonance imaging of the spinal cord in spinal dysraphisms. *J Pediatr Orthop* 1987; **7**: 541–545.

Theret E, Litre CF, Lefebvre F, et al. Huge intramedullar neurenteric cyst with intrathoracic development in a 1 month-old boy: excision though the anterior approach. A case report and review of the literature. *Acta Neurochir (Wien)* 2010; **152**: 481–483.

Till K. Spinal dysraphism. A study of congenital malformations of the lower back. *J Bone Joint Surg Br* 1969; **51**: 415–422.

Tokunaga S, Morioka T, Hashiguchi K, et al. Double lumbosacral lipomas of the dorsal and filar types associated with OEIS complex: case report. *Neurol Med Chir (Tokyo)* 2009; **49**: 487–490.

Tortori-Donati P, Rossi A, Cama A. Spinal dysraphism: a review of neuroradiological features with embryological correlations and proposal for a new classification. *Neuroradiology* 2000; **42**: 471–491.

Tubbs RS, Chambers MR, Smyth MD, et al. Late gestational intrauterine myelomeningocele repair does not improve lower extremity function. *Pediatr Neurosurg* 2003; **38**: 128–132.

Tucker A, Miyake H, Tsuji M, et al. Neurenteric cyst of the lower clivus. *Neurosurgery* 2010; **66**: E224–E225.

Tulipan N. Intrauterine closure of myelomeningocele: an update. *Neurosurg Focus* 2004; **16**: E2.

Tulipan N, Sutton LN, Bruner JP, Cohen BM, Johnson M, Adzick NS. The effect of intrauterine myelomeningocele repair on the incidence of shunt-dependent hydrocephalus. *Pediatr Neurosurg* 2003; **38**: 27–33.

Tulpius N. Observationes Medicae. Amsterdam: Elzevirium, 1641.

Unsinn KM, Geley T, Freund MC, Gassner I. US of the spinal cord in newborns: spectrum of normal findings, variants, congenital anomalies, and acquired diseases. *Radiographics* 2000; **20**: 923–938.

Urioste M, Garcia-Andrade Mdel C, Valle L, et al. Malignant degeneration of presacral teratoma in the Currarino anomaly. *Am J Med Genet A* 2004; **128**: 299–304.

Van Den Hof MC, Nicolaides KH, Campbell J, Campbell S. Evaluation of the lemon and banana signs in one hundred thirty fetuses with open spina bifida. *Am J Obstet Gynecol* 1990; **162**: 322–327.

Vandertop WP. Tethered cord. *J Neurosurg Spine* 2010; **12**: 334–335.

Verlinsky Y, Rechitsky S, Schoolcraft W, Kuliev A. Preimplantation diagnosis for homeobox gene HLXB9 mutation causing Currarino syndrome. *Am J Med Genet A* 2005; **134**: 103–104.

Wald NJ, Cuckle HS. Alpha fetoprotein in the antenatal diagnosis of open neural tube defects. *Br J Hosp Med* 1980; **23**: 473–480.

Walsh DS, Adzick NS, Sutton LN, Johnson MP. The rationale for in utero repair of myelomeningocele. *Fetal Diagn Ther* 2001; **16**: 312–322.

Woodhouse CR. Myelomeningocele: neglected aspects. *Pediatr Nephrol* 2008; **23**: 1223–1231.

Yamada S, Zinke DE, Sanders D. Pathophysiology of 'tethered cord syndrome'. *J Neurosurg* 1981; **54**: 494–503.

Yasuda M, Nakagawa H, Ozawa H, et al. Disseminated neurenteric cyst. *J Neurosurg Spine* 2008; **9**: 382–386.

Zenmyo M, Ishido Y, Yamamoto T, et al. Intradural neurenteric cyst—two case reports of surgical treatment. *Int J Neurosci* 2010; **120**: 625–629.

Zerah M, Roujeau T, Catala M, Pierre-Kahn A. In Memet Ozek M, Cinalli G, Maixner W, editors. The Spina Bifida. Management and Outcome. Springer, 2008: 445–474.

5
SPINAL CORD ABSCESS, HAEMORRHAGE, AND TRAUMA

Reza Yassari and John Houten

Injury to the spinal cord in the paediatric population is particularly devastating because of the emotional and economic impact it has on the patients and their families. The aetiology of injury can include a plethora of pathologies. In this chapter we discuss the clinical features, manifestation, diagnosis, and treatment algorithms of spinal cord abscess, spinal cord haemorrhage, and trauma to the spinal cord in the paediatric population.

Spinal cord abscess
EPIDEMIOLOGY AND RISK FACTORS IN PAEDIATRIC INTRASPINAL ABSCESS
Since the first case of an intramedullary spinal cord abscess was reported in 1830 by Hart, a total of 100 cases have been recorded in the literature (Hart 1830, Desai et al. 1999, Bunyaratavej et al. 2006). This rare pathology is far outnumbered by the more common epidural abscess in children and adults. In 1950, Courville reported a single incident of spinal cord abscess in 40,000 autopsies (Courville 1950). Analysis of the cases in the literature indicates that the mean age at presentation is 29 years, varying between 7 months and 72 years, with most cases falling between the first and third decade of life (Desai et al. 1999). In children the age of presentation is between 8 days and 17 years, with a median age of 36 months (Simon et al. 2003). A little more than half of these patients have an underlying anatomical defect, most commonly a dermal sinus.

ORGANISMS AND RISK FACTORS
Staphylococcus aureus is the most common causative organism, followed by streptococcal infections (23% and 16%, respectively) (Bartels et al. 1995). Other identified organisms included *Actinomyces, Brucella abortus* biotype 3, *Proteus, Escherichia coli, Pseudomonas, Listeria, Mycobacterium tuberculosis, Bacteroides, Nocardia, Enterococcus faecalis*, and *Candida albicans* (Menezes et al. 1977, King and Jeffree 1993, Candon and Frerebeau 1994, Cokca et al. 1994, Bartels et al. 1995, Lindner et al. 1995, Chu et al. 1996, Hanci et al. 1996, Menezes 1996, Cheng et al. 1997, Ushikoshi et al. 1998, Vora et al. 2004, Samkoff et al. 2008, Kurita et al. 2009). The incidence of negative microbacterial laboratory results ranges from 23 to 36%, particularly in chronic infections (Byrne et al. 1994, Bartels et al. 1995, Menezes 1996, Morandi et al. 1999, Tsurubuchi et al. 2002, Simon et al. 2003). The thoracic spine is most commonly involved (Menezes et al. 1977, Menezes 1996, Morandi

et al. 1999, Simon et al. 2003). The dorsal cord with its sluggish blood flow and watershed vascularity is more prone to hematogenous seeding of bacteria within the parenchyma of the spinal cord (Menezes 1996). The hematogenous route of infection is more common in adults than children and continues to be the case today, in part because of the incidence of infection resulting from intravenous drug use (Menezes 1996, Simon et al. 2003, Do-Dai et al. 2010). In children, however, an important additional source of the infection is a congenital dermal sinus, with its rare potential to lead to intramedullary contamination, accounting for 45% of cases of spinal cord abscess in this age group (Mount 1949, Courville 1950, el-Gindi and Fairburn 1969, Bean et al. 1979, Rogg et al. 1993, Chan and Gold 1998, Morandi et al. 1999, Simon et al. 2003, Al Barbarawi et al. 2009). Once the infection starts within the spinal cord, it can spread longitudinally within the fibre tracts (el-Gindi and Fairburn 1969, Desai et al. 1999). The extent of the abscess can range from three to six vertebrae (Byrne et al. 1994). Cases of holocord abscess have been reported in the literature with devastating neurological sequelae both in adults and children (Menezes 1996, Desai et al. 1999, Bunyaratavej et al. 2006).

CLINICAL PRESENTATION

Presentation may be acute (<1wk), subacute (1–6wk), or chronic (>6wk) (Foley 1949, Menezes et al. 1977, Menezes 1996). There is no literature that describes a relationship of acuteness of presentation or location of infection to the causative organism. Acute presentations will more reliably exhibit the typical signs of infection such as fever or leukocytosis; but even in these cases, the infectious laboratory parameters may lag behind the evolution of clinical neurological deficits. Neurological deterioration can be expected to be more precipitate and severe in patients with an acute presentation (Menezes et al. 1977).

Spinal cord abscesses present with a variable set of symptoms consisting of pain and neurological deficits referable to an acutely expanding lesion within the spinal cord (Menezes 1996). Most patients may have the signs and symptoms of an infectious process, such as fever, leukocytosis, and malaise. Specific neurological signs and symptoms typically consist of motor impairment (80%), sensory loss (43%), bowel/bladder symptoms (36%), and dorsal pain (10%) (Menezes 1996). The development of the neurological deficits of an acute abscess tends to be rapid, as seen in cases of an acute transverse myelitis, whereas more chronic abscesses will present with gradual onset of symptoms similar to that seen in spinal cord tumors (Byrne et al. 1994). Atypical clinical presentations may include the signs and symptoms of recurrent bacterial meningitis and, in this situation, detailed whole neuraxis magnetic resonance imaging (MRI) is mandatory to exclude distant seeding (Baradaran et al. 2008).

INVESTIGATION

MRI with gadolinium remains the criterion standard for the diagnosis of intra-medullary abscess (Murphy et al. 1998, Dorflinger-Hejlek et al. 2010). An important and reliable finding on MRI is high signal on the T_2-weighted sequence. On post-contrast T_1-weighted images, marginal enhancement with central low signal intensity may be appreciated (Do-Dai et al. 2010). With treatment, T_2 signal abnormalities usually decrease markedly and contrast-enhanced studies begin to more reliably show enhancement that gradually resolves with treatment over serial studies (Murphy et al. 1998).

Cerebrospinal fluid analysis is typically non-specific and is clinically similar to that found in cerebral abscesses, reflecting the fact that the infected mass is confined within the parenchyma and is not in direct contact with the surrounding cerebrospinal fluid. When present, abnormalities in the cerebrospinal fluid reflect the underlying causative agent and can mimic the findings of bacterial, viral, or atypical meningitis. Unlike patients with brain abscess in whom lumbar puncture is contraindicated because of the risk of downward herniation, spinal abscesses do not cause a pressure differential between the cranial and spinal compartments and, thus, lumbar puncture should be safe. No data, however, specifically addresses this question and, therefore, a lumbar puncture in the setting of spinal abscess should be approached in a manner similar to that of any expansive mass in the spinal cord: a small volume tap would be preferred while considering the requirements for adequate sampling for diagnosis.

An echocardiogram is generally indicated to rule out potential cardiac sources of distant seeding (Fernandez-Ruiz et al. 2009).

TREATMENT

Initiation of antibiotic and/or surgical treatment should never be delayed while awaiting cerebrospinal fluid or tissue analysis, and should be started on the basis of clinical and radiographic suspicion. In view of the potentially devastating neurological implication of an expanding mass within the spinal cord, surgical evacuation requires urgent consideration.

Untreated, an abscess will lead to neurological deterioration (Kamgarpour et al. 2008) and the outcome of conservative treatment with antibiotics alone that is reported in the literature is very poor (Pfadenhauer and Rossmanith 1995, Chu et al. 1996, Bingol et al. 1999, Lascaux et al. 2002, Novati et al. 2002, Crema et al. 2007, Kurita et al. 2009). In addition, the indication for medical treatment alone remains unclear: no data exist about the recommended duration of antibiotic treatment before surgery becomes indicated. Because there are no reliable guidelines to determine in whom medical treatment supersedes surgery or whether some patients with medical treatment have a better outcome than with surgery, the decision to operate remains dependent upon the specific clinical situation with the prevailing practice to drain these lesions surgically as soon as possible (Martin and Yuan 1996).

After surgery, antibiotic treatment can be adjusted based on the identification and sensitivity of the cultured organism (DiTullio 1977, Koppel et al. 1990, Menezes 1996). No data exist on using specific broad-spectrum antibiotics depending on an acute versus chronic presentation without a positive bacterial culture. The surgical mortality remains high in all age groups, reported in one study to be 13.6%, probably secondary to concomitant systemic illness such as congenital heart disease and septicaemia (Bartels et al. 1995). The importance of concurrent surgical and antibiotic treatment for spinal cord abscesses is illustrated by data available of patients with spinal cord abscess in the pre-antibiotic area: all cases succumbed to the disease without treatment (Bartels et al. 1995, Chan and Gold 1998). The prognosis has dramatically improved, however, after introduction of antibiotics

(Koppel et al. 1990, Menezes 1996, Chan and Gold 1998). The use of steroids in the setting of a spinal abscess is controversial, with the benefits of blunting cord oedema balanced by their depressive effects upon the immune system, and no level 1 data exist to confirm or refute their efficacy (Byrne et al. 1994).

The pathophysiology of the spinal cord injury includes possible venous infarction of the spinal cord due to the mass effect and engorgement of the spinal venous plexus. This makes prompt surgical and antibiotic treatment essential in order to try to preserve and restore as much function as possible, epecially in cases where the radiographic findings are equivocal (DiTullio 1977, Koppel et al. 1990, Candon and Frerebeau 1994, Menezes 1996). Most authors advocate surgical drainage through an open laminectomy and myelotomy over the full extent of the abscess (Mount 1949, Manfredi et al. 1970, Menezes et al. 1977, Bean et al. 1979, Maurice-Williams et al. 1980, Blacklock et al. 1982, Koppel et al. 1990, Benzil et al. 1992, Miranda Carus et al. 1992, Tewari et al. 1992, Rogg et al. 1993, Byrne et al. 1994, Bartels et al. 1995, Tacconi et al. 1995, Bavdekar et al. 1997, Morandi et al. 1999, Thome et al. 2001, Bruff and Sgouros 2002, Tsurubuchi et al. 2002, Morimoto et al. 2003, Simon et al. 2003). Alternatively, a catheter can be inserted into the abscess cavity for drainage, avoiding extensive bony decompression, especially for holocord spinal cord abscesses (el-Gindi and Fairburn 1969, Bunyaratavej et al. 2006). Catheter insertion is not recommended with loculated and non-contiguous abscess formation.

With a more extensive longitudinal spread of the abscess wherein multi-level laminectomies are required, iatrogenic spinal instability may be introduced requiring fusion with instrumentation for stabilization. Stabilization should be performed during the same procedure, especially in children (Cattell and Clark 1967, Lonstein 1977, Katsumi et al. 1989, Albert and Vacarro 1998). The likelihood of causing spinal instability that might lead to late kyphotic deformity depends upon the extent of laminectomy, the spinal level (thoracic vs cervical/lumbar), and the presence of any underlying structural defects. Cervical laminectomy carries the highest risk of postoperative deformity whereas the thoracic spine is considered relatively stable because of the presence of the rib cage, but the need for stabilization surgery must be determined by the surgeon on a case-by-case basis.

Clinical outcome after spinal abscess is variable and depends upon the duration and severity of the neurological deficit at presentation, the extent of the abscess, the promptness of treatment, and the virulence of the responsible organism.

Spinal cord haemorrhage
A compressive spinal cord haemorrhage, whether epidural, sub-dural, or sub-arachnoid in origin, is usually of acute onset and leads to rapidly progressive and devastating neurological deficits. Prompt recognition and treatment, therefore, is essential.

There is a paucity of data looking specifically at the paediatric population and the literature consists of lifespan data. The highest incidence of spinal haematoma occurs in two peaks between 15 and 20 years and 45 and 75 years (Kreppel et al. 2003). Epidural haematoma is the most prevalent type of haemorrhage of the spinal cord with almost 75% of all reported cases, followed by subarachnoid haematoma (16%) and subdural spinal haematoma (4%) (Kreppel et al. 2003). There is a male predominance of 2:1 for all types of spinal haemorrhage except for epidural haematoma for which the available literature consists of a total of 25 cases, limiting its statistical significance (Zuccarello et al. 1980, Williams and Nelson 1987, Kreppel et al. 2003).

The aetiology of the spinal haemorrhage is often unclear, with no identifiable cause determined even after a thorough imaging work up. It is probable that most adult cases occur spontaneously in the setting of anticoagulation or from procedures such as epidural injections (Arlecchini and Boriani 1981). In children, however, a haemorrhage is much more likely to be the result of an underlying vascular lesion including arteriovenous malformations and fistulas (Fig. 5.1). In all age groups, a coagulopathy such as haemophilia may be a significant risk factor. The underlying cause of a haemorrhage in most cases, however, is never determined (Harik et al. 1971, Ghanem and Ivan 1978, Beatty and Winston 1984, Kreppel et al. 2003).

There is a major concern about the risk of inducing a spinal haematoma with epidural or spinal anesthesia and lumbar puncture, especially in patients on anticoagulation (Owens et al. 1986, Bills et al. 1991). Although studies have indicated that the use of epidural analgesia in patients on anticoagulation, including aspirin and warfarin, does not appear to increase the risk of spinal haematoma (Odoom and Sih 1983, Dickman et al. 1990, Sage 1990, Horlocker et al. 1994, Horlocker et al. 1995, Kreppel et al. 2003), other papers recommend proceeding with intraspinal procedures in these patients only on a case-by-case basis (Horlocker et al. 1990, Maclean 1995). The authors recommend a more cautious approach, and avoiding any percutanous intraspinal intrusion or surgery without reversal of anticoagulation to achieve an INR of under 1.4 and verification of a platelet count of at least 100 000. In addition, the authors advise transfusion of platelets for patients on anti-platelet therapy within the previous week.

Less common but still important as a cause for paediatric spinal haemorrhage is trauma (Alderman 1956, Pecker et al. 1960, Posnikoff 1968, Kreppel et al. 2003). The infant is particularly predisposed to cervical injury because of the relative large weight of the head with respect to trunk and the immature features of the cervical spine. Adolescents are also at increased risk of trauma secondary to risk-taking activity and inexperience as car drivers.

A large majority of spinal haemorrhages extend beyond two spinal levels and are located dorsally (Posnikoff 1968, Pear 1972, Scott et al. 1976, Brawn et al. 1986, Groen and Ponssen 1990). The reasons may include the breadth and vascularization pattern of the dorsal epidural space (Maxwell and Puletti 1957, Post et al. 1982). A meta-analysis of 613 patients of all ages demonstrated that the spinal level of the haematoma varies with age: up to the age of 30, they occur predominantly in the cervical and superior thoracic region (Kreppel et al. 2003). In patients between the ages of 31 and 45, the entire cervical and thoracic area is affected. The pattern of haemorrhaging then descends further to the lower thoracic and lumbar spine for the 46 to 75 years age groups before changing back to the upper cervical and thoracolumbar region in the 76 to 95 years age group.

Presentation of non-traumatic spinal haemorrhage is typically marked by acute and severe pain at the level of haemorrhage and neurological deficit, including weakness, sensory loss, and bowel and bladder disturbances. This represents the classic 'coup de poignard' that was described in 1928 by Michon and is most commonly found with epidural

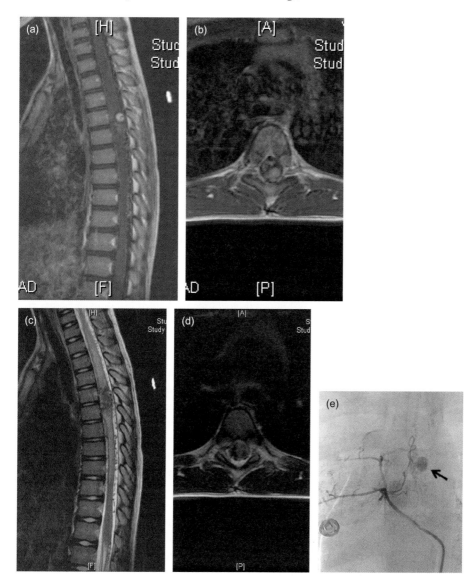

Fig. 5.1. Arterio-venous malformation at T5 to T6 in a 9-year-old child. Imaging modalities demonstrate the lesion on (a, b) sagittal and axial T_1-weighted MRI (c, d) sagittal and axial T_2-weighted MRI, and (e) angiography (arrow depicts the malformation). Surgery was performed for resection of the lesion.

haematoma (Michon 1928). Severe disruption or compression of the corticospinal fibres will result in flaccid paralysis and initial hyporeflexia (Markham et al. 1967). Blood in the subarachnoid space will result in cerebral signs including headache, vomiting, nausea, photophobia, and neck pain. Subdural haematoma presents in a similar but less fulminant fashion (Lao et al. 1993).

Computed tomography (CT) scans and plain radiographs are of very limited value in assessing spinal haematomas because of their poor ability to visualize soft tissue and the limited ability to discriminate blood and bone. Initial imaging investigation should be an MRI with and without gadolinium. MRI will localize the level of the bleed and any vascular lesions may be evident with contrast-enhanced sequences. Some vascular lesions will not be appreciable because of compression by haematoma. Thus, an MRI that fails to reveal any lesion should be repeated in 2 to 3 months. If there is any suggestion of an underlying vascular anomaly, a formal spinal angiogram is indicated.

Acute extrinsic compression of the spinal cord mandates rapid decompressive surgery. Haemorrhage in the intramedullary space may require urgent surgery if the spinal cord is significantly expanded, but smaller haematomas may be treated non-operatively. High-dose steroids are commonly used but this has not been substantiated by published evidence. The controversial high-dose spinal cord injury protocol recommended by some surgeons after trauma is not indicated in the paediatric population.

Spinal cord trauma in the paediatric population

Although most patients with spinal cord trauma are between the ages of 15 and 40, serious spinal trauma and spinal cord injuries are far less common in young children (Kewalramani et al. 1980, Kewalramani and Tori 1980, Reilly 2007, Parent et al. 2010). The base population-adjusted incidence of spinal cord injury in the paediatric population is 1 in 1 000 000 (Reilly 2007). The cervical spine is the most common site of injury, with between 60 and 80% of spinal cord injuries (Platzer et al. 2007, Parent et al. 2010). In comparison, thoracolumbar spine injuries in children have an incidence of only 5 to 34% (Dogan et al. 2007).

The immature spine and its biomechanical properties, including the relatively larger size of the head with respect to the neck and torso, predispose the paediatric spine to characteristic injury mechanisms that are distinct from trauma to the adult spine. Specific characteristics of the immature cervical spine are important in predisposing a child to injury. In children under 12, the upper cervical facets are orientated more horizontally, allowing for greater mobility and reduced resistance to rotational acceleration–deceleration. This accounts, for example, for a larger, normal dynamic characteristic of the atlanto-dental interval and the higher incidence of cervical pseudosubluxation (Bailey 1952, Penning 1978). These features explain a higher prevalence of cervical injury above the C4 level and a higher incidence of spinal cord injury without radiographic abnormality (SCIWORA) (Bailey 1952, Pang and Wilberger 1982, Hadley et al. 1988, Nitecki and Moir 1994).

Paediatric cord injuries include birth injury, non-accidental injury, road traffic accidents, falls, and sport injuries (Hubbard 1974, Anderson and Schutt 1980, Hadley et al. 1988, Reilly 2007). Birth trauma may result in spinal cord injury, especially in difficult deliveries with breech presentation, although such injury has even been reported after uncomplicated vaginal delivery (Ruggieri et al. 1999, Vialle et al. 2008, Goetz et al. 2010). Severe non-accidental trauma such as from the shaken-impact syndrome may result in spinal cord contusion and haematoma in the high cervical and cervicomedullary region (Hadley et al. 1988, Hadley et al. 1989). In a series of 13 patients who succumbed to the consequences of non-accidental trauma, almost 50% sustained upper cervical spinal cord injury: five out of six demonstrated cervical spine bleeding, four out of six also had a subdural component, whereas four out of six showed upper cervical spinal cord contusion (Hadley et al. 1989). Penetrating injury, however, a major cause of injury in the adult population, is unusual in the paediatric population (Reilly 2007).

SPINAL CORD INJURY WITHOUT RADIOGRAPHIC ABNORMALITY
SCIWORA was described as a distinct traumatic entity following the observation of patients with profound neurological dysfunction consistent with spinal cord injury in the absence of fracture on radiograph or CT (Pang and Wilberger 1982). The exact prevalence is uncertain but up to 33% of children with neurological signs and symptoms of spinal cord injury are diagnosed with SCIWORA (Pang and Wilberger 1982, Hadley et al. 1988). The advent of MRI has led to the realization that most patients with SCIWORA based upon CT scans or radiograph do have evidence of cord injury, most often because of ligamentous laxity in young children, usually in the cervical area, which allows for transient canal compromise and cord compression that reduces anatomical alignment without fracturing the facets or other bony elements. In some patients, MRI may show clear evidence of haematoma or oedema in the ligamentous elements (Pang 2004) The high head-to-body ratio in younger children described above may play a significant role in the aetiology of this entity. In older children, the incidence of SCIWORA decreases and patients present more and more with incomplete spinal cord injuries (Dickman et al. 1991) A practitioner needs to keep in mind the possibility of non-accidental injury, particularly in younger children, and to make the proper notification to relevant agencies whenever it is suspected. The prognosis of SCIWORA depends on the severity of the neurological deficit at presentation.

SPINAL FRACTURE MANAGEMENT
Bony fracture or disruption of ligamentous structures may undermine the stability of the spine and lead to abnormal movement. This, in turn, may cause injury to the spinal cord. Bony fractures are readily appreciated on either plain radiographs or a CT scan, but ligamentous disruption is better diagnosed on MRI. Flexion–extension radiographs are useful to demonstrate pathological movement between vertebral segments, but are only safe to perform in a neurologically intact patient old enough to cooperate fully with the study (Reilly 2007) The complete description of the management of cervical fractures is beyond the scope of this chapter, but fractures may be managed with a combination of surgical stabilization with fusion and instrumentation and/or the use of a variety of spinal braces. Upper cervical spine injuries are usually immobilized in a rigid, Philadelphia-type collar, whereas the lower cervical spine is braced in a Minerva-type orthosis, a rigid cervical collar attached to a chest brace.

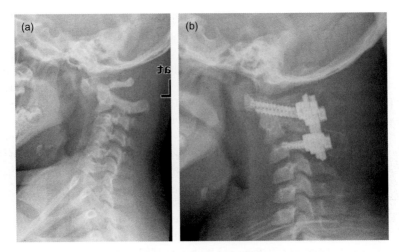

Fig. 5.2. Lateral cervical spine radiograph in a patient with Down synrome with C1 to C2 subluxation (a) before and (b) after instrumented fusion and correction of subluxation.

ATLANTO-OCCIPITAL INJURY

The anatomy and biomechanical characteristics of the paediatric cervical spine render it susceptible to atlanto-occipital injury (Pang et al. 2007). This type of injury is associated with high energy impact and is often fatal owing to coincident injury at the level of the cervico-medullary junction (Bucholz et al. 1979). As detailed in earlier sections, the relatively larger head-to-body relationship particularly predisposes newborns and very young children to cervico-medullary injury (Hadley et al. 1988, Pang et al. 2007).

Down syndrome results in abnormal ligamentous laxity at the occipital C1 and C1 to C2 levels and is a risk factor for injury (Fig. 5.2) (Hankinson and Anderson, Matsuda et al. 1995, Kattan and McDonald 1996). The diagnosis of occipito-cervical subluxation is more difficult in children under 3 years because the relation of the basion to the odontoid can be difficult to judge owing to the immature ossification of the odontoid. Assessing the extent of the neurological involvement can be challenging: typically patients have multiple injuries, including head trauma, and are intubated and sedated. If instability is detected, a halo can be applied until a definitive surgical stabilization through an occipito-cervical fusion can be done (Donahue et al. 1994, Sponseller and Cass 1997).

ATLANTAL FRACTURE AND TRAUMATIC ATLANTO-AXIAL INSTABILITY

Isolated atlas fracture is uncommon in children (Bohlman 1979, McGrory et al. 1993). It corresponds to the paediatric version of a Jefferson's fracture (Stauffer and Mazur 1982, Marlin et al. 1983). The atlas in children under the age of 6 years is composed of areas of cartilage, synchondrosis, that eventually ossify, resulting in a complete bony ring (Fig. 5.3) (Reilly and Leung 2005). When axial loading is applied to the ring, the synchondrosis can fail and push outward. Typically patients are neurologically stable because the spinal canal

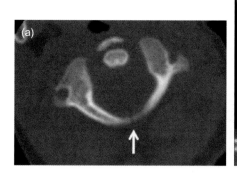
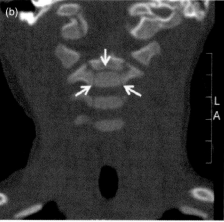

Fig. 5.3. (a) Axial and (b) coronal CT scan in a 2-year-old showing the synchondrosis at C1 and C2 (arrows). The difference from a fracture should be apparent once the patient's age is taken into account.

remains unobstructed. Treatment requires immobilization with a rigid cervical collar or halo-vest (Reilly 2007).

Isolated C1 to C2 ligamentous instability occurs with a tear of the transverse ligament and remains a rare injury (Bohlman 1979). The elasticity of the ligamentous apparatus in the paediatric spine allows a greater normal dynamic atlanto-dental interval; however, a tear of the transverse ligament may result in frank subluxation and compression of the spinal cord within the narrowed spinal canal (Dormans 2002). Flexion-extension radiographs detect any abnormal mobility between the C1 and C2 vertebrae and MRI best evaluates the integrity of the transverse ligament (Reilly 2007). In adults, the maximum atlanto-dental interval is 3mm, although flexibility of the ligamentous structures allows for an atlanto-dental interval up to 5mm in children under 6 years. If abnormal movement between C1 and C2 results in dynamic instability that causes pain or threatens spinal cord compression, surgical fusion for stabilization is indicated. Stabilization consists of laying bone graft upon the posterior aspect of C1 and C2 for fusion and placement of spinal instrumentation.

ODONTOID FRACTURE

Until the adolescent growth spurt, an odontoid fracture represents a disruption of the syn-chondrosis at the base of the odontoid (Sherk 1978, Sherk et al. 1978, Sanderson and Houten 2002). The most common cause for this injury is a road traffic accident (Odent et al. 1999). These fractures can be missed easily, especially in the younger population where ossification has not yet started (Sanderson and Houten 2002, Choit et al. 2005). Sagittal CT of the neck is the best modality to demonstrate radiographically an odontoid fracture (Fig. 5.4) (Fielding et al. 1980, Odent et al. 1999, Hernandez et al. 2004). In a setting of a significant mechanism of injury and complaint of neck pain, a CT scan should be obtained

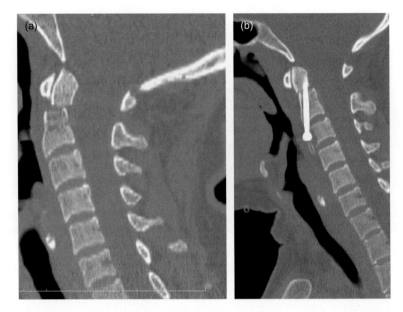

Fig. 5.4. Odontoid type II fracture seen on sagittal CT scan. (a) Retrolisthesis and distraction of the fractured dens is visible; (b) after odontoid screw placement.

if the diagnosis is unclear on a radiograph or if the anatomy of any fracture needs better definition before deciding on definitive treatment (Sanderson and Houten 2002). Non-displaced injuries can be managed effectively with a halo-vest as young children are usually poorly compliant with a hard cervical collar. If the odontoid is displaced, a closed reduction under fluoroscopic control and either fixation with spinal instrumentation or halo immobilization is indicated.

SUB-AXIAL CERVICAL SPINE INJURY

Sub-axial cervical spine fractures are rare under the age of 9 years, and, when they occur, are most often the result of road traffic accidents (Birney and Hanley 1989, Finch and Barnes 1998). Flexion and distraction moments of force may cause either unilateral or bilateral dislocation of the facet joints, also known as 'jumped facets'. Unilateral facet dislocations usually present with mild or no neurological deficit whereas bilateral facet dislocation typically is associated with severe neurological injury. In addition, burst fractures of the sub-axial cervical spine need to be ruled out with imaging studies (Fig. 5.5). Initial management is oriented to expeditious reduction of the dislocation to realign the spine and relieve any neural compression. Closed reduction under fluoroscopic control is successful in many patients, but is only possible in a cooperative patient. In patients in whom closed reduction is impossible or impractical, operative reduction from either an anterior or posterior approach with instrumentation is indicated. Halo immobilization for 2 to 3 months is indicated in most patients following successful closed reduction.

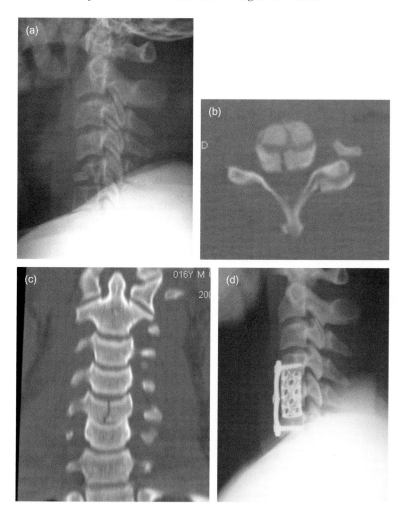

Fig. 5.5. C5 burst fracture in a 16-year-old after a motor vehicle accident. (a) Lateral cervical spine radiograph demonstrates a fractured C5 vertebra. (b) Axial and (c) coronal CT scan confirms the diagnosis. There is also a left lateral mass fracture at C2 visible on the coronal section. (d) Cervical spine radiograph after corpectomy, cage placement, and anterior instrumentation.

THORACO-LUMBAR INJURIES

Thoraco-lumbar and sacral injuries in the paediatric population are rare, mostly presenting as the result of non-accidental trauma or road traffic accident related to seat-belt injury (Miller and Smith 1991, Glassman et al. 1992, Rumball and Jarvis 1992, Dogan et al. 2007, Platzer et al. 2007). These injuries may be in association with chest or abdominal injuries and patients should be evaluated by the trauma team at presentation to the hospital. Neurological deficits are common as the typical fracture pattern is failure of the vertebral body in flexion, as occurs in seat-belt-type injury, resulting in retropulsion of bony elements into

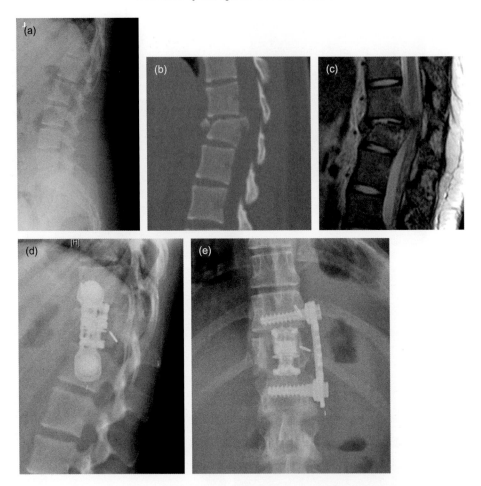

Fig. 5.6. (a) T12 vertebral fracture of a 17-year-old on lateral lumbar spine X-ray, (b) CT scan, and (c) MRI. At presentation the patient was neurologically stable. (d, e) Lateral and anterior–posterior radiographs after corpectomy, cage placement, and instrumentation.

the spinal canal (Rumball and Jarvis 1992). Treatment of thoracolumbar fractures is oriented towards decompression of the neural elements and stabilization of the spine, typically by placement of bone graft and spinal instrumentation from either an anterior or posterior approach (Fig. 5.6).

POST-TRAUMATIC AND POST-SURGICAL SPINAL DEFORMITY AND SEQUELAE
Spinal deformity following trauma almost invariably occurs in children whose injury occurred before the completion of growth (Andrews and Jung 1979, Lancourt et al. 1981, Dearolf et al. 1990, Parisini, Di Silvestre et al. 2002). Scoliosis, kyphosis, and lordosis are the most common deformities in descending order (Reilly 2007). Spinal bracing is an

effective treatment for mild deformities, but severe cases may warrant surgery. No convincing level 1 data exist, however, to support either the use of instrumentation or bracing in the paediatric population (Parent et al. 2010). For serious instances of spinal instability, surgery is generally performed to forestall the development of neural injury or paralysis even though the normal longitudinal growth of the spinal column may be adversely affected. Patients who have had serious spinal trauma are at risk of developing syringomyelia, which may lead to neurological deficit years after the traumatic event. The authors therefore recommend that paediatricians consider ordering an MRI early if these patients complain of any new symptoms of back pain, motor, or sensory disturbance (Gabriel and Crawford 1988).

REFERENCES

Al Barbarawi M, Khriesat W, Qudsieh S, Qudsieh H, Loai AA. Management of intramedullary spinal cord abscess: experience with four cases, pathophysiology and outcomes. *Eur Spine J* 2009; **18**: 710–717.

Albert TJ, Vacarro A. Postlaminectomy kyphosis. *Spine* 1998; **23**: 2738–2745.

Alderman DB. Extradural spinal-cord hematoma; report of a case due to dicumarol and review of the literature. *N Engl J Med* 1956; **255**: 839–842.

Anderson JM, Schutt AH. Spinal injury in children: a review of 156 cases seen from 1950 through 1978. *Mayo Clin Proc* 1980; **55**: 499–504.

Andrews LG, Jung SK. Spinal cord injuries in children in British Columbia. *Paraplegia* 1979; **17**: 442–451.

Arlecchini S, Boriani S. Acute spontaneous spinal epidural haematoma. *Ital J Orthop Traumatol* 1981; **7**: 245–250.

Bailey DK. The normal cervical spine in infants and children. *Radiology* 1952; **59**: 712–719.

Baradaran N, Ahmadi H, Nejat F, El Khashab M, Mahdavi A, Rahbarimanesh AA. Recurrent meningitis caused by cervico-medullary abscess, a rare presentation. *Childs Nerv Syst* 2008; **24**: 767–771.

Bartels RH, Gonera EG, van der Spek JA, Thijssen HO, Mullaart RA, Gabreels FJ. Intramedullary spinal cord abscess. A case report. *Spine* 1995; **20**: 1199–1204.

Bavdekar SB, Rao N, Kamat JR. Intramedullary spinal cord abscess. *Indian J Pediatr* 1997; **64**: 428–431.

Bean, J. R., J. W. Walsh, H. M. Blacker Cervical dermal sinus and intramedullary spinal cord abscess: case report. *Neurosurgery* 1979; **5** (1 Pt 1): 60–62.

Beatty RM, Winston KR. Spontaneous cervical epidural hematoma. A consideration of etiology. *J Neurosurg* 1984; **61**: 143–148.

Benzil DL, Epstein MH, Knuckey NW. Intramedullary epidermoid associated with an intramedullary spinal abscess secondary to a dermal sinus. *Neurosurgery* 1992; **30**: 118–121.

Bills DC, Blumbergs P, North JB. Iatrogenic spinal subdural haematoma. *Aust N Z J Surg* 1991; **61**: 703–706.

Bingol A, Yucemen N, Meco O. Medically treated intraspinal Brucella granuloma. *Surg Neurol* 1999; **52**: 570–576.

Birney TJ, Hanley EN Jr. Traumatic cervical spine injuries in childhood and adolescence. *Spine* 1989; **14**: 1277–1282.

Blacklock JB, Hood TW, Maxwell RE. Intramedullary cervical spinal cord abscess. Case report. *J Neurosurg* 1982; **57**: 270–273.

Bohlman HH. Acute fractures and dislocations of the cervical spine. An analysis of three hundred hospitalized patients and review of the literature. *J Bone Joint Surg Am* 1979; **61**: 1119–1142.

Brawn LA., Bergval UE, Davies-Jones GA. Spontaneous spinal epidural haematoma with spontaneous resolution. *Postgrad Med J* 1986; **62**: 885–887.

Bruff P, Sgouros S. Lumbar dermoid cyst causing pyomyelia in a child. *Pediatr Neurosurg* 2002; **36**: 162–163.

Bucholz RW, Burkhead WZ, Graham W, Petty C. Occult cervical spine injuries in fatal traffic accidents. *J Trauma* 1979; **19**: 768–771.

Bunyaratavej K, Desudchit T, Pongpunlert W. Holocord intramedullary abscess due to dermal sinus in a 2-month-old child successfully treated with limited myelotomy and aspiration. Case report. *J Neurosurg* 2006; **104** (4 Suppl.): 269–274.

Byrne RW, von Roenn KA, Whisler WW. Intramedullary abscess: a report of two cases and a review of the literature. *Neurosurgery* 1994; **35**: 321–326.

Candon E, Frerebeau P. [Bacterial abscesses of the spinal cord. Review of the literature (73 cases)]. *Rev Neurol* 1994; **150**: 370–376.

Cattell HS, Clark GL Jr. Cervical kyphosis and instability following multiple laminectomies in children. *J Bone Joint Surg Am* 1967; **49**: 713–720.

Chan CT, Gold WL. Intramedullary abscess of the spinal cord in the antibiotic era: clinical features, microbial etiologies, trends in pathogenesis, and outcomes. *Clin Infect Dis* 1998; **27**: 619–626.

Cheng KM, Ma MW, Chan CM, Leung CL. Tuberculous intramedullary spinal cord abscess. *Acta Neurochir* 1997; **139**: 1189–1190.

Choit RL, Jamieson DH, Reilly CW. Os odontoideum: a significant radiographic finding. *Pediatr Radiol* 2005; **35**: 803–807.

Chu JY, Montanera W, Willinsky RA. Listeria spinal cord abscess—clinical and MRI findings. *Can J Neurol Sci* 1996; **23**: 220–223.

Cokca F, Meco O, Arasil E, Unlu A. An intramedullary dermoid cyst abscess due to Brucella abortus biotype 3 at T11-L2 spinal levels. *Infection* 1994; **22**: 359–360.

Courville C. Pathology of the Central Nervous System. Mountain View, CA: Pacific Press, 1950.

Crema MD, Pradel C, Marra MD, Arrive L, Tubiana JM. Intramedullary spinal cord abscess complicating thoracic spondylodiscitis caused by Bacteroides fragilis. *Skeletal Radiol* 2007; **36**: 681–683.

Dearolf WW 3rd, Betz RR, Vogel LC, Levin J, Clancy M, Steel HH. Scoliosis in pediatric spinal cord-injured patients. *J Pediatr Orthop* 1990; **10**: 214–218.

Desai KI, Muzumdar DP, Goel A. Holocord intramedullary abscess: an unusual case with review of literature. *Spinal Cord* 1999; **37**: 866–870.

Dickman CA, Shedd SA, Spetzler RF, Shetter AG, Sonntag VK. Spinal epidural hematoma associated with epidural anesthesia: complications of systemic heparinization in patients receiving peripheral vascular thrombolytic therapy. *Anesthesiology* 1990; **72**: 947–950.

Dickman CA, Zabramski JM, Hadley MN, Rekate HL, Sonntag VK. Pediatric spinal cord injury without radiographic abnormalities: report of 26 cases and review of the literature. *J Spinal Disord* 1991; **4**: 296–305.

DiTullio MV Jr. Intramedullary spinal abscess: a case report with a review of 53 previously described cases. *Surg Neurol* 1977; **7**: 351–354.

Do-Dai DD, M. K. Brooks MK, Goldkamp A, Erbay S, Bhadelia RA. Magnetic resonance imaging of intramedullary spinal cord lesions: a pictorial review. *Curr Probl Diagn Radiol* 2010; **39**: 160–185.

Dogan, S., S. Safavi-Abbasi, N. Theodore, S. W. Chang, E. M. Horn, N. R. Mariwalla, H. L. Rekate, V. K. Sonntag Thoracolumbar and sacral spinal injuries in children and adolescents: a review of 89 cases. *J Neurosurg* 2007; **106**(6 Suppl.): 426–433.

Donahue DJ, Muhlbauer MS, Kaufman RA, Warner WC, Sanford RA. Childhood survival of atlantooccipital dislocation: underdiagnosis, recognition, treatment, and review of the literature. *Pediatr Neurosurg* 1994; **21**: 105–111.

Dorflinger-Hejlek E, Kirsch EC, Reiter H, Opravil M, Kaim AH. Diffusion-weighted MR imaging of intramedullary spinal cord abscess. *AJNR Am J Neuroradiol* 2010; **31**: 1651–1652.

Dormans JP. Evaluation of children with suspected cervical spine injury. *J Bone Joint Surg Am A* 2002; **84**: 124–132.

el-Gindi S, Fairburn B. Intramedullary spinal abscess as a complication of a congenital dermal sinus. Case report. *J Neurosurg* 1969; **30**: 494–497.

Fernandez-Ruiz M, Lopez-Medrano F, Garcia-Montero M, Hornedo-Muguiro J, Aguado JM. Intramedullary cervical spinal cord abscess by viridans group Streptococcus secondary to infective endocarditis and facilitated by previous local radiotherapy. *Intern Med* 2009; **48**: 61–64.

Fielding JW, Hensinger RN, Hawkins RJ. Os Odontoideum. *J Bone Joint Surg Am* 1980; **62**: 376–383.

Finch GD, Barnes MJ. Major cervical spine injuries in children and adolescents. *J Pediatr Orthop* 1998; **18**: 811–814.

Foley J. Intramedullary abscess of the spinal cord. *Lancet* 1949; **ii**: 193–195.

Gabriel KR, Crawford AH. Identification of acute posttraumatic spinal cord cyst by magnetic resonance imaging: a case report and review of the literature. *J Pediatr Orthop* 1988; **8**: 710–714.

Ghanem Q, Ivan LP. Spontaneous spinal epidural hematoma in an 8-year-old boy. *Neurology* 1978; **28**: 829–832.

Glassman SD, Johnson JR, Holt RT. Seatbelt injuries in children. *J Trauma* 1992; **33**: 882–886.

Goetz LL, Howard M, Cipher D, Revankar SG. Occurrence of candiduria in a population of chronically catheterized patients with spinal cord injury. *Spinal Cord* 2010; **48**: 51–54.

Groen RJ, Ponssen H. The spontaneous spinal epidural hematoma. A study of the etiology. *J Neurol Sci* 1990; **98**: 121–138.

Hadley MN, Sonntag VK, Rekate HL, Murphy A. The infant whiplash-shake injury syndrome: a clinical and pathological study. *Neurosurgery* 1989; **24**: 536–540.

Hadley MN, Zabramski JM, Browner CM, Rekate H, Sonntag VK. Pediatric spinal trauma. Review of 122 cases of spinal cord and vertebral column injuries. *J Neurosurg* 1988; **68**: 18–24.

Hanci M, Sarioglu AC, Uzan M, Islak C, Kaynar MY, Oz B. Intramedullary tuberculous abscess: a case report. *Spine* 1996; **21**: 766–769.

Hankinson TC, Anderson RC. Craniovertebral junction abnormalities in Down syndrome. *Neurosurgery* **66** (3 Suppl.): 32–38.

Harik SI, Raichle ME, Reis DJ. Spontaneously remitting spinal epidural hematoma in a patient on anticoagulants. *N Engl J Med* 1971; **284**: 1355–1357.

Hart J. A case of encysted abscess in the center of the spinal cord. *Dublin Hospital Report* 1830; **5**: 522–524.

Hernandez JA, Chupik C, Swischuk LE. Cervical spine trauma in children under 5 years: productivity of CT. *Emerg Radiol* 2004; **10**: 176–178.

Horlocker TT, Wedel DJ, Offord KP. Does preoperative antiplatelet therapy increase the risk of hemorrhagic complications associated with regional anesthesia? *Anesth Analg* 1990; **70**: 631–634.

Horlocker TT, Wedel DJ, Schlichting JL. Postoperative epidural analgesia and oral anticoagulant therapy. *Anesth Analg* 1994; **79**: 89–93.

Horlocker TT, Wedel DJ, Schroeder DR, et al. Wong Preoperative antiplatelet therapy does not increase the risk of spinal hematoma associated with regional anesthesia. *Anesth Analg* 1995; **80**: 303–309.

Hubbard DD. Injuries of the spine in children and adolescents. *Clin Orthop Relat Res* 1974; (100): 56–65.

Kamgarpour A, Izadfar MA, Razmkon A. Neglected intramedullary cord abscess in a 3-year old child: a case report. *Childs Nerv Syst* 2008; **24**: 153–155.

Katsumi Y, Honma T, Nakamura T. Analysis of cervical instability resulting from laminectomies for removal of spinal cord tumor. *Spine* 1989; **14**: 1171–1176.

Kattan H, McDonald P. Atlanto-occipital and atlanto-axial instability in children with Down syndrome. *Ann Saudi Med* 1996; **16**: 56–59.

Kewalramani LS, Kraus JF, Sterling HM. Acute spinal-cord lesions in a pediatric population: epidemiological and clinical features. *Paraplegia* 1980; **18**: 206–219.

Kewalramani LS, Tori JA. Spinal cord trauma in children. Neurologic patterns, radiologic features, and pathomechanics of injury. *Spine* 1980; **5**: 11–18.

King SJ, Jeffree MA. MRI of an abscess of the cervical spinal cord in a case of Listeria meningoencephalomyelitis. *Neuroradiology* 1993; **35**: 495–496.

Koppel BS, Daras M, Duffy KR. Intramedullary spinal cord abscess. *Neurosurgery* 1990; **26**: 145–146.

Kreppel D, Antoniadis G, Seeling W. Spinal hematoma: a literature survey with meta-analysis of 613 patients. *Neurosurg Rev* 2003; **26**: 1–49.

Kurita N, Sakurai Y, Taniguchi M, Terao T, Takahashi H, Mannen T. Intramedullary spinal cord abscess treated with antibiotic therapy—case report and review. *Neurol Med Chir* 2009; **49**: 262–268.

Lancourt JE, Dickson JH, Carter RE. Paralytic spinal deformity following traumatic spinal-cord injury in children and adolescents. *J Bone Joint Surg Am* 1981; **63**: 47–53.

Lao TT, Halpern SH, MacDonald D, Huh C. Spinal subdural haematoma in a parturient after attempted epidural anaesthesia. *Can J Anaesth* 1993; **40**: 340–345.

Lascaux AS, Chevalier X, Brugieres P, Levy Y. Painful neck stiffness secondary to an intramedullary abscess of the spinal cord in a HIV infected patient: a case report. *J Neurol* 2002; **249**: 229–230.

Lindner A, Becker G, Warmuth-Metz M, Schalke BC, Bogdahn U, Toyka KV. Magnetic resonance image findings of spinal intramedullary abscess caused by Candida albicans: case report. *Neurosurgery* 1995; **36**: 411–412.

Lonstein JE. Post-laminectomy kyphosis. *Clin Orthop Relat Res* 1977; **128**: 93–100.

Maclean A. Antiplatelet therapy, regional anesthesia, and spinal hematomas. *Anesth Analg* 1995; **81**: 1116.

Manfredi M, Bozzao L, Frasconi F. Chronic intramedullary abscess of the spinal cord. Case report. *J Neurosurg* 1970; **33**: 352–355.

Markham JW, Lynge HN, Stahlman GE The syndrome of spontaneous spinal epidural hematoma. Report of three cases. *J Neurosurg* 1967; **26**: 334–342.

Marlin AE, Williams GR, Lee JF. Jefferson fractures in children. Case report. *J Neurosurg* 1983; **58**: 277–279.

Martin RJ, Yuan HA Neurosurgical care of spinal epidural, subdural, and intramedullary abscesses and arachnoiditis. *Orthop Clin North Am* 1996; **27**: 125–136.

Matsuda Y, Sano N, Watanabe S, Oki S, Shibata T. Atlanto-occipital hypermobility in subjects with Down's syndrome. *Spine* 1995; **20**: 2283–2286.

Maurice-Williams RS, Pamphilon D, Coakham HB. Intramedullary abscess—a rare complication of spinal dysraphism. *J Neurol Neurosurg Psychiatry* 1980; **43**: 1045–1048.

Maxwell GM, Puletti F. Chronic spinal epidural hematoma in a child. *Neurology* 1957; **7**: 596–600.

McGrory BJ, Klassen RA, Chao EY, Staeheli JW, Weaver AL. Acute fractures and dislocations of the cervical spine in children and adolescents. *J Bone Joint Surg Am* 1993; **75**: 988–995.

Menezes AH, Graf CJ, Perret GE. Spinal cord abscess: a review. *Surg Neurol* 1977; **8**: 461–467.

Menezes AH, J V G. Spinal Cord Abscess. New York, NY: McGraw Hill, 1996.

Michon Le coup de poignard rachidien. [Initial symptoms of some sub-arachnoid hemorrhages. Essay on the spinal subarachnoid hemorrhage.] (In French.) *Press Med* 1928; **36**: 964–966.

Miller JA, Smith TH. Seatbelt induced chance fracture in an infant. Case report and literature review. *Pediatr Radiol* 1991; **21**: 575–577.

Miranda Carus ME, Anciones B, Castro A, Lara M, Isla A. Intramedullary spinal cord abscess. *J Neurol Neurosurg Psychiatry* 1992; **55**: 225–226.

Morandi X, Mercier P, Fournier HD, Brassier G. Dermal sinus and intramedullary spinal cord abscess Report of two cases and review of the literature. *Childs Nerv Syst* 1999; **15**: 202–206.

Morimoto K, Takemoto O, Nakamura H, Takeuchi M. Spinal dermal sinus associated with intramedullary abscess and dermoid. *Pediatr Neurosurg* 2003; **39**: 225–226.

Mount LA. Congenital dermal sinuses as a cause of meningitis, intraspinal abscess and intracranial abscess. *J Am Med Assoc* 1949; **139**: 1263–1268.

Murphy KJ, Brunberg JA, Quint DJ, Kazanjian PH. Spinal cord infection: myelitis and abscess formation. *AJNR Am J Neuroradiol* 1998; **19**: 341–348.

Nitecki S, Moir CR. Predictive factors of the outcome of traumatic cervical spine fracture in children. *J Pediatr Surg* 1994; **29**: 1409–1411.

Novati R, Vigano MG, de Bona A, Nocita B, Finazzi R, Lazzarin A. Neurobrucellosis with spinal cord abscess of the dorsal tract: a case report. *Int J Infect Dis* 2002; **6**: 149–150.

Odent T, Langlais J, Glorion C, Kassis B, Bataille J, Pouliquen JC. Fractures of the odontoid process: a report of 15 cases in children younger than 6 years. *J Pediatr Orthop* 1999; **19**: 51–54.

Odoom JA, Sih IL. Epidural analgesia and anticoagulant therapy Experience with one thousand cases of continuous epidurals. *Anaesthesia* 1983; **38**: 254–259.

Owens EL, Kasten GW, Hessel EA 2nd. Spinal subarachnoid hematoma after lumbar puncture and heparinization: a case report, review of the literature, and discussion of anesthetic implications. *Anesth Analg* 1986; **65**: 1201–1207.

Pang D. Spinal cord injury without radiographic abnormality in children, 2 decades later. *Neurosurgery* 2004; **55**: 1325–1342.

Pang D, Nemzek WR, Zovickian J. Atlanto-occipital dislocation—part 2: the clinical use of (occipital) condyle-C1 interval, comparison with other diagnostic methods, and the manifestation, management, and outcome of atlanto-occipital dislocation in children. *Neurosurgery* 2007; **61**: 995–1015.

Pang D, Wilberger JE Jr. Spinal cord injury without radiographic abnormalities in children. *J Neurosurg* 1982; **57**: 114–129.

Parent S, Dimar J, Dekutoski M, Roy-Beaudry M. Unique features of pediatric spinal cord injury. *Spine* 2010; **35** (21 Suppl): S202–S208.

Parisini P, Di Silvestre M, Greggi T. Treatment of spinal fractures in children and adolescents: long-term results in 44 patients. *Spine* 2002; **27**: 1989–1994.

Pear BL. Spinal epidural hematoma. *Am J Roentgenol Radium Ther Nucl Med* 1972; **115**: 155–164.

Pecker J, Javalet A, Le Menn G. [Ankylosing spondylarthritis and paraplegia due to traumatic extradural hematorrhachis.] *Presse Med* 1960; **68**: 183–184.

Penning L. Normal movements of the cervical spine. *AJR Am J Roentgenol* 1978; **130**: 317–326.

Pfadenhauer K, Rossmanith T. Spinal manifestation of neurolisteriosis. *J Neurol* 1995; **242**: 153–156.

Platzer P, Jaindl M, Thalhammer G, et al. Cervical spine injuries in pediatric patients. *J Trauma* 2007; **62**: 389–396.

Posnikoff J. Spontaneous spinal epidural hematoma of childhood. *J Pediatr* 1968; **73**: 178–183.

Post MJ, Seminer DS, Quencer RM. CT diagnosis of spinal epidural hematoma. *AJNR Am J Neuroradiol* 1982; **3**: 190–192.

Reilly CW. Pediatric spine trauma. *J Bone Joint Surg Am* 2007; **89** (Suppl. 1): 98–107.

Reilly CW, Leung F. Synchondrosis fracture in a pediatric patient. *Can J Surg* 2005; **48**: 158–159.

Rogg JM, Benzil DL, Haas RL, Knuckey NW. Intramedullary abscess, an unusual manifestation of a dermal sinus. *AJNR Am J Neuroradiol* 1993; **14**: 1393–1395.

Ruggieri M, Smarason AK, Pike M. Spinal cord insults in the prenatal, perinatal, and neonatal periods. *Dev Med Child Neurol* 1999; **41**: 311–317.

Rumball K, Jarvis J. Seat-belt injuries of the spine in young children. *J Bone Joint Surg Br* 1992; **74**: 571–574.

Sage DJ. Epidurals, spinals and bleeding disorders in pregnancy: a review. *Anaesth Intensive Care* 1990; **18**: 319–326.

Samkoff LM, Monajati A, Shapiro JL. Teaching NeuroImage: nocardial intramedullary spinal cord abscess. *Neurology* 2008; **71**: e5.

Sanderson SP, Houten JK. Fracture through the C2 synchondrosis in a young child. *Pediatr Neurosurg* 2002; **36**: 277–278.

Scott BB, Quisling RG, Miller CA, Kindt GW. Spinal epidural hematoma. *JAMA* 1976; **235**: 513–515.

Sherk HH. Fractures of the atlas and odontoid process. *Orthop Clin North Am* 1978; **9**: 973–984.

Sherk HH, Nicholson JT, Chung SM. Fractures of the odontoid process in young children. *J Bone Joint Surg Am* 1978; **60**: 921–924.

Simon JK, Lazareff JA, Diament MJ, Kennedy WA. Intramedullary abscess of the spinal cord in children: a case report and review of the literature. *Pediatr Infect Dis J* 2003; **22**: 186–192.

Sponseller PD, Cass JR. Atlanto-occipital fusion for dislocation in children with neurologic preservation. A case report. *Spine* 1997; **22**: 344–347.

Stauffer ES, Mazur JM. Cervical spine injuries in children. *Pediatr Ann* 1982; **11**: 502–508, 510–501.

Tacconi L, Arulampalam T, Johnston FG, Thomas DG. Intramedullary spinal cord abscess: case report. *Neurosurgery* 1995; **37**: 817–819.

Tewari MK, Devi BI, Thakur RC, Pathak A, Khandelwal N, Kak VK. Intramedullary spinal cord abscess: a case report. *Childs Nerv Syst* 1992; **8**: 290–291.

Thome C, Krauss JK, Zevgaridis D, Schmiedek P. Pyogenic abscess of the filum terminale. Case report. *J Neurosurg* 2001; **95** (1 Suppl.): 100–104.

Tsurubuchi T, Matsumura A, Nakai K, et al. Reversible holocord edema associated with intramedullary spinal abscess secondary to an infected dermoid cyst. *Pediatr Neurosurg* 2002; **37**: 282–286.

Ushikoshi S, Koyanagi I, Hida K, Iwasaki Y, Abe H. Spinal intrathecal actinomycosis: a case report. *Surg Neurol* 1998; **50**: 221–225.

Vialle R, Pietin-Vialle C, Vinchon M, Dauger S, Ilharreborde B, Glorion C. Birth-related spinal cord injuries: a multicentric review of nine cases. *Childs Nerv Syst* 2008; **24**: 79–85.

Vora YA, Raad II, McCutcheon IE. Intramedullary abscess from group F Streptococcus. *Surg Infect* 2004; **5**: 200–204.

Williams CE, Nelson M. The varied computed tomographic appearances of acute spinal epidural haematoma. *Clin Radiol* 1987; **38**: 363–365.

Zuccarello M, Scanarini M, D'Avella D, Andrioli GC, Gerosa M. Spontaneous spinal extradural hematoma during anticoagulant therapy. *Surg Neurol* 1980; **14**: 411–413.

6
TUMOURS OF THE SPINE IN CHILDREN

David A Chesler, Joseph Noggle, Gary Nicolin, John-Paul Kilday, and George I Jallo

Introduction

Tumours that affect the spinal canal and spinal cord are rare in children, accounting for 2 to 5% of all malignancies of childhood (Goh et al. 1997, Houten and Cooper 2000, Wilne et al. 2007). The diagnosis of these lesions can be challenging given the vague and insidious nature of symptoms in most patients, which often results in a prolonged symptom interval before diagnosis (Goh et al. 1997, Kothbauer 2007, Wilne et al. 2007). Long-term outcomes for patients can be poor because of the considerable neurological morbidity associated with these lesions and their treatment. A multidisciplinary approach is therefore important for establishing tumour diagnosis and management.

CLASSIFICATION

Tumours of the spine can encompass benign and malignant lesions. They can be classified into three broad categories according to their anatomical location within the spinal canal: intradural intramedullary, intradural extramedullary, or extradural (Table 6.1). Tumours may be primary (i.e. arising within the structures of the spinal cord or spinal canal), be a consequence of local invasion from a tumour extrinsic to the spinal canal, or be metastatic from a neoplasm originating within or outside the central nervous system (CNS).

CLINICAL PRESENTATION

The diagnosis of spinal cord tumours can be a complex and challenging endeavour for the clinician. Tumours may remain asymptomatic for prolonged periods or present with insidious, largely non-specific complaints that can delay or complicate the diagnosis. Nevertheless, early diagnosis is imperative for the preservation of neurological function and facilitating improved outcomes from surgical intervention when indicated.

Pain is most often the first symptom, the characteristics of which are frequently non-specific in both quality and distribution. Indeed, children may complain of abdominal pain rather than back pain. Dysaesthesia or sensory loss may also be present but are a rarely presenting symptom and are not easy to identify on examination in young children. In addition to pain or numbness, patients may present with motor deficits. These may be radicular in nature or alternatively present as progressive clumsiness, weakness, gait

TABLE 6.1
Classification of spinal tumours in children*

(a) Intradural tumours
    a. Intramedullary
        i.   Astrocytoma
            1. Pilocytic astrocytoma
            2. Ganglioglioma
            3. High-grade glioma
        ii.   Ependymoma
        iii. Primitive neuroectodermal tumour (PNET)
        iv. Lipoma
        v.   Haemangioblastoma
    b. Extramedullary
        i.   Neurofibroma
        ii.   Schwannoma
        iii. Meningioma
        iv. Malignant peripheral nerve sheath tumour
        v.   Myxopapillary ependymoma
        vi. Dermoid/epidermoid
        vii. Peripheral PNET (Ewing spectrum tumours)
        viii. Atypical teratoid/rhabdoid tumour
        ix. Lipoma
(b) Extradural tumours
    a. Epidural space
        i.   Leukaemia
        ii.   Lymphoma
        iii. Peripheral PNET
        iv. Germ cell tumours
        v.   Lipoma
    b. Bone/cartilage
        i.   Osteosarcoma
        ii.   Osteoid osteoma
        iii. Osteoblastoma
        iv. Langerhans cell histiocytosis
        v.   Aneurysmal bone cyst
        vi. Osteochondroma
        vii. Haemangioma
        viii. Sacrococcygeal teratoma
        ix. Lymphoma
        x.   Leukaemia
    c. Paravertebral tissue
        i.   Neuroblastoma
        ii.   Ganglioneuroma
        iii. Peripheral PNET

* Adapted from Wilne and Walker 2010.

disturbance, or frequency of falls. By contrast, children can present with paraplegia of rapid onset or, rarely, this may be present at birth.

Despite the clinical variability associated with paediatric spinal tumours, the anatomical compartment in which the tumours are located (intradural intramedullary, extramedullary, or extradural), the level and location of spinal cord involvement (cervical, thoracic, or lumbar as well as dorsal versus ventral), and the benign or malignant properties of a given process (insidious versus acute symptom onset) may guide the astute clinician to localize and differentiate particular lesions.

Intramedullary spinal cord tumours are often associated with a protracted clinical course, delaying diagnosis often until the disease is fairly advanced. Nevertheless, acute neurological deterioration can be encountered, typically with spontaneous intratumoural haemorrhage causing additional mass effect upon the surrounding cord, a feature seen occasionally with ependymomas. Intramedullary lesions most often arise in the central region of the spinal cord involving the spinothalamic tracts, sparing the dorsal columns early in the disease process. Accordingly, patients often initially present with poorly localized, dysaesthetic pain involving diffuse areas of the body. An exception to this can be seen in intramedullary haemangioblastomas because of their propensity to arise in a dorsal location, resulting in early dorsal column dysfunction and characteristic sensory ataxia due to impaired proprioception. Intramedullary tumour progression will eventually result in corticospinal involvement, causing spastic weakness which extends distally, reflecting the somatotopic organization of the spinal cord. Perhaps confusing the picture, early involvement of the anterior horns by centrally located tumours may also damage lower motor neurons causing muscle atrophy, fasciculations, and blunting of deep tendon reflexes. In addition to sensory and motor deficits, intramedullary tumours may present with autonomic dysfunction, which is highly dependent on the spinal level of involvement (e.g. isolated bowel and or bladder dysfunction associated with tumours of the conus medullaris). Scoliosis, kyphosis, or kyphoscoliosis may also be a presenting complaint, with up to a third of children and young adults diagnosed with any type of intramedullary cord tumour being initially found to have an abnormal curvature; this does not, however, appear to be the case with adults (Jallo 2001, Roonprapunt et al. 2001, Jallo et al. 2003).

The disease course seen with tumours of the intradural extramedullary and extradural spinal compartments is also often prolonged. Pain is again a central feature, frequently in conjunction with neurological deficits. However, in contrast to intramedullary tumours, the distribution of these findings tends to be ipsilateral, involving segmental motor or sensory nerve distributions consistent with an eccentric tumour location. Radicular pain is a common initial manifestation of these tumours compared with intramedullary counterparts. Weakness also tends to be unilateral, with patterns of unilateral radicular weakness, hemiparesis, or monoparesis being seen, depending on tumour size and locality.

A considered clinical examination can provide insight into the localization of specific spinal tumours in children. For lesions of the high cervical cord, specifically those involving the cervicomedullary junction, presenting symptoms may include vomiting, choking, dysphagia, recurrent pneumonias secondary to aspiration, dysarthria and or dysphonia, obstructive sleep apnoea, or failure to thrive (Robertson et al. 1994). Foramen magnum tumours can appear clinically similar to those of the high cervical cord but can also present with pain of the neck or occiput on movement, or features of hydrocephalus including headaches, nausea, vomiting, papilloedema, ataxia, and nystagmus (Symonds 1937). A classic feature of lesions compressing the foramen magnum is that of weakness of the ipsilateral arm, followed by the ipsilateral leg then contralateral extremities. Autonomic findings of tumours of the foramen magnum and high cervical cord include Horner syndrome (characterized by ptosis, miosis, and anhidrosis), and Ondine curse, a syndrome of central apnoeic hypoventilation when asleep, has also been described (Sanford and Smith 1986).

Tumours occurring distally in the sub-axial cervical spine can present with pain, sensory loss, motor weakness, and/or reflex abnormalities depending on both tumour location and degree of compression of the surrounding neural elements. Intramedullary tumours in this region can, moreover, result in bi-brachial involvement with sparing of the lower extremities (Shenkin 1944). Horner syndrome may again be observed, particularly with extradural tumours of the lower cervical and higher thoracic spine.

As with other levels, tumours of the thoracic spine are most often associated with pain, which can either be radicular or localize as back pain. Motor symptoms in this region typically spare the upper extremities and often involve the bilateral lower extremities, although a monoparesis can be seen with eccentrically located extramedullary tumours. Mass effect from spinal tumours of the thoracic spine may also present with sign or symptoms of myelopathy, as well as conus medullaris or cauda equina syndrome, particularly at more caudal levels.

Caudal tumours of the lumbosacral spine are associated with symptomatology that can be distinct from that of higher, cephalad levels. Anatomically in the normal term infant, the conus has already ascended to the level of T11/12 to L1/2, implying that most lumbosacral tumours involve primarily individual nerve roots or the cauda equina. Symptoms can include low back pain, radicular pain or weakness, stiffness of gait, saddle anaesthesia, or sphincter disturbances with associated bowel or bladder dysfunction. Hyperreflexia and hypertonic weakness are not classic signs.

Associated features from the patient's clinical evaluation may yield clues suggestive of an underlying diagnosis, and these should be carefully looked for during initial assessment. Findings in the history of weight loss, night sweats, and bone marrow suppression (lethargy, bruising, haemorrhaging, recurrent infections) may indicate the presence of a haematological malignancy or lymphomatous process. Likewise, a comprehensive family history may reveal inherited disorders associated with CNS neoplasms. These include the Li Fraumeni syndrome (a familial cancer predisposition disorder caused by a germline mutation of the *p53* tumour suppression gene), Turcot syndrome (caused by inherited *APC* gene mutations and characterized by the formation of adenomatous polyps, colorectal cancers in addition to CNS lesions), and the neurocutaneous syndromes including von Hippel–Lindau syndrome (caused by *VHL* gene mutations and associated with spinal haemangioblastomas, retinal detachment, café au lait patches, renal clear cell carcinomas, and phaeocromocytomas), tuberous sclerosis complex, and neurofibromatosis types 1 (NF1) and 2 (NF2).

The remaining examination may therefore be guided by an index of clinical suspicion. For instance, pallor, purpura, petechiae, lymphadenopathy, and hepatosplenomegaly may be sought if considering a leukaemia or lymphoma. Similarly, examination of the skin is appropriate to look for manifestations of NF1 (café au lait patches, axillary freckling, and neurofibroma) or tuberous sclerosis complex (adenoma sebaceum, ash leaf macules, shagreen patches, café au lait patches, and subungual fibromas). Ophthalmic sequelae of

Von Hippel–Lindau syndrome (retinal detachment) or the other neurocutaneous syndromes (Lisch nodules and optic glioma in NF1, juvenile subcapsular cataracts in NF2, and retinal phakomas in tuberous sclerosis complex) may also be apparent.

DIAGNOSTIC INVESTIGATIONS

The investigation of choice when a tumour of the spinal canal or cord is suspected is magnetic resonance imaging (MRI). When such an abnormality is noted on a spinal MRI, imaging should be extended to include the entire neuraxis. MRI should be performed with the administration of intravenous contrast-enhancing agents such as gadolinium with imaging series obtained in multiple anatomic planes. Though tumours cannot be definitively diagnosed by MRI alone, characteristic features may be identified including solid components, associated cysts, surrounding oedema, and the presence or absence of syrinxes.

Radiograph imaging of the spine, myelography, and computed tomography (CT) have limited use in investigating these tumours, although CT may delineate associated bone pathology more accurately.

Additional investigations may be performed to confirm any associated underlying aetiology. For instance, genetic blood analysis and pertinent imaging investigations for hereditary cancer predisposition syndromes above can be performed if clinically suspected. Likewise, very young children with paravertebral tumours extending into the extradural space (so-called dumb-bell tumours) in all likelihood have neuroblastomas and the diagnosis can be supported by thoracic or abdominal imaging, metaiodobenzylguanidine (MIBG) scanning and analysis of the urine for elevated levels of catecholamines. Abnormalities of a full blood count, blood film, or bone marrow aspirate may suggest a diagnosis of acute leukaemia, whereas lesions identified on imaging of other sites, for example the spleen, liver, lymphadenopathy, or multiple bony abnormalities, may point to a diagnosis of lymphoma. In these diseases, it may be possible to make a diagnosis, institute treatment, avoid surgery, and reduce potential long-term morbidity.

It is beyond the scope of this chapter to provide an exhaustive description of all the tumour types that involve the paediatric spine and their treatment. However, the more common and important entities will be described.

Intradural intramedullary tumours

Dr Anton von Eiselsberg was the first surgeon successfully to resect an intramedullary spinal cord tumour in Vienna, Austria, in 1907 (Von Eiselberg 1913). The first published report of this type of surgery emerged later in 1911, when Dr Charles Elsberg described a two-stage procedure in New York by which an initial midline myelotomy was followed a week later by the resection of a tumour that had partly extruded itself from the cord (Elsberg 1911). By 1912, the first successful resection of an intramedullary spinal cord haemangioblastoma had been reported (Schultze 1912). Multiple technical difficulties and complications in the aggressive surgical treatment of these tumours, such as CSF leaks, postoperative neurological deficits, infections, and death, dampened surgeons' enthusiasm for attempting the resection of intramedullary spinal cord tumours. The introduction and advancement of surgical intervention in the mid-20th century, including Yaşargil et al. reporting on the first series of intramedullary haemangioblastomas resected using microsurgical techniques, renewed interested in the treatment of these lesions among neurosurgeons (Yasargil et al. 1976, Jallo et al. 2001, Lonser and Oldfield 2005, Mandigo et al. 2009, Sciubba et al. 2009).

Using today's best practice modalities, the goal of treatment in intramedullary spinal cord tumours is, where possible, gross total resection while making every effort to preserve neurological function. As will be discussed in this chapter, the treatment of ependymomas and haemangioblastomas can frequently adhere to this goal, while the invasive nature of gliomas often precludes gross total resection because of the risk of permanent neurological deficit.

ASTROCYTOMAS

Astrocytomas are the most common intramedullary spinal cord tumours in children, accounting for approximately 55 to 60% of reported lesions (Reimer and Onofrio 1985, Epstein and Epstein 1981, Epstein et al. 1992, Epstein et al. 1993). In adults, the reported frequency can vary but is second only to ependymoma (Minehan et al. 1995, Houten and Cooper 2000). Predominantly low-grade lesions, they are primarily seen in the cervical spine (Fig. 6.1a–c) followed by the thoracic spine in frequency of occurrence. Holocord (whole cord length) tumours have also been reported (Fig. 6.1d, e) (Epstein and Epstein 1981, Houten and Cooper 2000). Categorized using the World Health Organization (WHO) histopathological classification scheme (Louis 2007), paediatric spinal cord astrocytomas are for the most part of the pilocytic subtype where, in comparison, low-grade lesions in adults are typically fibrillary (McCormick and Stein 1990, Allen et al. 1998, Houten and Cooper 2000).

Pilocytic spinal astrocytomas are relatively slow growing, frequently cystic, benign tumours. The peak incidence of these tumours is in the first two decades of life with a roughly equal sex distribution. Characterized as WHO grade I gliomas (Louis 2007), these are soft, grey, fleshy tumours on macroscopic inspection which may have sparse calcification or haemosiderin deposits. Histologically, these tumours appear biphasic with a mixture of compacted bipolar cells and associated Rosenthal fibres, interspersed alongside multi-polar cells with microcysts and eosinophilic granular bodies (Louis 2007). Rare mitoses may be seen along with occasional pleomorphic nuclei, glomeruloid vascular proliferation, and infarct-like necrosis; none of these are considered to be indications of malignancy in this context (Louis 2007). On MRI, pilocytic astrocytomas appear well circumscribed and enhance after intravenous contrast administration (Osborn 1994). As a rule, these lesions do not undergo malignant transformation to glioblastoma although sparse reports in the literature refer to the rare subsequent development of an anaplastic or atypical phenotype, often after radiation therapy (Tomlinson et al. 1994, Roessler et al. 2002).

When gross total resection can be effected, surgery can be curative. However, despite their seemingly circumscribed appearance, they do have the ability to invade surrounding tissues, thereby precluding total resection. Consequently, overall survival rates for spinal low-grade gliomas in children are excellent, yet progression-free survival data are less encouraging, cited as low as 44% at 5 years (Scheinemann et al. 2009). Long-term ortho-paedic and neurological morbidities are a frequent association of the tumours and their

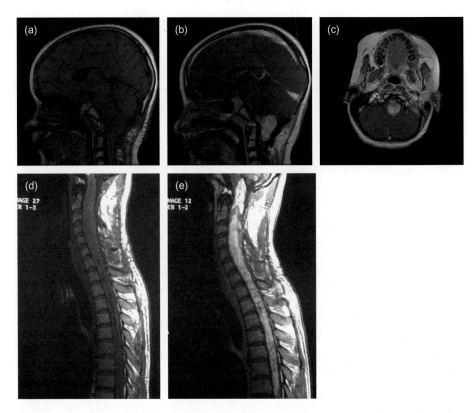

Fig. 6.1. MRI scans of spinal cord astrocytoma. (a) T_1-weighted sagittal image of the cervicomedullary junction demonstrating a hypodense eccentrically expansile mass. (b) T_1-weighted sagittal post-contrast image showing a heterogeneously enhancing tumour. (c) T_1-weighted axial post-contrast image demonstrating an eccentrically located, enhancing mass of the cervicomedullary junction. (d) T_1-weighted sagittal image from a patient with a holocord astrocytoma. (e) T_1-weighted sagittal post-contrast image of the same patient as in (d).

treatment, suggesting that future interventions should focus on improving functional outcome as opposed to survival alone (Scheinemann et al. 2009).

Diffuse or fibrillary astrocytomas (WHO grade II) (Louis 2007) are more frequent in the adult population than pilocytic astrocytomas, with peak incidences seen in the third to fourth decades of life and a slight predominance of affected males. They are typically eccentrically located and cause asymmetric expansion of the spinal cord (Houten and Cooper 2000). Compared with the pilocytic gliomas, grade II gliomas have a more invasive appearance, and are poorly enhancing on MRI (Osborn 1994). Indeed, enhancement is often considered an ominous feature, suggesting progression to a more aggressive phenotype. Microscopically, these tumours comprise fibrillary neoplastic astrocytes with marked nuclear atypia. The cytoplasm is usually scant giving the appearance of floating nuclei with infrequent mitoses. Consistent with the MRI appearance of invasiveness, fibrillary astrocytomas are known to invade the neural parenchyma causing distortion but not destruction of surrounding structures (Louis 2007). Genetically, grade II astrocytomas are characterized by p53 mutations (>60% of cases) as well as numerous chromosomal aberrations, although this information is primarily taken from studies of intracranial tumours (Reifenberger et al. 1996, Watanabe et al. 1997, Hirose et al. 2003, Okamoto et al. 2004, Louis 2007). Malignant degeneration into anaplastic astrocytomas or glioblastoma multiforme is a frequent consequence of these tumours, taking place over several years (Ohgaki et al. 2004, Okamoto et al. 2004, Ohgaki and Kleihues 2007).

Anaplastic astrocytomas (WHO grade III) and glioblastoma (WHO grade IV) (Louis 2007) represent the malignant spectrum of gliomas, comprising 10 to 20% of all spinal cord neoplasms (Allen et al. 1998, McCormick and Stein 1990, Houten and Cooper 2000). In contrast to lower-grade tumours, time to diagnosis is much shorter as symptomatic progression is typically accelerated because of the increased aggressiveness of these tumours. Histologically, anaplastic astrocytomas show marked nuclear atypia and mitoses but lack microvascular proliferation or necrosis. Glioblastomas, in comparison, demonstrate the features of anaplastic astrocytomas with the addition of pseudopallisading necrosis (Louis 2007). Macroscopically, anaplastic astrocytomas appear similar to grade II lesions, although often more differentiated from surrounding tissues. Glioblastomas are yellow to grey in appearance, reflecting tumour bulk as well as areas of necrosis (Louis 2007). On MRI both anaplastic astrocytoma and glioblastomas strongly enhance, demonstrate invasiveness into surrounding tissues, and show marked surrounding oedema (Osborn 1994). Moreover, glioblastomas demonstrate central necrosis represented by areas of hypodensity on T_1-weighted imaging (Osborn 1994). Surgical management of these tumours is primarily limited to tissue diagnosis and central debulking with attention to the avoidance of neurological insult. As with their intracranial counterparts, survival is measured in months both for anaplastic astrocytoma and glioblastomas, with surgery having limited effect on their clinical course (Garces-Ambrossi et al. 2009, Raco et al. 2010).

In addition to the astrocyte lineage-derived neoplasms discussed above, tumours of mixed glioneuronal origin have also been described. Gangliogliomas are well differentiated, slowly growing tumours of such mixed glial-neuronal origin. Comprising mature ganglion cells in combination with neuroplastic glial cells, these tumours are considered grade I neoplasms by WHO criteria (Louis 2007). Primarily tumours of paediatric and young adult populations, they have a peak incidence in the second and third decades of life (Louis 2007). Radiographically, gangliogliomas are well circumscribed T_1-dark, T_2-bright masses with variable enhancement intensity and patterns (Osborn 1994). As with astrocytomas, these tumours do not necessarily have clean planes differentiating between tumour and spinal cord.

EPENDYMOMAS

Thought to arise from the ependymal lining of the ventricles, ependymomas are known to involve both the brain and spinal cord. These tumours represent the most common primary intramedullary spinal cord tumours in adults, although they are less frequently observed in the paediatric population (Helseth et al. 1989, Schwartz and McCormick 2000). Most of these tumours are sporadic, but an increased incidence is seen in children with

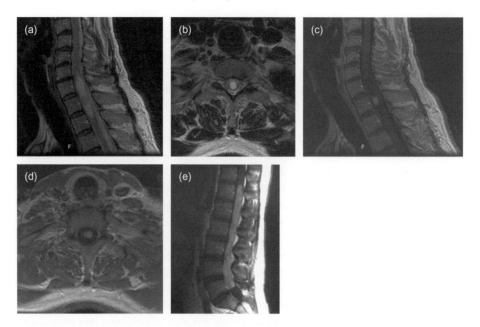

Fig. 6.2. Representative MRI of spinal ependymomas. (a) T_2-weighted sagittal image demonstrating a nodular tumour at the level of C7 with a surrounding syrinx-like cavity. (b) T_2-weighted axial imaging showing central fluid collection isodense to cerebrospinal fluid (CSF) consistent with tumour-associated syrinx. (c) T_1-weighted sagittal post-contrast image showing brightly enhancing nodular mass surrounded by a syrinx-like cavity. (d) T_1-weighted axial post-contrast image showing centrally located, enhancing tumour. (e) T_1-weighted sagittal post-contrast image on the lumbar spine demonstrating a myxopapillary ependymoma involving the cauda equina.

neurofibromatosis type 2 (NF2) (Chi et al. 2006). Although occurring at any site along the ventricular system and spinal canal, most intramedullary spinal ependymomas occur in the cervical region, particularly those that are NF2 related (Nakasu et al. 1992, Chi et al. 2006). Ependymomas are usually slow-growing tumours which, in the spinal cord, classically adopt a central location causing symmetric expansion of the cord (unlike the grade II astrocytomas discussed previously) (Fig. 6.2). Based on the WHO classification scheme, these tumours can be divided into four subtypes: subependymoma (grade I), myxopapillary ependymoma (grade I), classic ependymoma (grade II), and anaplastic ependymoma (grade III) (Louis 2007).

Subependymomas are slowly growing benign lesions most often associated with the fourth ventricle. When found in the spinal cord, they are frequently in the cervical cord. On MRI they are poorly to non-enhancing lesions which are well demarcated with occasional haemorrhage. They are variable in their appearance on T_1- and T_2-weighted sequences and, in contrast to the classic ependymoma, can be eccentric in their intramedullary location (Osborn 1994, Louis 2007). Visually, they appear to be greyish, nodular tumours, usually 1 to 2cm in diameter with well-demarcated surgical tumour borders. On histopathology, subependymomas are characterized by clusters of nuclei in a dense fibrillary matrix with occasional pseudorosettes; mitoses are rare to absent, and sporadic calcifications or haemorrhage can be seen (Louis 2007). Total resection of subependymomas is considered curative with occasional recurrences reported, often because of incomplete resection.

Myxopapillary ependymoma, also a WHO grade I lesion, occurs almost exclusively in the distal spinal cord involving the conus medullaris and the nerve roots of the cauda equina. With a slight male predilection, these tumours are seen across a wide age-range, with patients being reported from 6 to 82 years (Cervoni et al. 1997, Yoshii et al. 1999). On MRI these tumours are sharply demarcated, brightly enhancing lesions in which cystic components or haemorrhage may be observed (Fig. 6.2e). Macroscopically these tumours are sausage-like, grey- to tan-coloured lesions. Histologically they are characterized by glial fibrillary acidic protein (GFAP)-expressing, cuboidal to elongated tumour cells radially arranged around stromal or vascular cores. A myxoid matrix accumulating between cells and blood vessels of the tumour can be appreciated with Alcian-blue staining; mitotic indices, as evidenced by Ki67 or MIB1, are low to absent (Louis 2007). The genetics of myxopapillary ependymomas remain undefined. The prognosis for this tumour group is excellent with gross total resection, although late recurrences, both local and distant, after subtotal resections have been described both in adult and paediatric patient populations (Sonneland et al. 1985, Epstein et al. 1993, Akyurek et al. 2006).

Classic ependymomas (WHO grade II) are the most common neuroepithelial neoplasm of the spinal cord in adults, comprising 50 to 60% of spinal gliomas (Louis 2007). Similar to subependymomas, these tumours are most often found in the cervical cord. Red or greyish-purple in appearance, they are soft, and friable with a clearly definable surgical plane between tumour and surrounding tissues, typically not invading the normal spinal cord (Goh et al. 1997, Parsa et al. 2004, 2005). Microscopically, these tumours are characterized by glial fibrillary acidic protein immunoreactivity and both by true and pseudorosette formation. Non-pallisading necrosis may occasionally be seen. Mitotic rates are low and typically lower than that seen with intracranial tumours (Louis 2007). Several pathological variants of the classic grade II ependymoma have now been identified, including papillary, clear cell, and tanycytic ependymomas. On diagnosis, papillary and tanycytic tumours can be mistaken for oligodendrogliomas and pilocytic astrocytomas respectively (Louis 2007). Radiologically, grade II ependymomas are variable in the degree of contrast enhancement seen on MRI although they are well demarcated lesions; cystic components, intratumoural haemorrhage, and associated syrinxes may also be seen, although peritumoural oedema is not common (Fig. 6.2a–d) (Osborn 1994). Genetically, classic spinal ependymomas have been found to be associated with *NF2* gene mutations as well as increased expression of *HOX*-family members (Rodriguez and Berthrong 1966, Martuza and Eldridge 1988, Korshunov et al. 2003). As with the other ependymal variants described above, gross total resection of classic ependymomas of the spinal cord can be curative although late recurrences have been described.

Although most ependymoma variants are benign tumours with slowly progressive clinical courses, a malignant variant, the anaplastic ependymoma (grade III), has been described and is known to occur both in the brain and spinal cord (Louis 2007). In contrast to grade II ependymomas, anaplastic lesions are much more aggressive with increased mitotic mitoses, microvascular proliferation, and pseudopallisading necrosis seen on histopathology (Louis 2007). On MRI, these tumours appear similar to their classic counterparts, with the exception of more consistent contrast enhancement (Osborn 1994). The origin of grade III ependymomas is unclear although it has been suggested that they are likely to be due to malignant transformation of previously undiagnosed grade II lesions (Reni et al. 2007).

The reported survival rates for patients with spinal cord ependymomas is variable between studies, often limited by small cohort numbers. Long-term progression-free survival rates range between 46% and over 90% (Sonneland et al. 1985, Whitaker et al. 1991, Gomez et al. 2005), with equally broad overall survival rates (Sonneland et al. 1985, Whitaker et al. 1991, Waldron et al. 1993, Stuben et al. 1997, McLaughlin et al. 1998, Isaacson 2000, Gomez et al. 2005). Purported independent prognostic factors include histological grade (Whitaker et al. 1991, Waldron et al. 1993) and degree of surgical resection (Whitaker et al. 1991, Gomez et al. 2005), yet neither have been established consistently.

HAEMANGIOBLASTOMAS

Haemangioblastomas are highly vascular lesions of the CNS. Seen throughout the neuraxis, these lesions are found predominantly in the cerebellum, brainstem, and spinal cord. Although commonly associated with von Hippel–Landau disease, an autosomal-dominant disease of variable penetrance involving the *VHL* tumour suppressor gene located on chromosome 3p25, most spinal cord haemangioblastomas are in fact sporadic, isolated lesions (accounting for 70–80% of cases) (Latif et al. 1993, Van Velthoven et al. 2003, Catapano et al. 2005, Lonser and Oldfield 2006, Mandigo et al. 2009). Despite being histologically benign lesions, haemangioblastomas can cause significant neurological deficit, particularly when located in the spinal cord where they comprise between 1.5 and 5% of all intramedullary spinal cord tumours.

Haemangioblastomas are well-circumscribed masses, easily discerned from surrounding tissues. In both sporadic and von Hippel–Landau-associated disease, these tumours have an extensive vascular network interspersed with pockets of stromal cells often described as 'clear cell' in appearance. Capillaries comprising the vascular network of these tumours are benign in appearance with normal endothelial cells and associated pericytes. The stromal component of haemangioblastomas have large pleomorphic, and often hyperchromic, nuclei surrounded by numerous lipid-filled vacuoles. Mitotic rates are usually low in these tumours, reinforcing their benign nature (Kumar 2009).

On MRI, haemangioblastomas are typically well-circumscribed, appearing hypo- to isointense on T_1-weighted sequences. The appearance of these lesions on T_2-weighted sequences is more variable, tending towards an increased intensity. On post-contrast T_1-weighted imaging, these tumours are brightly enhancing most frequently in a homogenous pattern; heterogeneity in enhancement frequently correlates with vascular flow-voids. Haemangioblastomas are often dorsally located, predominantly intramedullary, and almost invariably found to have associated syringomyelia and/or significant oedema (Fig. 6.3) (Chu et al. 2001). Spinal angiography can be a valuable adjuvant imaging modality, particularly in surgical planning, to assist in delineating patterns of arterial and venous supply to tumours, particularly in the case of larger lesions.

130

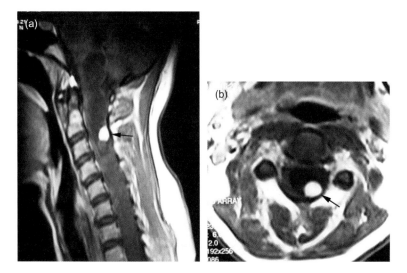

Fig. 6.3. MRI of a patient with a cervical intramedullary haemangioblastoma. (a) T_1-weighted sagittal post-contrast image with gadolinium demonstrates a small, dorsally situated, enhancing tumour abutting the pial surface with an associated syrinx (arrow). (b) Axial T_1-weighted post-contrast image demonstrating the same tumour (arrow) as in (a).

All patients with a tissue diagnosis of haemangioblastoma should undergo work-up for von Hippel–Landau disease, which includes a detailed family history, ophthalmologic examination, and complete imaging of the neuraxis and abdomen with molecular screening for identification of the *VHL* mutation on chromosome 3 (Catapano et al. 2005).

Surgery for patients diagnosed with a sporadic lesion needs no additional follow-up apart from that considered standard postoperative care; total resection is curative. With patients harbouring a mutation in the *VHL* gene, however, annual surveillance screening is indicated. In such cases, surgical resection is again curative for a given lesion, but these patients have a bleaker prognosis for declining functional status as they are predisposed to multiple lesions arising throughout the neuraxis (Wind et al. 2011).

LIPOMAS

Spinal cord lipomas are exceedingly rare, benign lesions that comprise fewer than 1% of intraspinal tumours and can be found in intramedullary, extramedullary, and extradural compartments of the spinal cord (Caram et al. 1957, Lee et al. 1995). Intramedullary lipomas are a subset of the intradural entities often reported at the conus medullaris and cauda equina. As with most other intramedullary lesions, these tumours present with slow, indolent courses, with diagnosis often coming months to years after symptom onset. Interestingly, patients with these tumours frequently have an acceleration of symptoms in the weeks to months leading up to diagnosis (Lee et al. 1995). On MRI, lipomas are T_1-bright, T_2-dark and non-enhancing, consistent with fat (Fig. 6.4). Pathologically, these tumours comprise mostly mature adipocytes admixed with connective tissues, often grossly with a

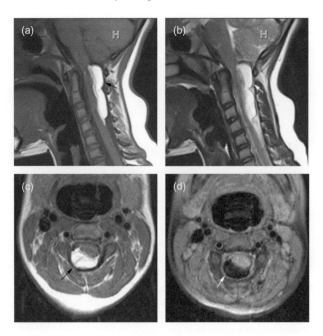

Fig. 6.4. MRI of a cervical lipoma. (a) T_1-weighted sagittal image of a cervical lipoma originating from the dorsal aspect of the spinal cord. (b) T_2-weighted sagittal image from the same patient as in (a). (c) T_1-weighted axial image of the cervical spine demonstrating a exophytic lipoma extending dorsally from the spinal cord (arrow). (d) T_1-weighted fat saturated imaging showing at approximately the same level as in (c) demonstrating suppression of the lesion's hyperintensity consistent with a lipoma (arrow).

lobulated appearance (Kumar 2009). Though appearing well circumscribed, these tumours can be densely adherent to surrounding neural tissues, placing the spinal cord at high risk of injury during resection; for this reason, limiting surgery to central debulking of the tumour is recommended.

Intradural extramedullary tumours

TUMOURS ASSOCIATED WITH NEUROFIBROMATOSIS

NF1 and NF2 are inherited autosomal dominant neurocutaneous syndromes which demonstrate high penetrance but variable phenotypic expression. NF1 is far more common than NF2, accounting for approximately 90% of all neurofibromatosis cases.

NF1 occurs in 1:3500 births and arises from a mutation of the gene *neurofibromin 1* (*NF1*), a tumour suppressor gene on chromosome 17q12 which encodes a negative regulator protein member of the Ras pathway. Mutational absence of the *NF1* gene results in uncontrolled cellular proliferation and tumour formation (Feldkamp et al. 1999). Clinically, the disorder produces an overgrowth syndrome associated with a range of dermatological, skeletal, and ophthalmological stigmata, comprising café au lait patches, freckling of the axillae or groin, bone dysplasia, neurofibromas, and Lisch nodules of the iris. In the CNS, the syndrome can be associated with hydrocephalus, areas of high signal on T_2 MRI (foci of abnormal signal intensity), and an increased incidence of several neoplasms. Such tumours include optic pathway tumours and other low-grade gliomas, neurofibromas, schwannomas, meningiomas, myxopapillary ependymomas, and malignant peripheral nerve sheath tumours. Excluding malignant peripheral nerve sheath tumours, which have a high mortality and can grow rapidly, most of these lesions are very slow growing and are often observed on serial imaging, if they arise in the spine, well before specific treatment is required. The optimal treatment in most cases is complete resection, although this is not always possible when they occur in the spine. Individual cases are best discussed by a multidisciplinary team of clinicians expert in the management of these often complicated lesions.

NF2 has a lower frequency than NF1, occurring in 1:25,000 births (Plotkin et al. 2009). It is seen rarely in the paediatric population, being diagnosed most commonly in early adulthood. NF2 results from a mutation of the tumour suppressor gene *Merlin*, found on chromosome 22q12, which encodes the schwannomin protein product. The development of bilateral vestibulocochlear schwannomas is the hallmark of the condition, causing tinnitus, vertigo, and progressive hearing loss if untreated. As with NF1, the syndrome is characterized by ocular and skin manifestations (subcapsular cataracts, café au lait patches), and an increased frequency of CNS lesions, such as meningiomas, spinal ependymomas and nerve sheath tumours.

Bevacizumab, an anti-angiogenic monoclonal antibody inhibitor of vascular endothelial growth factor, has shown recent efficacy against the pathognomonic vestibulocochlear schwannomas of patients with NF2 in small studies, causing both a reduction in tumour volume and hearing improvement in a substantial proportion of patients (Plotkin et al. 2009, Mautner et al. 2010). The agent appears well tolerated, although reported side effects included poor wound healing, proteinuria, and hypertension (Plotkin et al. 2009, Mautner et al. 2010). Although encouraging, larger trials will be required to establish the effect profile for bevacizumab (duration of efficacy, long-term adverse events, etc.) and to verify whether this agent may have extended applicability to spinal lesions in this context.

NERVE SHEATH TUMOURS (NEUROFIBROMAS AND SCHWANNOMAS)
Nerve sheath tumours typically arise from the dorsal sensory roots of the spine (Halliday et al. 1991). Broadly these tumours can be divided into two categories: schwannomas and neurofibromas. On MRI, both tumour types appear as homogenously enhancing extramedullary lesions. Extension through the neuroforamina can occasionally be seen, conferring a dumb-bell appearance on imaging. Pathologically, neurofibromas are composed of densely cellular portions (Antoni A) with adjacent hypocellular regions (Antoni B). Verocay bodies (pallisading nuclei) and positive immunostaining for S100 are also a frequent feature. In contrast, schwannomas contain a benign stroma composed of axons, Schwann cells, fibroblasts, and perineural cells (Kumar 2009). Both tumour types are benign, although malignant transformation has been described in rare cases (Foley et al. 1980). Clinically, pain or numbness in a radicular distribution is the most frequent complaint associated with these tumours. More pronounced sequelae may be found with larger lesions, particularly in the cervical or thoracic region, where a Brown-Séquard picture can be observed. Treatment for symptomatic lesions is gross total resection, which is frequently achievable. In the case of

schwannomas, a plane can often be established between the nerve and tumour, facilitating nerve-sparing resection. Neurofibromas tend to involve the associated nerve intimately, obligating the surgeon to sacrifice the sensory root in most cases. As mentioned above, some nerve sheath tumours may extend into the extradural space through the neural foramen, requiring a separate extraspinal resection to address the remaining tumour bulk (Jallo 2003, Safavi-Abbasi et al. 2008). Radiation has been reserved for plexiform lesions not amenable to surgical resection. However, concern does exist in the literature for malignant transformation after radiotherapy (Foley et al. 1980) and the development of vasculopathy post-irradiation of patients with NF1, as discussed later (Desai et al. 2006).

MENINGIOMAS

Meningiomas represent only 5% of spinal cord tumours in the paediatric population (Yamamoto 1999, Fortuna et al. 1981). Occurring most frequently in the thoracic spine, the average age at presentation is between 12 and 15 years. As stated above, an increased incidence is found in patients with neurofibromatosis, particularly those with NF2. Radiographically, meningiomas are variable in appearance on T_1- and T_2-weighted sequences, but homogenously enhance on post-contrast imaging. These benign lesions represent a histologically diverse tumour group, with more than 25 different subtypes being recognized (Louis 2007). Nevertheless, most meningiomas stain positively for expression of vimentin and epithelial membrane antigen by immunohistochemistry (Louis 2007, Kumar 2009). Grossly, these tumours are globular, encapsulated tumours attached to the dura, ventral to the dentate ligament in most instances, causing compression of the adjacent spinal cord and nerve roots without invasion. Surgically, a clear plane is easily developed from the pia mater, making resection curative; however, care must be taken to minimize manipulation of the spinal cord given the degree of compression associated with these tumours.

Extradural tumours

BENIGN VERTEBRAL COLUMN TUMOURS

Osteoid osteoma and osteoblastomas are benign bony lesions, which primarily affect the long bones and spine. Most frequently seen in the second decade of life, osteoid osteoma is more common than osteoblastoma. Osteoid osteoma is traditionally associated with night pain particularly sensitive to treatment with salicylates. In contrast, osteoblastoma is often associated with more constant pain or discomfort (Janin et al. 1981, Pettine and Klassen 1986, Raskas et al. 1992, Gupta 2003, Burn et al. 2009).

Radiographically, osteoid osteoma is described as having a central nidus, less than 2cm in diameter, encompassed by a lucent ring. On visual inspection, the nidus appears as a red nodule, often surrounded by a layer of sclerotic white bone. Microscopically, the nidus comprises irregular trabeculae of variably ossified osteoid with a layer of osteoblasts. Osteoblastomas are visibly larger lesions on imaging (often greater than 2cm in diameter), which appear to have a nidus with surrounding cortical expansion. In some instances osteoblastomas may have more aggressive features, demonstrating cortical destruction and expansion beyond the anatomical limits of the involved bone. Histologically similar to osteoid osteomas, osteoblastoma can have a variable appearance with epithelioid appearing osteoblasts, degenerative atypia, and invasion into adjacent bone (Osborn 1994, Kumar 2009).

Treatment of osteoid osteoma is largely aimed at symptomatic relief using anti-inflammatory medications. In cases of non-remitting pain, surgical excision is the treatment of choice. Instrumented fusion is typically not required unless instability is encountered as a consequence of the surgical approach or the location and size of the lesion. Percutaneous ablation of osteoid osteoma has also been described as an alternative modality to open resection in children failing symptomatic management (Gangi et al. 2007, Donkol et al. 2008). Osteoblastoma is most preferentially treated by surgical excision with clean margins whenever possible as these tumours have a predilection for recurrence, particularly with subtotal resection (up to 15% of cases, compared with 4.5% in osteoid osteoma) (Jackson et al. 1977, Mitchell and Ackerman 1986, Bloem and Kroon 1993, Lucas et al. 1994, Cerase and Priolo 1998). As these tumours preferentially involve the posterior spinal elements, a need for instrumented fusion is more common compared with osteoid osteoma. There is poor evidence for the use of adjuvant chemoradiation in subtotal resections or recurrences in osteoblastoma (Harrop et al. 2009).

Aneurysmal bone cysts are considered non-neoplastic vascular lesions composed of lytic regions with blood products of variable age. Primarily a disease of paediatric patients, more than 80% of lesions are found in persons younger than 20 years. Radiographically, these lesions are cystic with highly variable associated features including cortical sclerosis, fibrosis, or destruction; variably aged blood products as seen on MRI are a distinguishing feature (Kransdorf and Sweet 1995). In contrast to the above-mentioned entities, rapid expansion of aneurysmal bone cysts can occur, resulting in the sudden onset or worsening of neurological deficits and requiring prompt decompression and resection. Curative treatment involves complete surgical resection, which may require instrumented stabilization of the spine depending on the extent of resection. Additionally, extensive haemorrhaging may be encountered in the resection of these tumours, which is generally controllable through packing of the resection cavity; preoperative embolization can be used to minimize blood loss during resection (Hay et al. 1978). The prognosis for aneurysmal bone cysts is excellent, with an overall survival of 90 to 95% (Papagelopoulos et al. 1998, Gibbs et al. 1999). Recurrence has been associated with a younger patient age at diagnosis (Gibbs et al. 1999).

Vertebral haemangiomas are often solitary lesions involving the paediatric spine. Most frequently found as incidental lesions, they are largely asymptomatic and do not usually require clinical intervention or surveillance. In instances where lesions are associated with uncontrolled pain or neurological deficit, excision is indicated. Histologically these lesions appear as clusters of thin-walled vessels, which as a consequence are associated with substantial blood loss intraoperatively. Perioperative embolization is therefore advocated in the treatment of these tumours (Raco et al. 1990, Lonser et al. 1998, Goyal et al. 1999). Radiotherapy has also been described as effective for the treatment and control of recurrence of vertebral haemangiomas although care should be exercised in using radiotherapy in the growing spine, particularly in the setting of a benign lesion (Heyd et al. 2010).

Eosinophilic granuloma of the bone is a benign and localized form of Langerhans cell histiocytosis. Characterized by lytic lesions in early life, vertebral body collapse results in the classic radiological appearance of vertebra plana (Osborn 1994, Floman et al. 1997). Isolated lesions have a predilection for the cervical spine in the paediatric population (MRI and CT demonstrate a lytic lesion with surrounding sclerotic bone); the oedema associated with the central soft tissue core is appreciable although not as substantial as that seen with infectious or malignant processes. The long-term prognosis for Langerhans cell histiocytosis of the spine is excellent (Bertram et al. 2002, Tan et al. 2004, Peng et al. 2009). Therapy is usually indicated for lesions compromising spinal stability or associated with neurological deficit. Institutional treatment regimens have included immobilization, surgery, steroid monotherapy, and chemotherapy, the last for children with soft-tissue extension from the primary spinal lesion (Bertram et al. 2002, Tan et al. 2004, Peng et al. 2009). Historically, low-dose radiotherapy was also used (Nesbit et al. 1969, Womer et al. 1985), although concerns about impaired spinal growth, scatter toxicity, and the initiation of secondary neoplasms have curtailed its use.

Spinal teratomas, most commonly found in the sacrococcygeal spine, are benign tumours simultaneously possessing components of endodermal, ectodermal, and mesodermal origin. They are often diagnosed in utero or in the immediate post-partum period. Treatment of these lesions is radical resection, which can be curative in mature, benign teratomas. More aggressive variants have been described, including immature and malignant teratomas which carry higher risks of metastasis and poorer prognoses (Sharma et al. 1993, Sciubba et al. 2008). Nevertheless, with radical surgery (including coccygectomy) and platinum-based chemotherapy regimens, long-term overall survival rates for malignant lesions are above 80% (Rescorla et al. 1998, Marina et al. 1999, Gobel et al. 2001, Gabra et al. 2006).

MALIGNANT EXTRADURAL TUMOURS
Neuroblastoma
Neuroblastomas are embryonal tumours that predominantly occur in young children below 3 years of age (and can present at birth), although they are also described in adolescents and young adults (Young and Miller 1975). Thought to originate from neural crest cell precursors, these tumours can arise from the adrenal glands (35%), or from the paravertebral sympathetic nervous chain, anywhere from the neck to the pelvis (abdomen 30%, thorax 20%, neck 10%, pelvis 5%). When they arise paravertebrally, neuroblastomas can extend through the intervertebral foramina and into the spinal canal forming so called 'dumb-bell' tumours. When the latter occur, spinal cord compression is a common mode of presentation. Histologically, neuroblastomas are characterized by the appearance of tightly packed small round blue cells in a fibrovascular stroma and dense core neurosecretory granules on electron microscopy (Louis 2007). The diagnosis can be supported by the detection of raised levels of catecholamines in the urine and findings from compatible imaging. These tumours are T_1- and T_2-variable by MRI, and on CT often show an enhancing mass with stippled calcifications (Abramson et al. 1993, Osborn 1994). Alongside imaging to characterize the extent of spinal involvement, nuclear medicine techniques such as MIBG uptake can be useful in determining the systemic tumour burden (or 'stage') at the time of diagnosis. Indeed, the current international staging criteria for neuroblastoma takes into account the

degree of tumour dissemination and the presence of biological and image-defined risk factors (Cohn et al. 2009). A biopsy is not required to make a diagnosis with paravertebral lesions but is usually done to look for a particular adverse biological marker (amplification of the *MYCN* oncogene), which is highly prognostic and used to risk-stratify therapy (Bown et al. 1999, Cohn et al. 2009).

There still remains some controversy about the optimal management of a child who has presented with neurological signs indicative of spinal cord compression where a diagnosis of neuroblastoma has been made. Initially, high-dose steroids can be used to reduce any oedema associated with compression. The current evidence would suggest that if appropriate chemotherapy is then started promptly, the chances of neurological recovery is just as good as formal neurosurgical decompression, thereby avoiding the potential long-term adverse sequelae of laminotomies or laminectomies (Poretti and Grotzer 2012). Age at diagnosis plays a role in survival, with 5-year overall survival rates being reported as approximately 83% for infants, 55% for children aged 1 to 5 years, and 40% for children older than 5 years (Sciubba et al. 2008).

Peripheral primitive neuroectodermal tumours (Ewing spectrum tumours)
Peripheral primitive neuroectodermal tumours (pPNETs) should be distinguished from the central PNETs that arise intrinsically from the CNS (also called medulloblastomas when occurring in the cerebellum). Central PNETs can occur as primary intramedullary tumours but, more commonly, occur in the spine as leptomeningeal-based metastases from a primary cerebellar lesion.

Peripheral PNETS can also be called Ewing spectrum tumours, which may cause less confusion to the unwary. The pPNETs can arise from bone (Ewing sarcoma), classically involving the vertebral body ventral to the neural arch, or from soft tissue adjacent to the bone (Burgert et al. 1990). The most frequent site of occurrence for Ewing sarcoma is the sacrococcygeal region, followed by lumbar and thoracic regions (Saito et al. 2008). Metastatic spinal deposits from another bone or soft tissue primary site are seen more frequently than primary spinal disease (Mukherjee et al. 2011). When arising from the posterior chest wall (a relatively common site), Ewing sarcoma can extend through the intervertebral foramina and into the spinal canal, causing spinal cord compression.

Grossly these tumours are cystic, necrotic, and frequently haemorrhagic. Genetically, t(11:22) transpositions are typical of Ewing sarcoma (Casha 2006). On histological examination these tumours comprise small, round, blue cells divided by abundant collagen and accompanied by regions of osteonecrosis (Kumar 2009). MRI characteristically reveals T_1-dark, T_2-bright lesions with moderate, heterogenous enhancement. Lytic destructive process of the vertebral bodies sparing the disc space can be appreciated with conventional radiograph or CT modalities (Osborn 1994).

In addition to the clinical presentation common to tumours involving the spinal column, systemic manifestations including fever and weight loss, in combination with non-specific laboratory markers of inflammation such as leukocytosis and elevation of C-reactive protein or erythrocyte sedimentation rate, can be seen. Unlike neuroblastomas, a diagnosis of Ewing sarcoma would require a biopsy and, as response to chemotherapy is less predictable and probably slower, neurosurgeons should consider a spinal cord decompression both for diagnostic material and to safeguard the spinal cord. Because of the frequently extensive involvement, gross total resection is often unobtainable.

Further treatment for pPNETs involves chemotherapy, second-look surgery to attempt a delayed complete resection, and/or radiotherapy. In the absence of combined adjuvant chemo-radiation, Ewing sarcoma is universally fatal; however, 41 to 49% and 31 to 36% survival rates have been reported at 5 and 10 years respectively with multimodal therapy (Marco et al. 2005, Mukherjee et al. 2011).

Leukaemia and lymphoma
The acute leukaemias in childhood (particularly acute myeloid leukaemia) can occasionally present with bulky/solid disease: sometimes these lesions are termed chloromas. They can rarely occur in the spinal canal. The diagnosis may be made on the peripheral blood film or bone marrow analysis and immunophenotyping, thereby avoiding the need for biopsy. Chemotherapy usually results in a rapid shrinkage of disease and it would be rare to require the services of a neurosurgeon. Although outcome can vary between the different biological subgroups of acute myeloid leukaemia (M0–M7), overall survival rates for children with acute myeloid leukaemia have improved over the past 30 years. Indeed 5-year rates are now cited between 55 and 65% (Gibson et al. 2005, Kaspers and Creutzig 2005, Ries 2007, Creutzig et al. 2008, Lange et al. 2008). Remission can be achieved after induction chemotherapy in approximately 85 to 90% of cases, whereas event-free survival rates range between 45 and 55% (Gibson et al. 2005, Kaspers and Creutzig 2005, Creutzig et al. 2008, Lange et al. 2008).

The lymphomas (usually non-Hodgkin lymphomas) may present with solid disease affecting the spine or cord. CNS involvement by non-Hodgkin lymphoma is an adverse prognostic marker and is typically associated with a higher stage of disease (Wong et al. 1996). As a result, there are often other disease sites (bones, spleen, lymph nodes, liver, skin, pleural effusion, ascites, bone marrow) which may be identified on accompanying imaging modalities (technetium total bone scintigraphy, positron emission tomography) and yield diagnostic tissue. Response to chemotherapy is also usually rapid and neurosurgery is rarely required.

Overall survival for children and adolescents with non-Hodgkin lymphoma has generally improved over recent decades, with 10-year rates now cited above 85% (Pulte et al. 2008). Nevertheless, CNS involvement in this age group is less encouraging, with 5 year estimated event-free survival rates reported at 64% (Salzburg et al. 2007).

Management of spinal tumours
EXTRADURAL TUMOURS
Therapy for malignant extradural lesions is dependent on tumour type and adheres to treatment packages involving either chemotherapy (acute myeloid leukaemia, non-Hodgkin lymphoma, primary paraspinal neuroblastoma) or chemo-radiotherapy (pPNET), with surgery reserved for obtaining histological diagnosis and spinal cord decompression.

Describing the variety of specific therapies adopted in this setting is beyond the scope of this chapter and will not be discussed.

EXTRAMEDULLARY TUMOURS

As previously stated, although it is justifiable to monitor asymptomatic extramedullary lesions serially without intervention, treatment for symptomatic lesions remains gross surgical resection of the lesion. In the case of neurofibromas, this unfortunately results in sacrificing the implicated sensory nerve root.

INTRAMEDULLARY TUMOURS

Surgical management

The aim of surgical treatment of intramedullary spinal cord tumours is gross total resection. As is discussed below, the extent to which this goal can be obtained is partly dictated by the type of tumour being addressed, the anatomy of the tumour, and the results of intraoperative electrophysiological monitoring. For instance, a recent single-institution series analysis correlated tumour histology and definable tissue planes with gross total resection and progression-free survival in ependymomas and haemangioblastomas but not astrocytomas (Garces-Ambrossi et al. 2009).

After induction of anaesthesia, intubation, and establishment of the appropriate intravenous and arterial access, the patient is positioned prone on the operating table with gel rolls supporting the chest in an effort to reduce venous hypertension. The head is positioned using a Mayfield horseshoe or foam doughnut with careful attention paid to the pressure points such as the maxillary prominences and the eyes; in the instance of tumours located in the cervical or high-thoracic region, three-point fixation is used by a Mayfield skull clamp. Sufficient padding of extremity pressure-points is accomplished using a foam egg-crate, and the arms are tucked at the side for cervical or high-thoracic approaches or placed in the 'Superman' position with arm boards for mid- and lower-thoracic tumours. High-dose dexamethasone is given before surgery, and then weaned over the next 4 to 7 days, while perioperative antibiotics are also administered. As discussed below, somatosensory and motor evoked potential baseline readings are obtained before incision.

A plain radiograph or fluoroscopic image is used to localize the intended spinal level with correlation made to the preoperative MRI, after which the area is prepped and draped in the standard fashion. A sharp, midline incision is made with the dissection carried out in the midline with attention made to minimizing blood loss along with a subperiosteal reflection of the paraspinal musculature using a combination of blunt and electrocautery dissection. In patients without previous history of spinal surgery, a laminectomy designed to expose the rostral-caudal extent of the solid tumour is made with preservation of the facet joints laterally to maintain stability; it is our practice, particularly in children, to perform this laminectomy using a craniotome attachment of a pneumatic drill to allow for post-resection laminoplasty. In the case of patients with previous laminectomy, a re-opening of the prior bony defect is made with extension to the bone above and below to identify normal anatomy and facilitate easy extension of the exposure if necessary. Before opening the dura, ultrasound imaging is often used to visualize the tumour and confirm appropriate level and extent of the laminectomy with adjustments made as needed; exposure of rostral or caudally associated syrinxes or cystic components is not necessary for resection. Epidural electrodes are placed rostral and caudal to the planned site of tumour resection for measurement of D-wave motor evoked potentials (see below), the operative microscope is brought into the field, and the dura is sharply incised in the midline and tacked to the paraspinal musculature with braded nylon sutures. Saline-dampened cottonoids are used to line the gutters of the laminectomy to reduce the introduction of blood into the intradural space.

Depending on the type of lesion being treated, the goals of surgery vary. Gliomas both of low and high-grade pathology are highly invasive, lacking clear planes between normal spinal cord tissue and tumour; overt manipulation by the surgeon in these cases in an attempt to define this border should be avoided as a high risk of injury to the spinal cord is inherent in this manoeuvre. With these lesions, an initial midline myelotomy is made via a sharp dissection to expose the tumour; because of the distortion of the spinal cord by tumour expansion the midline may not be readily apparent, in this case the relationship of the supposed midline to the bilateral dorsal root entry zones or the identification of the midline dorsal vasculature can be used as an indicator. Pial sutures can be placed to help provide traction facilitating definition of tumour–tissue interfaces. Once the tumour is exposed, a biopsy should be obtained for immediate histological examination. In the case of a high-grade lesion, the goal of surgery should be a limited debulking of readily discernible tumour with preservation of neurological function based on intraoperative monitoring, as the prognosis for this entity remains poor despite the extent of resection (Garces-Ambrossi et al. 2009). To address low-grade astrocytomas and gangliogliomas, the resection starts with internal debulking of the tumour via ultrasonic aspiration (e.g. CUSA) starting at the mid-portion of the tumour as opposed to the cephalad or caudal poles where the tumour volume is the least and places the spinal cord at greatest risk of injury from manipulation. Though a clear cleavage plain is often absent in these tumours, the lesion can be gently removed from surrounding spinal cord tissue with gentle suction keeping in mind that motor tracts are often displaced anteriorly and laterally. The surgery in these cases is carried out with the goal of gross total resection as allowed for by the measured neuro-evoked potentials.

Ependymomas in contrast to astrocytomas, are typically located in the centre of the spinal cord, have a clearly definable cleavage plane facilitating surgical resection, and often are associated with a rostral or caudal cyst. Following the midline myelotomy, the cleavage plane is most easily identified at the poles of the tumour. Adhesions to the surrounding tumour can be cut either sharply or with the contact laser. Internal debulking can be used in the case of larger tumours, although en bloc removal should be considered to reduce the likelihood of subsequent development of drop metastases.

In the case of haemangioblastomas, most are well circumscribed, vascular lesions and are associated with the pial surface in a dorsal or dorsolateral location. The resection is started by bipolar coagulation of the feeding and draining vessels, along with the tumour surface, to facilitate manipulation of the tumour and reduce intra-operative haemorrhaging. Careful circumferential dissection of the tumour–parenchymal interface is then undertaken to separate the mass from the surrounding spinal tissue. In contrast to surgical resection of other tumours such as ependymomas or gliomas, these tumours cannot and should not be internally debulked as unacceptable and potentially uncontrollable haemorrhaging will be encountered. Also unlike the surgical management of glial tumours, although sensory and motor evoked potentials are closely monitored, this information is used to predict functional outcome rather than guide resection as leaving residual tumour predisposes the patient to a greatly increased risk of subsequent spinal cord haemorrhage.

After resection of the tumour, the intradural compartment is copiously irrigated and the dural edges re-approximated and closed primarily with prolene sutures. If appropriate, a laminoplasty is performed, bone is secured in place using titanium dog bone fixation plates and screws, while the paraspinal muscles and fascia are re-approximated and secured in the standard fashion. Finally, the skin is approximated with a running nylon suture or surgical staples at the surgeon's discretion.

Intraoperative electrophysiological monitoring
Intraoperative electrophysiological monitoring has become readily available for use in neurosurgical procedures and should be considered a standard of care in the treatment of intramedullary spinal cord tumours. In today's operating room, a combination of somato-sensory evoked potentials, muscle motor evoked potentials, and epidural electrode D-wave monitoring can be used to monitor the integrity of the spinal cord during the resection of intramedullary tumours.

First reported in 1978 as being used in spinal surgery, somatosensory evoked potentials measure afferent conduction of impulses from peripheral sites, such as the tibial or median nerve, to the brainstem or cerebral cortex depending on electrode placement; degradation in these signals indicate sensory pathway insults (involving the dorsal column and antero-lateral tracts) but cannot define injury to the motor pathways. Additionally, monitoring of somatosensory evoked potentials relies on signal averaging, which can delay detection of changes, thereby impacting on the surgeon's ability to alter their surgical plan based on these results alone. In contrast to somatosensory evoked potentials, motor evoked potentials and epidural electrodes can be used in real-time to assess the integrity of motor pathways during manipulation of the spinal cord. D-wave monitoring uses epidural electrodes, which measure the number of intact descending motor units as represented by the amplitude of the wave. In conjunction with motor evoked potentials, which provide an 'all or-none' assessment of peripheral motor function in a given distribution, inferences can made in real-time about impending irreversible damage to the spinal cord, and even transient post-operative deficits can be anticipated (Sciubba et al. 2009, Hsu et al. 2010).

Surgical complications
In the early postoperative period, it is not uncommon to see mild, transient exacerbation of preoperative symptoms or even the onset of new neurological findings. These symptoms are, however, typically mild and short lived in nature. Immediately postoperatively, patients may be found to have mild weakness or spasticity, bladder dysfunction, and sensory dis-turbances. Despite the finding of early neurological sequelae, more than 80 to 90% of

patients are found to have stable to improved long-term neurological function after resection of spinal cord tumours (Roonprapunt et al. 2001, Lonser and Oldfield 2005, Garces-Ambrossi et al. 2009, Mandigo et al. 2009).

As with all intradural spinal procedures, CSF leak with its associated risk of meningitis and wound breakdown is also of concern. This is a relatively uncommon occurrence, being seen primarily in patients who have been previously operated on. As mentioned above, the dura is closed in a watertight fashion with a running, non-absorbable suture; placement of a dural graft or patch using several dural substitutes, although not frequently employed, is used as appropriate. Additionally, the fascia is also closed in a watertight, tension-free manner, and the patient is kept flat in bed for 24 to 48 hours postoperatively.

ADJUVANT THERAPY
Prospective, randomized analyses of adjuvant therapy for specific intramedullary tumour types in children are lacking. This reflects the relative rarity of these lesions in the paediatric population and, in most cases, the protracted time to progression or recurrence that is observed. To have sufficient cohort sizes, most retrospective studies have historically combined paediatric and adult age groups, different tumour grades, or even grouped different spinal tumour types together. As a result, conclusions on the role of adjuvant radiotherapy and chemotherapy in this setting must be considered with a degree of caution.

Radiotherapy
The use of postoperative irradiation in the management strategy of paediatric intramedullary spinal tumours remains controversial. As stated, this is in part due to a paucity of randomized trials comparing adjuvant radiotherapy against primary spinal tumour surgery in children.

Newer conformal irradiation techniques, such as three-dimensional conformal radiotherapy, proton therapy, and immune-modulated radiation therapy, allow more precise dose administration such that doses exceeding 50Gy can now be administered with a reduction of scatter dosage to surrounding normal tissues. Nevertheless, potential adverse sequelae of radiotherapy have limited its widespread use as an adjuvant modality across paediatric spinal cord tumours. These include an increased risk of secondary malignancies (Inskip 2006), abnormal curvature of the spine secondary to impairment of spinal growth (Barrena et al. 2011), an increased incidence of moyamoya disease and ischaemic vasculopathies in patients with NF1(Desai et al. 2006) and a predisposition to radiation-induced myelopathy and subsequent neurological impairment (Nagasawa et al. 2011).

Despite these potential effects, conformal irradiation remains the standard adjuvant therapy in most institutions for high-grade gliomas (WHO grade III or IV), irrespective of the extent of primary tumour excision. This follows initial findings from randomized controlled trials of adult CNS high-grade gliomas, which found that when compared with surgery alone, postoperative radiotherapy improved survival rates (Laperriere et al. 2002). Current paediatric studies are now evaluating the efficacy of adding both concomitant and subsequent maintenance chemotherapy to current radiotherapy schedules, as highlighted in the chemotherapy discussion below.

For children with spinal low-grade gliomas, complete resection is deemed curative, thereby negating the need for adjuvant therapy. For cases of incomplete resection, radiotherapy was historically used as the primary adjuvant modality (Schmandt and Packer 2000, Mishra et al. 2006), whereas chemotherapy was used to delay the initiation of radiation therapy for very young patients (Packer et al. 1997). This stemmed from the view of some oncologists that the effects of chemotherapy were less durable, and the relative risks of radiotherapy were lower for older children (Packer et al. 1997, Kortmann et al. 2003). Nevertheless, concerns over the sequelae of radiation therapy in the past two decades have resulted in a major shift towards using chemotherapy as the primary postoperative therapy for paediatric low-grade gliomas anywhere in the CNS. Even at symptomatic recurrence, several institutions now favour re-operation and secondary courses of chemotherapy rather than administering radiotherapy (Massimino et al. 2002, Gururangan et al. 2007), although this practice is not universally adhered to, particularly for older patients.

As with spinal low-grade gliomas, most existing literature proposes that radiotherapy should not be administered after complete surgical excision of intramedullary ependymomas, given that they are low grade, slow-growing lesions that are often amenable to removal (Nagasawa et al. 2011). However, the use of primary adjuvant radiotherapy for spinal ependymomas remains apparent, irrespective of surgical resection (Benesch et al. 2010), based on reports that irradiation may delay the onset of ependymoma recurrence or progression (Akyurek et al. 2006, Chao et al. 2011). In contrast, most studies advocate the use of spinal radiotherapy after incomplete resections as evidence from predominantly adult studies suggests that it may prolong progression-free survival and even lead to functional improvement (Nagasawa et al. 2011).

Chemotherapy

As stated previously, chemotherapy is now most frequently used as first-line adjuvant therapy in the management of symptomatic or progressive paediatric CNS low-grade gliomas not amenable to complete tumour removal. Despite this, literature reporting the use of chemotherapy exclusively in spinal cord low-grade lesions is limited (Bouffet et al. 1997, Packer et al. 1997, Fort 1998, Grill 1998, Lowis et al. 1998, Doireau et al. 1999, Hassall et al. 2001). Evidence from a relatively large single institutional series of 29 such childhood tumours demonstrated that chemotherapy was as effective as radiotherapy at producing sustained disease control, even in cases of recurrence, and did not impair functional outcome (Scheinemann et al. 2009), a finding reinforced by other groups (Grill et al. 2005). The intravenous chemotherapeutic regimens that have been reported to be of value in this setting include vincristine in combination with carboplatin, single-agent vinblastine, carboplatin monotherapy, and thioguanine, procarbazine, lomustine, and vincristine (TPCV) (Lowis et al. 1998, Doireau et al. 1999, Hassall et al. 2001, Scheinemann et al. 2009). These agents appear well tolerated when used for periods up to and beyond 1 year, with toxicity profiles that rarely require discontinuation of therapy. Noteworthy associated adverse effects include allergy (carboplatin), peripheral neuropathy (vincristine and vinblastine), haematological toxicity (all regimens), and seizures (TPCV) (Scheinemann et al. 2009, Ater et al. 2012, Bouffet et al. 2012). Some clinicians are reluctant to use TPCV because of concerns about the potential for this combination to impair fertility (secondary to procarbazine) and increase the risk of secondary malignancy, although there is no definitive evidence for the latter effect from the paediatric literature (Ater et al. 2012).

Although radiotherapy appears marginally to improve survival and delay progression in CNS high-grade gliomas, such that it remains the standard adjuvant therapy, there is little evidence to suggest that incorporating postoperative chemotherapy after radiotherapy significantly improves outcome from this devastating disease (Hardison et al. 1987, Cohen et al. 1989). Historically, combinations of agents such as PCV (prednisolone, vincristine, and lomustine) or the '8 in 1 day' regimen (vincristine, hydroxyurea, procarbazine, lomustine, cisplatin, cytarabine, methylprednisolone, and either dacarbazine or cyclophosphamide) have yielded inconsistent or disappointing results (Sposto et al. 1989, Allen et al. 1998). Recent class I evidence from adult data revealed that the alkylating agent temozolomide, used with irradiation as concomitant and subsequent maintenance oral chemotherapy for a duration of 1 year, improves overall survival rates (2 year rates of 26% vs 10% without temozolomide), with minimal additional toxicity (fatigue, bone marrow suppression) (Stupp et al. 2005). Consequently, this regime has now been extrapolated and adopted as the best-known therapy for children aged above 3 years with a CNS malignant glioma. An international clinical trial co-ordinated by the Children's Oncology Group of North America (ACNS 0821), is now evaluating whether other novel therapies, administered in addition to or in substitution of temozolomide, will confer an additional survival advantage for these children, including those with intramedullary spinal lesions. Such chemotherapeutic agents under investigation include the antiangiogenic monoclonal antibody bevacizumab and the histone deacetylase inhibitor vorinostat.

The role of chemotherapy as a primary adjuvant therapy for childhood intramedullary ependymomas is not established. No prospective randomized controlled trial of its efficacy compared with surgery alone has ever been undertaken. Most data reporting chemotherapy use in spinal ependymoma have been in adult recurrent disease (Nagasawa et al. 2011), where case reports have purported the use of several agents including oral etoposide, intravenous carboplatin, the oral platelet-derived growth factor inhibitor imatinib, and subcutaneous interferon- 2b (Dorr et al. 1988, Chamberlain 2002, Fakhrai et al. 2004, Iunes et al. 2011). An evaluation of certain chemotherapies in the management of paediatric recurrent spinal ependymoma may therefore also merit consideration.

Summary
Tumours of the spine in children represent a diverse number of entities, ranging from benign lesions curable through surgical resection to malignant pathologies that can be fatal despite current best treatment practices. Surgical resection, however, remains the best treatment option for most of these tumours. The combination of improved microsurgical instruments, imaging, intraoperative neurophysiological monitoring, and spinal instrumentation has allowed more aggressive, radical resection of these tumours. Preoperative functional status and a clear intraoperative plane are the strongest indicators of complete resection and favourable progression-free survival in most tumours; the importance of preoperative function argues for earlier surgical intervention before worsening of neurological status (Cooper

1989, McCormick and Stein 1990, McCormick et al. 1990, Houten and Cooper 2000, Jallo et al. 2003, Garces-Ambrossi et al. 2009). No randomized trials of adjuvant therapy in the exclusive management of childhood intramedullary tumours have, as yet, been published, precluding definitive conclusions on their efficacy in this setting.

REFERENCES

Abramson SJ, Berdon WE, Ruzal-Shapiro C, Stolar C, Garvin J. Cervical neuroblastoma in eleven infants—a tumor with favorable prognosis. Clinical and radiologic (US, CT, MRI) findings. *Pediatr Radiol* 1993; **23**: 253–257.

Akyurek S, Chang EL, Yu TK, et al. Spinal myxopapillary ependymoma outcomes in patients treated with surgery and radiotherapy at MD Anderson Cancer Center. *J Neurooncol* 2006; **80**: 177–183.

Allen JC, Aviner S, Yates AJ, et al. Treatment of high-grade spinal cord astrocytoma of childhood with "8-in-1" chemotherapy and radiotherapy: a pilot study of CCG-945 Children's Cancer Group. *J Neurosurg* 1998; **88**: 215–220.

Ater JL, Zhou T, Holmes E, et al. Randomized study of two chemotherapy regimens for treatment of low-grade glioma in young children: a report from the Children's Oncology Group. *J Clin Oncol* 2012; **30**: 2641–1647.

Barrena S, Miguel M, De La Torre CA, et al. Late surgery for spinal deformities in children previously treated for neural tumors. *Eur J Pediatr Surg* 2011; **21**: 54–57.

Benesch M, Weber-Mzell D, Gerber NU, et al. Ependymoma of the spinal cord in children and adolescents: a retrospective series from the HIT database. *J Neurosurg Pediatr* 2010; **6**: 137–144.

Bertram C, Madert J, Eggers C. Eosinophilic granuloma of the cervical spine. *Spine* 2002; **27**: 1408–1413.

Bloem JL, Kroon HM. Osseous lesions. *Radiol Clin North Am* 1993; **31**: 261–278.

Bouffet E, Amat D, Devaux Y, Desuzinges C. Chemotherapy for spinal cord astrocytoma. *Med Pediatr Oncol* 1997; **29**: 560–562.

Bouffet E, Jakacki R, Goldman S, et al. Phase II study of weekly vinblastine in recurrent or refractory pediatric low-grade glioma. *J Clin Oncol* 2012; **30**: 1358–1363.

Bown N, Cotterill S, Lastowska M, et al. Gain of chromosome arm 17q and adverse outcome in patients with neuroblastoma. *N Engl J Med* 1999; **340**: 1954–1961.

Burgert EO Jr, Nesbit ME, Garnsey LA, et al. Multimodal therapy for the management of nonpelvic, localized Ewing's sarcoma of bone: intergroup study IESS-II. *J Clin Oncol* 1990; **8**: 1514–1524.

Burn SC, Ansorge O, Zeller R, Drake JM. Management of osteoblastoma and osteoid osteoma of the spine in childhood. *J Neurosurg Pediatr* 2009; **4**: 434–438.

Caram PC, Carton CA, Scarcella G. Intradural lipomas of the spinal cord; with particular emphasis on the intramedullary lipomas. *J Neurosurg* 1957; **14**: 28–42.

Casha S, Phan N, Rutka J. In Dickman C, Fehlings MG, Gokaslan ZL, editors. Spinal Cord and Spinal Column Tumors. New York, NY: Thieme, 2006: 187–203.

Catapano D, Muscarella LA, Guarnieri V, Zelante L, D'Angelo VA, D'Agruma L. Hemangioblastomas of central nervous system: molecular genetic analysis and clinical management. *Neurosurgery* 2005; **56**: 1215–1221.

Cerase A, Priolo F. Skeletal benign bone-forming lesions. *Eur J Radiol* 1998; **27** (Suppl. 1): S91–S97.

Cervoni L, Celli P, Caruso R, Gagliardi FM, Cantore GP. [Neurinomas and ependymomas of the cauda equina. A review of the clinical characteristics.] (In Italian.) *Minerva Chir* 1997; **52**: 629–633.

Chamberlain MC. Salvage chemotherapy for recurrent spinal cord ependymoma. *Cancer* 2002; **95**: 997–1002.

Chao ST, Kobayashi T, Benzel E, et al. The role of adjuvant radiation therapy in the treatment of spinal myxopapillary ependymomas. *J Neurosurg Spine* 2011; **14**: 59–64.

Chi JH, Cachola K, Parsa AT. Genetics and molecular biology of intramedullary spinal cord tumors. *Neurosurg Clin N Am* 2006; **17**: 1–5.

Chu BC, Terae S, Hida K, Furukawa M, Abe S, Miyasaka K. MR findings in spinal hemangioblastoma: correlation with symptoms and with angiographic and surgical findings. *AJNR Am J Neuroradiol* 2001; **22**: 206–217.

Cohen AR, Wisoff JH, Allen JC, Epstein F. Malignant astrocytomas of the spinal cord. *J Neurosurg* 1989; **70**: 50–54.

Cohn SL, Pearson AD, London WB, et al. The International Neuroblastoma Risk Group (INRG) classification system: an INRG Task Force report. *J Clin Oncol* 2009; **27**: 289–297.

Cooper PR. Outcome after operative treatment of intramedullary spinal cord tumors in adults: intermediate and long-term results in 51 patients. *Neurosurgery* 1989; **25**: 855–859.

Creutzig U, Buchner T, Sauerland MC, et al. Significance of age in acute myeloid leukemia patients younger than 30 years: a common analysis of the pediatric trials AML-BFM 93/98 and the adult trials AMLCG 92/99 and AMLSG HD93/98A. *Cancer* 2008; **112**: 562–571.

Desai SS, Paulino AC, Mai WY, Teh BS. Radiation-induced moyamoya syndrome. *Int J Radiat Oncol Biol Phys* 2006; **65**: 1222–1227.

Doireau V, Grill J, Zerah M, et al. Chemotherapy for unresectable and recurrent intramedullary glial tumours in children. Brain Tumours Subcommittee of the French Society of Paediatric Oncology (SFOP). *Br J Cancer* 1999; **81**: 835–840.

Donkol RH, Al-Nammi A, Moghazi K. Efficacy of percutaneous radiofrequency ablation of osteoid osteoma in children. *Pediatr Radiol* 2008; **38**: 180–185.

Dorr RT, Salmon SE, Robertone A, Bonnem E. Phase I-II trial of interferon-alpha 2b by continuous subcutaneous infusion over 28 days. *J Interferon Res* 1988; **8**: 717–725.

Elsberg CA, Beer R. The operability of intramedullary tumors of the spinal cord. A report of two operations with remarks upon the extrusion of intraspinal tumors. *Am J Med Sci* 1911; **142**: 636.

Epstein F, Epstein N. Surgical management of holocord intramedullary spinal cord astrocytomas in children. *J Neurosurg* 1981; **54**: 829–832.

Epstein FJ, Farmer JP, Freed D. Adult intramedullary astrocytomas of the spinal cord. *J Neurosurg* 1992; **77**: 355–359.

Epstein FJ, Farmer JP, Freed D. Adult intramedullary spinal cord ependymomas: the result of surgery in 38 patients. *J Neurosurg* 1993; **79**: 204–209.

Fakhrai N, Neophytou P, Dieckmann K, et al. Recurrent spinal ependymoma showing partial remission under Imatimib. *Acta Neurochir (Wien)* 2004; **146**: 1255–1258.

Feldkamp MM, Angelov L, Guha A. Neurofibromatosis type 1 peripheral nerve tumors: aberrant activation of the Ras pathway. *Surg Neurol* 1999; **51**: 211–218.

Floman Y, Bar-On E, Mosheiff R, Mirovsky Y, Robin GC, Ramu N. Eosinophilic granuloma of the spine. *J Pediatr Orthop B* 1997; **6**: 260–265.

Foley KM, Woodruff JM, Ellis FT, Posner JB. Radiation-induced malignant and atypical peripheral nerve sheath tumors. *Ann Neurol* 1980; **7**: 311–318.

Fort DW, Packer RJ, Kirkpatrick GB, Kuttesch JF Jr, Ater JL. Carboplatin and vincristine for pediatric spinal cord astrocytomas. Abstract presented at the 8th International Neuro-Oncology Symposium. *Childs Nerv Syst* 1998; **14**: 484.

Fortuna A, Nolletti A, Nardi P, Caruso R. Spinal neurinomas and meningiomas in children. *Acta Neurochir (Wien)* 1981; **55**: 329–341.

Gabra HO, Jesudason EC, McDowell HP, Pizer BL, Losty PD. Sacrococcygeal teratoma—a 25-year experience in a UK regional center. *J Pediatr Surg* 2006; **41**: 1513–1516.

Gangi A, Alizadeh H, Wong L, Buy X, Dietemann JL, Roy C. Osteoid osteoma: percutaneous laser ablation and follow-up in 114 patients. *Radiology* 2007; **242**: 293–301.

Garces-Ambrossi GL, McGirt MJ, Mehta VA, et al. Factors associated with progression-free survival and long-term neurological outcome after resection of intramedullary spinal cord tumors: analysis of 101 consecutive cases. *J Neurosurg Spine* 2009; **11**: 591–599.

Gibbs CP Jr, Hefele MC, Peabody TD, Montag AG, Aithal V, Simon MA. Aneurysmal bone cyst of the extremities. Factors related to local recurrence after curettage with a high-speed burr. *J Bone Joint Surg Am* 1999; **81**: 1671–1678.

Gibson BE, Wheatley K, Hann IM, et al. Treatment strategy and long-term results in paediatric patients treated in consecutive UK AML trials. *Leukemia* 2005; **19**: 2130–2138.

Gobel U, Schneider DT, Calaminus G, et al. Multimodal treatment of malignant sacrococcygeal germ cell tumors: a prospective analysis of 66 patients of the German cooperative protocols MAKEI 83/86 and 89. *J Clin Oncol* 2001; **19**: 1943–1950.

Goh KY, Velasquez L, Epstein FJ. Pediatric intramedullary spinal cord tumors: is surgery alone enough? *Pediatr Neurosurg* 1997; **27**: 34–39.

Gomez DR, Missett BT, Wara WM, et al. High failure rate in spinal ependymomas with long-term follow-up. *Neuro-oncol* 2005; **7**: 254–259.

Goyal M, Mishra NK, Sharma A, et al. Alcohol ablation of symptomatic vertebral hemangiomas. *AJNR Am J Neuroradiol* 1999; **20**: 1091–1096.

Grill J, Chastagner P, et al. Chemotherapy for intramedullary glial tumours. Abstract presented at the 8th International Neuro-Oncology Symposium. *Childs Nerv Syst* 1998; **14**: 484–485.

Grill J, Kalifa C, Doireau V. Intramedullary spinal cord astrocytomas in children. *Pediatr Blood Cancer* 2005; **45**: 80.

Gupta N, Frim D. In Winn, HR, editor. Youmans Neurological Surgery (5th edition). Philadelphia, PA: Saunders, 2003: 3587–3588.

Gururangan S, Fisher MJ, Allen JC, et al. Temozolomide in children with progressive low-grade glioma. *Neuro-oncol* 2007; **9**: 161–168.

Halliday AL, Sobel RA, Martuza RL. Benign spinal nerve sheath tumors: their occurrence sporadically and in neurofibromatosis types 1 and 2. *J Neurosurg* 1991; **74**: 248–253.

Hardison HH, Packer RJ, Rorke LB, Schut L, Sutton LN, Bruce DA. Outcome of children with primary intramedullary spinal cord tumors. *Childs Nerv Syst* 1987; **3**: 89–92.

Harrop JS, Schmidt MH, Boriani S, Shaffrey CI. Aggressive "benign" primary spine neoplasms: osteoblastoma, aneurysmal bone cyst, and giant cell tumor. *Spine* 2009; **34**: S39–S47.

Hassall TE, Mitchell AE, Ashley DM. Carboplatin chemotherapy for progressive intramedullary spinal cord low-grade gliomas in children: three case studies and a review of the literature. *Neuro-oncol* 2001; **3**: 251–257.

Hay MC, Paterson D, Taylor TK. Aneurysmal bone cysts of the spine. *J Bone Joint Surg Br* 1978; **60B**: 406–411.

Helseth A, Mork SJ, Johansen A, Tretli S. Neoplasms of the central nervous system in Norway IV A population-based epidemiological study of meningiomas. *APMIS* 1989; **97**: 646–654.

Heyd R, Seegenschmiedt MH, Rades D, et al. [The significance of radiation therapy for symptomatic vertebral hemangiomas (SVH).] (In German.) *Strahlenther Onkol* 2010; **186**: 430–435.

Hirose Y, Aldap D, Chan S, Lamborn K, Berger MS, Feuerstein BG. Grade II astrocytomas are subgrouped by chromosome aberrations. *Cancer Genet Cytogenet* 2003; **142**: 1–7.

Houten JK, Cooper PR. Spinal cord astrocytomas: presentation, management and outcome. *J Neurooncol* 2000; **47**: 219–224.

Hsu W, Bettegowda C, Jallo GI. Intramedullary spinal cord tumor surgery: can we do it without intraoperative neurophysiological monitoring? *Childs Nerv Syst* 2010; **26**: 241–245.

Inskip PD, Heineman EF, In: Cutis RE, Freedman DM, Ron E, Ries LAG, et al. editors. New Malignancies among Cancer Survivors: SEER Cancer Registries, 1973–2000. NIH Publication number 05-5302. Bethseda, MD: National Cancer Institute, 2006.

Isaacson SR. Radiation therapy and the management of intramedullary spinal cord tumors. *J Neurooncol* 2000; **47**: 231–238.

Iunes EA, Stavale JN, De Cassia Caldas Pessoa R, et al. Multifocal intradural extramedullary ependymoma. Case report. *J Neurosurg Spine* 2011; **14**: 65–70.

Jackson RP, Reckling FW, Mants FA. Osteoid osteoma and osteoblastoma. Similar histologic lesions with different natural histories. *Clin Orthop Relat Res* 1977; **128**: 303–313.

Jallo GI, Freed D, Epstein F. Intramedullary spinal cord tumors in children. *Childs Nerv Syst* 2003; **19**: 641–649.

Jallo GI, Kim B, Epstein F. The current management of intramedullary neoplasms in children and young adults. *Ann Neurosurg* 2001; **1**: 1–13.

Jallo GI, Kothbauer KF, Epstein FJ. Intrinsic spinal cord tumor resection. *Neurosurgery* 2001; **49**: 1124–1128.

Jallo GI, Kothbauer KF, Epstein F. In Winn, HR, editor. Youmans Neurological Surgery (5th edition). Philadelphia, PA: Saunders, 2003: 3616–3707.

Janin Y, Epstein JA, Carras R, Khan A. Osteoid osteomas and osteoblastomas of the spine. *Neurosurgery* 1981; **8**: 31–38.

Kaspers GJ, Creutzig U. Pediatric acute myeloid leukemia: international progress and future directions. *Leukemia* 2005; **19**: 2025–2029.

Korshunov A, Neben K, Wrobel G, et al. Gene expression patterns in ependymomas correlate with tumor location, grade, and patient age. *Am J Pathol* 2003; **163**: 1721–1727.

Kortmann RD, Timmermann B, Taylor RE, et al. Current and future strategies in radiotherapy of childhood low-grade glioma of the brain. Part I: treatment modalities of radiation therapy. *Strahlenther Onkol* 2003; **179**: 509–520.

Kothbauer KF. Neurosurgical management of intramedullary spinal cord tumors in children. *Pediatr Neurosurg* 2007; **43**: 222–235.

Kransdorf MJ, Sweet DE. Aneurysmal bone cyst: concept, controversy, clinical presentation, and imaging. *AJR Am J Roentgenol* 1995; **164**: 573–580.

Kumar V, Abbas A, Fausto N, Aster J, editors. Robbins and Cotran Pathologic Basis of Disease. Philadelphia, PA: WB Saunders, 2009.

Lange BJ, Smith FO, Feusner J, et al. Outcomes in CCG-2961, a children's oncology group phase 3 trial for untreated pediatric acute myeloid leukemia: a report from the children's oncology group. *Blood* 2008; **111**: 1044–1053.

Laperriere N, Zuraw L, Cairncross G. Radiotherapy for newly diagnosed malignant glioma in adults: a systematic review. *Radiother Oncol* 2002; **64**: 259–273.

Latif F, Tory K, Gnarra J, et al. Identification of the von Hippel-Lindau disease tumor suppressor gene. *Science* 1993; **260**: 1317–1320.

Lee M, Rezai AR, Abbott R, Coelho DH, Epstein FJ. Intramedullary spinal cord lipomas. *J Neurosurg* 1995; **82**: 394–400.

Lonser RR, Heiss JD, Oldfield EH. Tumor devascularization by intratumoral ethanol injection during surgery. *J Neurosurg* 1998; **88**: 923–924.

Lonser RR, Oldfield EH. Microsurgical resection of spinal cord hemangioblastomas. *Neurosurgery* 2005; **57**: 372–6.

Lonser RR, Oldfield EH. Spinal cord hemangioblastomas. *Neurosurg Clin N Am* 2006; **17**: 37–44.

Louis DH, Ohgaki H, Wiestler OD, et al. editors. WHO Classification of Tumours of the Central Nervous System (4th edition). Lyons: International Agency for Research on Cancer, 2007.

Lowis SP, Pizer BL, Coakham H, Nelson RJ, Bouffet E. Chemotherapy for spinal cord astrocytoma: can natural history be modified? *Childs Nerv Syst* 1998; **14**: 317–321.

Lucas DR, Unni KK, McLeod RA, O'Connor MI, Sim FH. Osteoblastoma: clinicopathologic study of 306 cases. *Hum Pathol* 1994; **25**: 117–134.

Mandigo CE, Ogden AT, Angevine PD, Mccormick PC. Operative management of spinal hemangioblastoma *Neurosurgery* 2009; **65**: 1166–1177.

Marco RA, Gentry JB, Rhines LD, et al. Ewing's sarcoma of the mobile spine. *Spine* 2005; **30**: 769–773.

Marina NM, Cushing B, Giller R, et al. Complete surgical excision is effective treatment for children with immature teratomas with or without malignant elements: a Pediatric Oncology Group/Children's Cancer Group Intergroup study. *J Clin Oncol* 1999; **17**: 2137–2143.

Martuza RL, Eldridge R. Neurofibromatosis 2 (bilateral acoustic neurofibromatosis). *N Engl J Med* 1988; **318**: 684–688.

Massimino M, Spreafico F, Cefalo G, et al. High response rate to cisplatin/etoposide regimen in childhood low-grade glioma. *J Clin Oncol* 2002; **20**: 4209–4216.

Mautner VF, Nguyen R, Kutta H, et al. Bevacizumab induces regression of vestibular schwannomas in patients with neurofibromatosis type 2. *Neuro-oncol* 2010; **12**: 14–18.

McCormick PC, Stein BM. Intramedullary tumors in adults. *Neurosurg Clin N Am* 1990; **1**: 609–630.

McCormick PC, Torres R, Post KD, Stein BM. Intramedullary ependymoma of the spinal cord. *J Neurosurg* 1990; **72**: 523–532.

McLaughlin MP, Marcus RB Jr, Buatti JM, et al. Ependymoma: results, prognostic factors and treatment recommendations. *Int J Radiat Oncol Biol Phys* 1998; **40**: 845–850.

Minehan KJ, Shaw EG, Scheithauer BW, Davis DL, Onofrio BM. Spinal cord astrocytoma: pathological and treatment considerations. *J Neurosurg* 1995; **83**: 590–595.

Mishra KK, Puri DR, Missett BT, et al. The role of up-front radiation therapy for incompletely resected pediatric WHO grade II low-grade gliomas. *Neuro-oncol* 2006; **8**: 166–174.

Mitchell ML, Ackerman LV. Metastatic and pseudomalignant osteoblastoma: a report of two unusual cases. *Skeletal Radiol* 1986; **15**: 213–218.

Mukherjee D, Chaichana KL, Gokaslan ZL, Aaronson O, Cheng JS, McGirt MJ. Survival of patients with malignant primary osseous spinal neoplasms: results from the Surveillance, Epidemiology, and End Results (SEER) database from 1973 to 2003. *J Neurosurg Spine* 2011; **14**: 143–150.

Nagasawa DT, Smith ZA, Cremer N, Fong C, Lu DC, Yang I. Complications associated with the treatment for spinal ependymomas. *Neurosurg Focus* 2011; **31**: E13.

Nakasu S, Nakasu Y, Saito A, Handa J. Intramedullary subependymoma with neurofibromatosis—report of two cases. *Neurol Med Chir (Tokyo)* 1992; **32**: 275–280.

Nesbit ME, Kieffer S, D'Angio GJ. Reconstitution of vertebral height in histiocytosis X: a long-term follow-up. *J Bone Joint Surg Am* 1969; **51**: 1360–1368.

Ohgaki H, Dessen P, Jourde B, et al. Genetic pathways to glioblastoma: a population-based study. *Cancer Res* 2004; **64**: 6892–6899.

Ohgaki H, Kleihues P. Genetic pathways to primary and secondary glioblastoma. *Am J Pathol* 2007; **170**: 1445–1453.

Okamoto Y, Di Patre PL, Burkhard C, et al. Population-based study on incidence survival rates and genetic alterations of low-grade diffuse astrocytomas and oligodendrogliomas. *Acta Neuropathol* 2004; **108**: 49–56.

Osborn A. Diagnostic Neuroradiology. St Louis, MO: Mosby, 1994.

Packer RJ, Ater J, Allen J, et al. Carboplatin and vincristine chemotherapy for children with newly diagnosed progressive low-grade gliomas. *J Neurosurg* 1997; **86**: 747–754.

Papagelopoulos PJ, Currier BL, Shaughnessy WJ, et al. Aneurysmal bone cyst of the spine Management and outcome. *Spine* 1998; **23**: 621–628.

Parsa AT, Chi JH, Acosta FL Jr, Ames CP, McCormick PC. Intramedullary spinal cord tumors: molecular insights and surgical innovation. *Clin Neurosurg* 2005; **52**: 76–84.

Parsa AT, Lee J, Parney IF, Weinstein P, McCormick PC, Ames C. Spinal cord and intradural-extraparenchymal spinal tumors: current best care practices and strategies. *J Neurooncol* 2004; **69**: 291–318.

Peng XS, Pan T, Chen LY, Huang G, Wang J. Langerhans' cell histiocytosis of the spine in children with soft tissue extension and chemotherapy. *Int Orthop* 2009; **33**: 731–736.

Pettine KA, Klassen RA. Osteoid-osteoma and osteoblastoma of the spine. *J Bone Joint Surg Am* 1986; **68**: 354–361.

Plotkin SR, Stemmer-Rachamimov AO, Barker FG II, et al. Hearing improvement after bevacizumab in patients with neurofibromatosis type 2. *N Engl J Med* 2009; **361**: 358–367.

Poretti A, Grotzer MA. Neuroblastoma with spinal cord compression: is there an emergency treatment of choice? *Dev Med Child Neurol* 2012; **54**: 297–298.

Pulte D, Gondos A, Brenner H. Trends in 5- and 10-year survival after diagnosis with childhood hematologic malignancies in the United States 1990–2004. *J Natl Cancer Inst* 2008; **100**: 1301–1309.

Raco A, Ciappetta P, Artico M, Salvati M, Guidetti G, Guglielmi G. Vertebral hemangiomas with cord compression: the role of embolization in five cases. *Surg Neurol* 1990; **34**: 164–168.

Raco A, Piccirilli M, Landi A, Lenzi J, Delfini R, Cantore G. High-grade intramedullary astrocytomas: 30 years' experience at the Neurosurgery Department of the University of Rome "Sapienza". *J Neurosurg Spine* 2010; **12**: 144–153.

Raskas DS, Graziano GP, Herzenberg JE, Heidelberger KP, Hensinger RN. Osteoid osteoma and osteoblastoma of the spine. *J Spinal Disord* 1992; **5**: 204–211.

Reifenberger J, Ring GU, Gies U, et al. Analysis of p53 mutation and epidermal growth factor receptor amplification in recurrent gliomas with malignant progression. *J Neuropathol Exp Neurol* 1996; **55**: 822–831.

Reimer R, Onofrio BM. Astrocytomas of the spinal cord in children and adolescents. *J Neurosurg* 1985; **63**: 669–675.

Reni M, Gatta G, Mazza E, Vecht C. Ependymoma. *Crit Rev Oncol Hematol* 2007; **63**: 81–89.

Rescorla FJ, Sawin RS, Coran AG, Dillon PW, Azizkhan RG. Long-term outcome for infants and children with sacrococcygeal teratoma: a report from the Childrens Cancer Group. *J Pediatr Surg* 1998; **33**: 171–176.

Ries LAG, Melbert D, Krapcho M, et al. SEER Cancer Statistics Review 1975–2005. Betheda, MD: National Cancer Institute, 2007.

Robertson PL, Allen JC, Abbott IR, Miller DC, Fidel J, Epstein FJ. Cervicomedullary tumors in children: a distinct subset of brainstem gliomas. *Neurology* 1994; **44**: 1798–803.

Rodriguez HA, Berthrong M. Multiple primary intracranial tumors in von Recklinghausen's neurofibromatosis. *Arch Neurol* 1966; **14**: 467–475.

Roessler K, Bertalanffy A, Jezan H, et al. Proliferative activity as measured by MIB-1 labeling index and long-term outcome of cerebellar juvenile pilocytic astrocytomas. *J Neurooncol* 2002; **58**: 141–146.

Roonprapunt C, Silvera VM, Setton A, Freed D, Epstein FJ, Jallo GI. Surgical management of isolated hemangioblastomas of the spinal cord. *Neurosurgery* 2001; **49**: 321–327.

Safavi-Abbasi S, Senoglu M, Theodore N, et al. Microsurgical management of spinal schwannomas: evaluation of 128 cases. *J Neurosurg Spine* 2008; **9**: 40–47.

Saito Y, Matsuzaki A, Suminoe A, et al. Congenital Ewing sarcoma in retroperitoneum with multiple metastases. *Pediatr Blood Cancer* 2008; **51**: 698–701.

Salzburg J, Burkhardt B, Zimmermann M, et al. Prevalence clinical pattern and outcome of CNS involvement in childhood and adolescent non-Hodgkin's lymphoma differ by non-Hodgkin's lymphoma subtype: a Berlin-Frankfurt-Munster Group Report. *J Clin Oncol* 2007; **25**: 3915–3922.

Sanford RA, Smith RA. Hemangioblastoma of the cervicomedullary junction. Report of three cases. *J Neurosurg* 1986; **64**: 317–321.

Scheinemann K, Bartels U, Huang A, et al. Survival and functional outcome of childhood spinal cord low-grade gliomas. *J Neurosurg Pediatr* 2009; **4**: 254–261.

Schmandt SM, Packer RJ. Treatment of low-grade pediatric gliomas. *Curr Opin Oncol* 2000; **12**: 194–198.

Schultze F, Weiterer Beitrag Zur. Diagnose und operativen Behandlung von Geschwülsten der Rückenmarkshäute und des Rückenmarks. *Deutsch Med Wochenschr* 1912; **38**: 1676–1679.

Schwartz TH, McCormick PC. Intramedullary ependymomas: clinical presentation surgical treatment strategies and prognosis. *J Neurooncol* 2000; **47**: 211–218.

Sciubba DM, Hsieh P, McLoughlin GS, Jallo GI. Pediatric tumors involving the spinal column. *Neurosurg Clin N Am* 2008; **19**: 81–92.

Sciubba DM, Liang D, Kothbauer KF, Noggle JC, Jallo GI. The evolution of intramedullary spinal cord tumor surgery. *Neurosurgery* 2009; **65**: 84–91.

Sharma AK, Sharma CS, Gupta AK, Sarin YK, Agarwal LD, Zaffar M. Teratomas in pediatric age group: experience with 75 cases. *Indian Pediatr* 1993; **30**: 689–694.

Shenkin HA, Alpers BJ. Clinical and pathologic features of gliomas of the spinal cord. *Archives of Neurology Psychiatry* 1944; **52**: 87–105.

Sonneland PR, Scheithauer BW, Onofrio BM. Myxopapillary ependymoma. A clinicopathologic and immunocytochemical study of 77 cases. *Cancer* 1985; **56**: 883–893.

Sposto R, Ertel IJ, Jenkin RD, et al. The effectiveness of chemotherapy for treatment of high grade astrocytoma in children: results of a randomized trial. A report from the Childrens Cancer Study Group. *J Neurooncol* 1989; **7**: 165–177.

Stuben G, Stuschke M, Kroll M, Havers W, Sack H. Postoperative radiotherapy of spinal and intracranial ependymomas: analysis of prognostic factors. *Radiother Oncol* 1997; **45**: 3–10.

Stupp R, Mason WP, Van Den Bent MJ, et al. Radiotherapy plus concomitant and adjuvant temozolomide for glioblastoma. *N Engl J Med* 2005; **352**: 987–996.

Symonds CP, Meadows SP. Compression of the spinal cord in the neighbourhood of the foramen magnum. *Brain* 1937; **60**: 52–84.

Tan G, Samson I, De Wever I, Goffin J, Demaerel P, Van Gool SW. Langerhans cell histiocytosis of the cervical spine: a single institution experience in four patients. *J Pediatr Orthop B* 2004; **13**: 123–126.

Tomlinson FH, Scheithauer BW, Hayostek CJ, et al. The significance of atypia and histologic malignancy in pilocytic astrocytoma of the cerebellum: a clinicopathologic and flow cytometric study. *J Child Neurol* 1994; **9**: 301–310.

Van Velthoven V, Reinacher PC, Klisch J, Neumann HP, Glasker S. Treatment of intramedullary hemangioblastomas with special attention to von Hippel-Lindau disease. *Neurosurgery* 2003; **53**: 1306–13.

Von Eiselberg AF, Ranzi E. Uber die chirurgische Behandlung der Hirnund Ruckermarkstumoren. *Arch Klin Chir* 1913; **102**: 309–468.

Waldron JN, Laperriere NJ, Jaakkimainen L, et al. Spinal cord ependymomas: a retrospective analysis of 59 cases. *Int J Radiat Oncol Biol Phys* 1993; **27**: 223–229.

Watanabe K, Sato K, Biernat W, et al. Incidence and timing of p53 mutations during astrocytoma progression in patients with multiple biopsies. *Clin Cancer Res* 1997; **3**: 523–530.

Whitaker SJ, Bessell EM, Ashley SE, Bloom HJ, Bell BA, Brada M. Postoperative radiotherapy in the management of spinal cord ependymoma. *J Neurosurg* 1991; **74**: 720–728.

Wilne S, Collier J, Kennedy C, Koller K, Grundy R, Walker D. Presentation of childhood CNS tumours: a systematic review and meta-analysis. *Lancet Oncol* 2007; **8**: 685–695.

Wilne S, Walker D. Spine and spinal cord tumours in children: a diagnostic and therapeutic challenge to healthcare systems. *Arch Dis Child Educ Pract Ed* 2010; **95**: 47–54.

Wind JJ, Bakhtian KD, Sweet JA, et al. Long-term outcome after resection of brainstem hemangioblastomas in von Hippel-Lindau disease. *J Neurosurg* 2011; **114**: 1312–1318.

Womer RB, Raney RB Jr, D'Angio GJ. Healing rates of treated and untreated bone lesions in histiocytosis X. *Pediatrics* 1985; **76**: 286–288.

Wong ET, Portlock CS, O'Brien JP, Deangelis LM. Chemosensitive epidural spinal cord disease in non-Hodgkins lymphoma. *Neurology* 1996; **46**: 1543–1547.

Yamamoto M, Raffel C. In: Albright, A, Pollack, I, Adelson, P, editors. Principles and Practice of Pediatric Neurosurgery. New York, NY: Thieme, 1999.

Yasargil MG, Antic J, Laciga R, De Preux J, Fideler RW, Boone SC. The microsurgical removal of intramedullary spinal hemangioblastomas. Report of twelve cases and a review of the literature. *Surg Neurol* 1976; 141–148.

Yoshii S, Shimizu K, Ido K, Nakamura T. Ependymoma of the spinal cord and the cauda equina region. *J Spinal Disord* 1999; **12**: 157–161.

Young JL Jr, Miller RW. Incidence of malignant tumors in U S children. *J Pediatr* 1975; **86**: 254–258.

7
INFLAMMATORY, METABOLIC, VASCULAR, AND DEMYELINATING DISORDERS

Michael Absoud, Ming J Lim, and Evangeline Wassmer

A diverse range of disorders (other than trauma and tumour) can result in an acquired myelopathy, and may be classified as inflammatory, metabolic, vascular, and demyelinating in aetiology. A review of the clinical features of these conditions and the characteristics specific to childhood presentation are discussed in this chapter.

Acute transverse myelitis

INTRODUCTION

Childhood acute transverse myelitis (ATM) is an inflammatory disorder of the spinal cord and is a subgroup of the non-compressive transverse myelopathies (Transverse Myelitis Consortium Working Group 2002). It is a potentially devastating condition with variable outcome (Banwell 2007). ATM may be differentiated into (1) idiopathic ATM and (2) ATM associated with other diseases. Specifically, ATM may be the result of an underlying systemic autoimmune disease (e.g. systemic lupus erythematosus), infection (e.g. varicella zoster), or it may be the first presentation of relapsing demyelinating inflammatory diseases such as neuromyelitis optica (NMO) or multiple sclerosis.

EPIDEMIOLOGY

Idiopathic ATM has been more commonly reported in adults, but occurs in children in approximately 20% of cases (Pidcock et al. 2007). Most published studies on transverse myelitis are retrospective case series reviews. Two prospective ATM paediatric surveillance studies in Canada (Banwell et al. 2009) and in UK neurology centres (De Goede et al. 2010) showed the incidence of ATM to be 2 per million and 1.7 per million children respectively. In recent literature (2007–2010), there has been a trend that male children are more likely to present with ATM, with ratios of 1.04:1 to 1.6:1 reported (Pidcock et al. 2007, Dajusta et al. 2008, Banwell et al. 2009, De Goede et al. 2010, Alper et al. 2011). There appears to be a bimodal distribution, with children predominantly affected under 5 years and older than 10 years (Pidcock et al. 2007, De Goede et al. 2010). In the Canadian and UK population studies, mean ages were 11.0 years (range 0.66–17.35) and median 9 years (0.5–15.9) respectively. The adult literature has also reported another peak between 30 and 39 years of age (Bhat et al. 2010). Idiopathic ATM represents approximately 14 to 22% of all first inflammatory demyelination syndromes of the central nervous system (CNS) (Mikaeloff et al. 2004, Banwell et al. 2009) and there appears to be no seasonal influence or difference in ethnicity prevalence.

DEFINITIONS

Although reports of ATM date back to 1882 (Quain 1882, Krishnan and Kerr 2005) there has been a recent interest and effort in classifying and defining this condition to facilitate biomarker discovery and clinical trials. The Transverse Myelitis Consortium Working Group (2002) published diagnostic criteria for idiopathic transverse myelitis. These criteria have to include all of the following:

1. Development of sensory, motor, or autonomic dysfunction attributable to the spinal cord
2. Bilateral signs and/or symptoms (although not necessarily symmetric)
3. Clearly defined sensory level
4. Inflammation within the spinal cord demonstrated by cerebrospinal fluid (CSF) pleocytosis or elevated immunoglobulin G (IgG) index or gadolinium enhancement
5. If none of the inflammatory criteria are met at symptom onset, repeat magnetic resonance imaging (MRI) and lumbar puncture evaluation between days 2 and 7 after symptom onset may be used to meet criteria
6. Progression to nadir between 4 hours and 21 days after the onset of symptoms (if patient awakens with symptoms, symptoms must become more pronounced from point of awakening)
7. (a) Exclusion of extra-axial compressive aetiology by neuroimaging (MRI; computed tomography [CT] of spinal cord not adequate)
   (b) Other presentations to be excluded are the following:
   - History of previous radiation to the spinal cord within the past 10 years
   - Clear arterial distribution of clinical deficit consistent with occlusion of the anterior spinal artery
   - Abnormal flow voids on the surface of the spinal cord consistent with arteriovenous malformation.

In 2007, The International Paediatric Multiple Sclerosis Study Group (IPMSSG) classified ATM as in adult literature as a subtype of clinically isolated syndrome, which is defined as a first acute-clinical episode of CNS symptoms with a presumed inflammatory demyelinating cause (Krupp et al. 2007).

Since the publication of the ATM criteria (Transverse Myelitis Consortium Working Group 2002), seven paediatric case series (Table 7.1) have been published with a total of 190 cases. Five studies are retrospective, and hence subject to confounding factors and selection bias to the more severe cases. Two studies were prospective in nature and included ascertainment from neurology centres only (where milder cases may not be seen) with relatively short follow-up. None of the studies used similar criteria, investigative procedures, or outcome measures at the outset. There is hence a need to standardize core outcome measurement, and for prospective longitudinal large population-based study designs. Nevertheless, data derived from these studies are informative and are reviewed in the subsequent sections.

CLINICAL FEATURES

The clinical features of ATM depend on the location and extent of the spinal cord lesion. The spinal cord dysfunction presents with a varied and sometimes asymmetric combination of motor (weakness of the limbs), sensory, and sphincter disturbance of diverse severity. Clinically, neurological signs are caused by interruption of neuroanatomical pathways in the transverse plane of the cord, and a resulting sensory level is characteristic (Frohman and Wingerchuk 2010). However, in very young children, sensory deficits may be difficult to determine. Additionally, MRI lesions do not always result in a corresponding clinical sensory level (Dajusta et al. 2008). When myelitis also occurs in the context of encephalopathy, and polyfocal neurological symptoms with inflammatory demyelinating lesions in the brain, acute disseminated encephalomyelitis is diagnosed. Table 7.1 summarizes the recent case series in children with ATM highlighting the cardinal clinical features. Most children reach a nadir within the first 1 to 2 weeks of presentation (most common symptoms being pain, lower limb weakness, and bladder dysfunction). In most children a sensory level was detectable (75–95%). More than half of patients have a thoracic clinical sensory level, and the rest have a cervical or lumbosacral level. A 'plateau' typically lasts for approximately 1 week before ongoing recovery begins. The recovery period may extend to several years after the initial insult. Motor deficits tend to recover before bladder dysfunction.

For adults, the American Spinal Injury Association scale of myelopathy rates patients according to severity:

A. Complete: no motor or sensory function is preserved in the sacral segments S4 to S5
B. Incomplete: sensory but not motor function is preserved below the neurological level and includes the sacral segments S4 to S5.
C. Incomplete: motor function is preserved below the neurological level, and more than half of key muscles below the neurological level have a muscle grade less than 3.
D. Incomplete: motor function is preserved below the neurological level, and at least half of key muscles below the neurological level have a Medical Research Council grade of 3 or more.
E. Normal: motor and sensory function are normal.

DIFFERENTIAL DIAGNOSIS

The three main categories in the differential diagnosis of ATM are inflammatory demyelination (multiple sclerosis, acute disseminated encephalomyelitis, NMO, and idiopathic acute transverse myelitis), infection (e.g. herpes), and other inflammatory disorders such as systemic lupus erythematosus. The following summary may be useful in the differential of

ATM associated with other diseases (Transverse Myelitis Consortium Working Group 2002):

1. Serological or clinical evidence of connective tissue disease (such as systemic lupus erythematosus, sarcoidosis, Behçet disease, Sjogren syndrome, mixed connective tissue disorder)
2. CNS manifestations of *Mycoplasma* pneumonia, Lyme disease, viral infection (e.g. human T-cell lymphotropic virus-1 [HTLV-1]; human immunodeficiency virus [HIV]; herpes simplex virus; enteroviruses; varicella zoster virus; Epstein–Barr virus; cytomegalovirus; human herpes virus)
3. Brain MRI abnormalities meeting multiple sclerosis diagnostic criteria for dissemination in space
4. Presentation (polyfocal neurological deficits and encephalopathy) and MRI findings consistent with acute disseminated encephalomyelitis
5. A history of concomitant optic neuritis, or relapsing ATM should raise the suspicion of NMO.

As ATM is only one of the causes of an acute myelopathy the differentials of acute compressive myelopathy (e.g. trauma, tumour) and vascular disorders (e.g. haemorrhage, infarction) are also important considerations. Clinical presentation, MRI, and CSF findings should appropriately guide the clinician. The conditions mentioned are considered in other chapters.

PATHOGENESIS

Idiopathic ATM is an inflammatory demyelinating condition with immune mediated mechanisms implicated. Numerous case series have reported many patients having CSF pleocytosis and raised CSF proteins (Defresne et al. 2003, Pidcock et al. 2007, Yiu et al. 2009, De Goede et al. 2010, Alper et al. 2011). Histopathological studies have demonstrated focal infiltration of the spinal cord by monocytes and lymphocytes as well as astroglial activation (Krishnan and Kerr 2005). Grey and white matter have been observed to be equally affected, confirming recent MRI observations (Alper et al. 2011).

Several immune mechanisms have been postulated. In healthy CNS, immune surveillance involves immune cells both entering and possibly leaving the CNS, and antigen draining from the CNS into the periphery (reviewed in Hickey 2001, Bailey et al. 2006). Activated T cells can migrate across the blood–brain barrier, facilitated by a host of endothelial and local factors (Carrithers et al. 2002). Under normal conditions this lymphocyte surveillance activity does not lead to inflammation or alter blood–brain barrier integrity (Brabb et al. 2000, Hickey 2001). However, when patrolling lymphocytes, in the context of local infection or autoimmune disease, re-encounter their specific antigens in the CNS (presented through perivascular antigen-presenting cells), they may initiate a classic 'autoinflammatory' response. The response promotes blood–brain barrier disruption and invasion of high numbers of activated lymphocytes into CNS parenchyma (Becher et al. 2006). These mechanisms form the cornerstone of our current thinking on the induction of disease in CNS autoimmune disorders (reviewed in Goverman 2009).

TABLE 7.1
Summary of recent largest case series for clinical features of acute transverse myelitis in children

Reference	Alper et al. 2010	De Goede et al. 2010	Kalra et al. 2009	Yiu et al. 2009	Dajusta et al. 2008	Pidcock et al. 2007	Defresne et al. 2003
Setting, design, and follow up	USA, Pittsburgh; 1 centre retrospective MRI study review; 1985–2008; 5.2y mean follow-up 0.04–13.1)	UK, 14 regional paediatric neurology centres; prospective surveillance; 2002–2004; 0.5y follow-up	India; prospective case-control One centre 2003–2007 1y follow-up	Australia; One centre retrospective comparison with ADEM 1997–2004 1.0y median follow-up (0.3–8.5y)	USA; New Jersey; Retrospective review 1995–2004 Mean follow-up 2.3y	USA, Baltimore; One centre retrospective review: idiopathic ATM 2000–2004 3.2 yr median follow-up	France; retrospective review; single centre 1965–1995 6.5y median follow-up (1–20y)
Demographics	27 cases Mean age 9.5y (0.5–16.9) M:F 1.07	41 cases Median age 9y (0.5–15.9) M:F 1.56	15 cases Mean age 7.9y (3.5–14). M: F 1.5:1	22 cases Median age 7.5y (0.3–15) M:F 1.6:1	14 cases Mean age 11.2y (0.7–18) M:F 1.3:1	47 cases Mean age 8.3y, clustering 0–3, 5–17y M:F 1.04:1	24 cases Mean age 8y (2–14) M:F 0.85:1
Transverse Myelitis Consortium Working Group criteria used/ exclusions	Yes; 14 definite ATM, and 13 probable Two excluded with NMO, none multiple sclerosis	No: all probable ATM except two: vascular myelopathy. No relapse at 6mo	No, but all probable ATM	Yes Excluded: One NMO, one CTD, one radiation myelitis	Yes	Yes Two had recurrent ATM, one NMO, one multiple sclerosis, one ADEM	No, but all probable ATM None developed MS

Table 7.1 continues

Table 7.1 continued

Clinical features	Four monoparesis, 20 paraparesis, three tetraparesis	27 sensory (22 with level), 34 motor (15 flaccid legs, 13 arms and legs involved), 26 sphincter; six cerebral involvement One had ON and ATM	Mean time to nadir 3.9d (0.5–14). Two required mechanical ventilation. Motor improved before sphincter. At 3mo, eight ambulatory (four with support)	Weakness in limbs: lower 100%, upper 41% Bladder disturbance 68% Sensory 55% Pain 64%	All lower limb motor deficits and bladder dysfunction Sensory; 35% cervical, 65% thoracic	At nadir (mean 2d): 89% could not walk and/or ventilated; 85% sphincter dysfunction; sensory level cervical 25%, thoracic 53%, lumbar 5%, sacral 3% (1/36), unclear in 14%	Nadir of 5d Pain (88%), motor loss (1/2 bilateral, lower limbs and/or upper) preceded sphincter dysfunction (15/24) 12% cervical, 88% thoracic
Treatment	N/a	30/36 high-dose steroids	All received high dose IV steroids for 5 days	21/22 High dose IV steroids mean 5d and tapering oral prednisolone 4wk	All high-dose IV steroids ± IVIG	70% IV steroids 33% IVIG 15% PLEX	High-dose steroids, six no treatment
Outcome/disability	N/a	80% started recovery<2wk; 19 complete, eight good, three fair, six poor*; 17 had continuing bladder problems	Eight full recovery, three non-ambulatory, Seven bladder disturbances *One death	61% complete, 21% good, 6% fair, 6% poor Bladder dysfunction (14% moderate/severe)	4/14 full motor and bladder recovery 4/14 Non-ambulant and intermittent catheterization (cervical levels)	At median 3.2y: 43% were unable to walk 30 feet and 21% required a walker or other support; 50% required bladder catheterization *Two deaths	2/16 (13%) children had severe motor sequelae 5/15 had severe sphincter dysfunction *One death

* Normal, complete recovery; good, insignificant sequelae; fair, sequelae but not interfering with daily life; poor, sequelae interfering with daily life. ATM, acute transverse myelitis; ADEM, acute disseminated encephalomyelitis; CTD, connective tissue disease; IV, intravenous; IVIG, intravenous immunoglobulin; M:F, male to female ratio; MS, multiple sclerosis; NMO, neuromyelitis optica; ON, optic neuritis; PLEX, plasmapheresis; N/a, not available.

Additionally, although many reports have quoted childhood infections and immunizations as temporal associations, studies have not included an appropriate design such as large case–control studies. If these associations are confirmed, it remains uncertain whether the link with ATM is a result of molecular mimicry (immune targeting of infection/vaccine-related proteins that bear molecular similarity to neuronal proteins), or whether the heightened immunity increases the pool of T or B cell clones that possess the ability to recognize neuronal proteins (Banwell 2007) or a combination of the two.

MRI FINDINGS IN ATM

Imaging of the spinal cord should be conducted using MRI with gadolinium contrast, and brain MRI should be included. Central cord hyperintensity involving grey matter and neighbouring white matter, with inflammation extending over three or more segments (longitudinally extensive transverse myelitis), is the most frequent finding in ATM (Alper et al. 2011). Longitudinally extensive transverse myelitis, however, is a feature not unique to ATM: it also occurs in NMO and multiple sclerosis (Banwell et al. 2008, Pidcock et al. 2007). Early ATM MRIs may be reported as normal, with a few children (usually with poor outcome) having later scans showing atrophy of the cord, highlighting the importance of follow-up imaging, particularly where early imaging is inconclusive (De Goede et al. 2010, Alper et al. 2011). Table 7.2 highlights the main MRI findings recently reported in the literature.

INVESTIGATIVE FINDINGS IN ATM

Approximately half of the children reported in the literature have CSF pleocytosis and/or raised protein levels. In isolated monophasic ATM, CSF oligoclonal bands are normally absent (Table 7.2). In children, the Transverse Myelitis Consortium Working Group criteria may be too stringent, repeat investigations to confirm inflammatory criteria may not be appropriate, and hence a diagnosis of probable ATM may be made based on clinical presentation, investigation, and MRI findings. Testing for NMO-IgG antibodies should also be considered at the outset for all children presenting with ATM (see NMO section on page 160).

TREATMENT

There are no controlled trials for the treatment of ATM in children or adults; however, early recognition and treatment remain important. Data are mainly extrapolated from case series or data from clinical trials for the treatment of exacerbations of adult multiple sclerosis (Transverse Myelitis Consortium Working Group 2002, Greenberg et al. 2007, Frohman and Wingerchuk 2010). In adults, treatment of relapses with intravenous methylprednisolone shortened relapse duration and sped up recovery. High doses of intravenous methylprednisolone (more than 500mg/d for at least 3d in adults) are superior to lower doses (Oliveri et al. 1998). A retrospective uncontrolled review (Greenberg et al. 2007) of 122 adults with idiopathic ATM evaluated therapies given acutely at one centre between 2001 and 2005. Patients who did not have a level A disability at nadir according to the American Spinal Injury Association scale, or a history of autoimmune disease, benefited from the addition of plasmapharesis but not cyclophosphamide. In patients who were level A at

TABLE 7.2

Summary of investigative and magnetic resonance imaging features of acute transverse myelitis

Reference	Alper et al. 2010	DeGoede et al. 2010	Kalra et al. 2009	Dajusta et al. 2008	Yiu et al. 2008	Pidcock et al. 2007	Defresne et al. 2003
CSF pleocytosis/ raised protein	10/27 (37%)	16/36 pleocytosis (44%), 11/36 protein >0.4g/l	3/6 pleocytosis, 4/6 raised proteins	N/a	CSF (in 74%): 67% pleocytosis; 38% raised protein	50% pleocytosis (17/34) Raised protein in 48% (14/29)	15/24 pleocytosis 3/14 raised protein;
CSF OGB positive/ IgG index	0/22 OGB positive, 2/21 IgG index raised	4/27 OGB positive	N/a	N/a	N/a	OGB positive or raised IgG index in <5%	0/14 OGB positive
NMO-IgG/other antibody tests	0/5 positive	N/a	Anti-GM1 Abs in 46% with ATM vs 6.6% control ($p=0.035$)	N/a	N/a	N/a	N/a
MRI spine; segment lengths affected	Segments (mean 6.4)	7/39 > six segments	13/15 had > three segments (two entire cord)	N/a	68% had at least three segments (mean eight segments)	Mean segments=6 (one multifocal, one entire cord)	4/6 had > two segments
MRI spine; regions affected	10 cervical ± thoracic, six thoracic, one lumbar, 4 other multiregional	14 cervical, 19 thoracic, seven lumbrosacral	thoracic cord most common; one multiregional	Cervical 57%, thoracic 43%	N/a	cervical 19/38, thoracic 15/38, lumbar/conus 2/38, 2/38 normal	2/6 normal
MRI spine; GAD enhancement	4/21	N/a	2/4	N/a	N/a	74% (26/35)	3/6
MRI brain features	1/25 patchy T_2 hyperintensity	17/26 abnormalities (six symptomatic)	N/a	N/a	3/10 abnormal (two asymptomatic, one brainstem extension)	N/a	One of four multiple T_2 lesions in cortex and basal ganglia

bs, Anti-GM1 antiganglioside immunoglobulin G antibodies; CSF, cerebrospinal fluid; GAD, gadolinium; IV, steroids; Neuromyelitis Optica; OGB, oligoclonal band; igG, lin-G; N/a, not available.

159

presentation, a combination of intravenous cyclophosphamide with plasmapharesis showed benefit compared with plasmapharesis alone. These conclusions, although they provide useful data, have the significant limitations of an uncontrolled retrospective analysis, as well as inherent biases as part of clinician treatment choices for patients. An evidence-based review of the treatment of ATM in adults was published by Scott et al. (2011), which also advocates for more therapeutic trials.

In a multi-centre review, 12 children with severe ATM were treated with intravenous methylprednisolone and compared with a historical group of 17 patients. The treatment had a significant effect on the proportion of patients walking independently at 1 month and on the proportion with full recovery at 1 year, with no differences in the frequency of complications between the groups (Defresne et al. 2001).

Children are usually treated with high-dose intravenous steroids for 3 to 5 days to attenuate inflammation (Table 7.1). In children who do not respond to steroids, intravenous immunoglobulin is often used, although the data to support this are limited to small case series and single case reports (Banwell et al. 2007). Plasmapharesis is increasingly used as rescue therapy based on its efficacy in a small randomized controlled trial in adults with acute CNS demyelination (Weinshenker et al. 1999).

OUTCOME
Children are thought to have a better outcome than adults (Dunne et al. 1986, Defresne et al. 2003, De Goede et al. 2010), with approximately half making a complete recovery. However, a group of children have severe disabilities. Additionally deaths have been reported, mainly because of respiratory failure associated with a high cervical cord lesion (Defresne et al. 2003, Pidcock et al. 2007, Kalra et al. 2009). The most common sequelae affecting children are sensory disturbances and bladder dysfunction (15–50%). Approximately one-quarter are non-ambulant or require an aid for walking. A group of children never regain mobility or bladder function (10–20%). Several studies have attempted to correlate presenting clinical and laboratory features with clinical outcome (Table 7.3). A higher spinal level is the only consistent poor prognostic feature across these studies. An identifiable trigger (intercurrent illness or vaccination) does not appear to predict clinical outcome. The influence of age, rapidity to nadir of symptoms, and late start of recovery in predicting clinical outcome appear to vary between studies.

ATM may be isolated or part of a polyfocal clinically isolated syndrome. It can be monophasic, or later relapse and hence be the first presentation of a relapsing NMO spectrum (Fig. 7.1) disorder or multiple sclerosis (Fig. 7.2). Patients with ATM should be followed up longitudinally irrespective of initial outcome, in part to clarify the diagnosis and to provide continuing multidisciplinary support into rehabilitation (motor, sphincter, psychological, and educational).

NMO
NMO is a severe immune mediated inflammatory demyelinating condition characterized by the presence of both optic neuritis and transverse myelitis occurring simultaneously or separated in time and distinct from multiple sclerosis. It is also characterized by the presence of

TABLE 7.3

Summary of poor prognostic factors reported in recent case series for paediatric acute transverse myelitis

Reference	Older age (>10)?	Rapid onset to nadir <1d?	Late start of recovery >1wk	Higher spinal levels?	Sphincter involvement?	Flaccid legs at presentation?	Many spinal segments?	Cerebrospinal fluid pleocytosis?	Intercurrent illness/ vaccination?
DeGoede et al. 2010	Yes	Yes	Yes	Yes	Yes	Yes	N/a	N/a	No
Yiu et al. 2009	No: younger age	No	N/a	Respiratory failure requiring ventilation	N/a	Yes	No	N/a	N/a
Pidcock et al. 2007	No: younger age	No	N/a	Yes	N/a	N/a	Yes	Yes	No
Defresne et al. 2003	N/a	Yes	N/a	N/a	N/a	Complete paraplegia	N/a	N/a	N/a
Miyazawa et al. 2003*	No: younger age	No	N/a	N/a	N/a	No Babinski's reflex	N/a	N/a	No

*Compilation of 50 case reports from Japan (1987–2001). N/a, not available

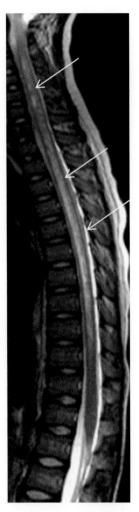

Fig. 7.1. MRI scan of spinal cord changes in a child with relapsing acute transverse myelitis (neuromyelitis optica-immunoglobulin-G positive), demonstrating high signal cervical to lower thoracic level lesion (arrows). The patient presented at 7 years of age, with relapses after 6 months and 11 months. The patient was treated with azathioprine 75mg once daily and 5mg oral prednisolone alternate days. At 2 years the patient was relapse free with no disability or bladder dysfunction.

the NMO-IgG antibody directed against the astrocytic water channel protein aquaporin-4 (Lennon et al. 2004); this discovery has broadened the disease spectrum. NMO-IgG appears to be a specific test as it is invariably negative in paediatric multiple sclerosis (Banwell et al. 2008, Huppke et al. 2010). NMO may initially present as an isolated optic neuritis (with abnormal visual evoked potentials) in adults (see Collongues et al. 2010a) and in childhood (Absoud et al. 2011) or as ATM before further relapses reveal the underlying diagnosis (Collongues et al. 2010a). It can be a monophasic illness but is usually a relapsing remitting disorder in the paediatric population. NMO is a very rare disorder, comprising 3 to 8% of childhood CNS inflammatory demyelinating diseases (Banwell et al. 2008). Longitudinally extensive transverse myelitis is a feature of NMO but can also occur in monophasic ATM and paediatric multiple sclerosis (Pidcock et al. 2007, Banwell et al. 2008, Verhey et al. 2010).

In 2007, the IPMSSG defined NMO as having all of the following criteria:

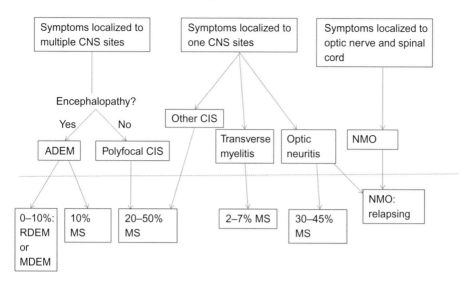

Fig. 7.2. Risk of childhood muliple sclerosis (MS) after a first attack of inflammatory demyelination in the central nervous system (CNS). ADEM, acute disseminated encephalomyelitis; RDEM, recurrent ADEM; MDEM, multiphasic ADEM; CIS, clinically isolated syndrome; NMO, neuromyelitis optica.

1. Optic neuritis and acute myelitis
2. Either a spinal MRI lesion extending over three or more segments or be NMO positive on antibody testing.

Two recent adult diagnostic criteria were developed on the basis of the most recent clinical, MRI, and aquaporin-4 antibody results:

A. Revised diagnostic criteria (Wingerchuk et al. 2006); two absolute criteria:
   (i) optic neuritis
   (ii) myelitis
   and at least two of three supportive criteria:
   (i) spinal cord MRI lesion extending more than two vertebral segments
   (ii) MRI criteria not satisfying the revised McDonald diagnostic criteria (Polman et al. 2005) for multiple sclerosis
   (iii) aquaporin-4 antibody in serum.
B. The US National MS Society task force on differential diagnosis of multiple sclerosis (Miller et al. 2008); major criteria (all are required, but may be separated by an unspecified interval):
   (i) Optic neuritis in one or two eyes
   (ii) Transverse myelitis, clinically complete or incomplete, but associated with MRI evidence of spinal cord lesion extending more than two spinal segments on T_2-weighted MRI images and hypointensities on T_1-weighted images when obtained during acute episode of myelitis, and

163

(iii) No evidence for sarcoidosis, vasculitis, clinically manifest systemic lupus ery-thematosus, or Sjögren syndrome, or other explanation of the syndrome.

Minor criteria, of which at least one must be fulfilled:

1. Most recent brain MRI scan of the head must be normal or may show abnormalities not fulfilling the Barkhof criteria used for McDonald diagnostic criteria including
    (i) non-specific brain T_2-signal abnormalities not satisfying the Barkhof criteria for dissemination in space used in the revised McDonald criteria,
    (ii) lesions in the dorsal medulla, either in contiguity or not in contiguity with a spinal cord lesion,
    (iii) hypothalamic and/or brainstem lesions,
    (iv) linear periventricular/corpus callosum signal abnormality, but not ovoid, not extending into the parenchyma of the cerebral hemispheres in Dawson finger configuration.
2. Positive test in serum or CSF for NMO-IgG/aquaporin-4 antibodies.

Table 7.4 summarizes the clinical features in the three recent case series of paediatric NMO using diagnostic criteria. Although the current diagnostic criteria are as recommended by the IPMSSG, it is likely that modifications need to be considered with the evolution of new evolving MRI criteria such as those in Miller et al. (2008). Further prospective studies are needed to clarify the spectrum of these diseases.

Out of the 38 NMO cases described in the three studies, 16 (42%) tested negative for NMO-IgG. In children, as in adults (see Sellner et al. 2010), NMO-IgG positivity is associated with recurrence and higher risk syndromes; however, larger international prospective studies are required with standardization of antibody testing.

MRI BRAIN ABNORMALITIES IN NMO
In children in particular, the presence of brain lesions should not exclude NMO as a diagnosis because lesions located in the hypothalamus, brainstem, or cerebral white matter have been described in children who have typical features of NMO (as defined in Wingerchuk et al. 2006) (Fig. 7.3). Brain lesions in paediatric NMO hence appear to occur more commonly (50–100%) compared with adult NMO (25%) (Collongues et al. 2010a). A recent case series (Collongues et al. 2010b) showed that the first brain MRI in paediatric NMO (as defined in Wingerchuk et al. 2006) can show a diffuse inflammatory process, such as multiple-sclerosis-like (two patients) or acute disseminated encephalomyelitis-like lesions (one patient). Brain lesions in another series (Lotze et al. 2008) also confirmed this observation and demonstrated that MRI brain changes in paediatric NMO frequently involve the diencephalon. In another series (Banwell et al. 2008) nine out of 17 children with NMO (Wingerchuk et al. 2006) had brain lesions. It is important to recognize the spectrum of brain abnormalities in NMO, as the occurrence of such lesions and sometimes the presence of encephalopathy and polyfocal neurological deficits may resemble acute disseminated encephalomyelitis, with misleading implications as to prognosis and therapy (Table 7.4).

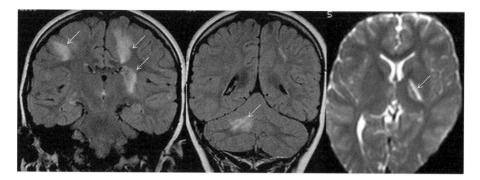

Fig. 7.3. MRI brain fluid-attenuated inversion recovery (FLAIR) sequences in a 5-year-old child with relapsing NMO showing, from left to right, multiple large, diffuse juxtacortical, and deep white matter lesions. There is also a left internal capsule lesion with restricted diffusion. This relapse was characterized by acute-onset encephalopathy and right-sided hemiplegia. The patient was treated with plasma exchange and on recovery was ambulatory with mild residual motor deficits. The patient had severe visual impairment from previous attacks of optic neuritis with onset at 3 years of age and persistently high NMO-IgG levels.

PAEDIATRIC NMO SPECTRUM DISORDERS

Cases that are NMO-IgG positive but not fulfilling current criteria have been described as NMO spectrum disorders in the literature, and the spectrum of these disorders is expanding both in adults and children (Belman et al. 2007).

The largest series on paediatric NMO spectrum disorders involved a cross-sectional study from one laboratory (USA), where 88 consecutive NMO-IgG seropositive paediatric patients were ascertained and followed up for a median of 1 year (McKeon et al. 2008). Clinical information was available for 58 (66%) children, with 88% being female and nearly three-quarters non-white, hence highlighting the female predominance and ethnic variation. The median age at symptom onset was 12 years (range 4–18). Presenting symptoms involved the brain in nine patients (16%). Median duration between attacks was 3 months (range 1–87). All but one (98%) had at least one attack of optic neuritis (78%) or transverse myelitis (78%). Other attack-related symptoms involved the brain or brainstem in 26 patients (45%). Thirty-eight (66%) cases fulfilled NMO diagnostic criteria (Wingerchuk et al. 2006) at follow-up. The median longitudinal extent of attack-related spinal cord MRI abnormalities was 10 vertebral segments. Thirty-eight (68%) had brain MRI abnormalities, predominantly involving periventricular areas and (in descending order of frequency) the medulla, supratentorial and infratentorial white matter, midbrain, cerebellum, thalamus, and hypothalamus. Surprisingly, additional autoantibodies were detected in 57 out of 75 patients (76%), and 16 out of 38 (42%) had a coexisting autoimmune disorder recorded (systemic lupus erythematosus, Sjogren syndrome, juvenile rheumatoid arthritis, Graves disease). Although this study provides useful information, conclusions cannot be universally extrapolated given the many limitations, including that the lack of information on a third of patients (possibly because of a milder course), the relatively short follow-up period, and the referral-centre-based retrospective laboratory ascertainment.

TABLE 7.4
Summary of recently described paediatric neuromyelitis optica case series

Reference	Setting, design and criteria used	Demographics	NMO-IgG and CSF OGB	First attack and course / Time to first relapse / ARR	MRI brain features	Disease modifying treatment	Outcome/disability
Collongues et al. 2010a	Multicentre (mainly adult). retrospective. France. Mean follow-up 19.3y. Wingerchuk et al. 2006 criteria.	12 cases. Median age 14.5y (4.1–17.9) 3F:1M	8/12 NMO-IgG positive	First attack: 6ON/5SC/1OS. All relapsing-remitting. First attack interval 17mo (7–154).	6/12 MRI brain abnormal (1–10 lesions). Three MS radiological criteria positive (two MS/one ADEM) 0 Barkhof	All treatments used: azathioprine; cyclophosphamide; glatiramer acetate; IVIG; interferon; mitoxantrone; MMF; rituximab.	Median time to EDSS 4, 20.7y. Vision: residual visual loss +1 logMAR or 20/200 Snellen=1.3y.
Lotze et al. 2008	Retrospective single centre. USA. Follow-up median 4y (0.6–9). Wingerchuk et al. 2006 criteria.	Nine cases. Median age 14y (1.9–16). All female.	6/9 NMO-IgG positive (one had recurrent ATM only)	First attack: 5OS/1TM/2ON. All relapsing. ARR=2.6.	9/9 MRI brain abnormal (five symptomatic).	All treatments used: six steroids + MMF; five rituximab; one had monthly IVIG; one had azathioprine, glatiramer, and monthly PLEX.	Median EDSS 3 (range 0–8)
Banwell et al. 2008	Selected prospective cohort. Canada and Argentina. Median follow-up 36mo (1.2–126). Wingerchuk et al. 1999.	17 cases. Median age 10.4y (4.4–15.2). 3.2F:1M.	8/17 NMO-IgG positive. 13 CSG OGB negative. (One recurrent ON, and one recurrent ATM NMO-IgG positive; 68 other CNS inflammatory demyelination were negative).	Nine relapsing (NMO-IgG positive). Eight monophasic (NMO-IgG positive).	9/17 MRI brain abnormal	At time of serum: seven prednisone, one glatiramer acetate, one interferon-1α, two had monthly IV cyclophosphamide.	One non-ambulant, one gait limited aid not required. Vision: 12/18 decreased visual acuity or severe visual impairment (4/18).

ADEM, acute disseminated encephalomyelitis; ARR, annualized relapse rate; EDSS, Expanded Disability Status Scale; IVIG, intravenous immunoglobulin; MMF, mycophenolate mofetil; MRI, magnetic resonance imaging; MS, multiple sclerosis; NMO-IgG, neuromyelitis optica antibodies; ON, optic neuritis; OS, optico-spinal; PLEX, plasmapharesis; SC, spinal cord; M:F, male to female ratio.

TREATMENT AND OUTCOME IN NMO

It is important to recognize NMO early in the course of the disease as permanent disability is more attack-related in NMO than in multiple sclerosis (Sellner et al. 2010). Hence, early and aggressive intensive treatment with disease-modifying treatment may be beneficial in reducing the disability and ameliorating the course of disease in children (see Banwell et al. 2008, Lotze et al. 2008, Miller et al. 2008, Collongues et al. 2010b, Sellner et al. 2010). There have been no large randomized trials in children or adults and current practice is based on case series and expert opinion. Recent adult European consensus guidelines have been published (Sellner et al. 2010). In children, acute exacerbations are usually treated with 5 days of intravenous steroids with or without intravenous immunoglobulin (Table 7.4). Severe exacerbations are treated with plasmapheresis. A wide variety of disease modifying drugs have recently been used (Table 7.4) but recent reports show that drugs used to treat multiple sclerosis (interferons, glatiramer) may exacerbate NMO (Palace et al. 2010). Future clinical trials incorporating children are needed in this condition.

Paediatric NMO appears to have a better prognosis than adult NMO in terms of disability. In one study, median time from onset to Expanded Disability Status Scale 4 ([significant disability but self-sufficient and able to walk without aid for approximately 500m] 20.7 vs 5.3y; $p<0.01$) and Expanded Disability Status Scale 6 ([requires a walking aid to walk about 100m] 26 vs 8.5y; $p<0.01$) was largely explained by the increased severity of the first myelitis in the adult NMO group (Collongues et al. 2010b). In contrast, the US paediatric NMO spectrum series showed residual disability in 43 out of 48 patients (90%), with 54% having visual impairment (27% blind) and 44% motor deficits (median Expanded Disability Status Scale 4.0) at 12 months (McKeon et al. 2008). Further prospective longitudinal studies are needed to clarify these findings.

Multiple sclerosis

The IPMSSG defined paediatric multiple sclerosis as requiring multiple episodes of CNS inflammatory demyelination separated in time and space as in adults. Dissemination in time can be met if new T_2- or gadolinium-enhancing lesions develop 3 months or more after the initial clinical event. Dissemination in space can be met by one of the following:

(1) The revised McDonald criteria for a 'positive MRI' are applied; with three of the following: (1) more than eight white matter lesions or one gadolinium enhancing lesion, (2) more than two periventricular lesions, (3) a juxtacortical lesion, (4) an infratentorial lesion
(2) The combination of an abnormal CSF (oligoclonal bands or elevated IgG index) and two lesions on the MRI (at least one in brain).

Compared with other presentations of a clinically isolated syndrome, isolated ATM carries the lowest risk of progression to multiple sclerosis (Defresne et al. 2003, Mikaeloff et al. 2004). Studies comparing ATM with a polyfocal clinically isolated syndrome and multiple sclerosis are sparse. Case series in ATM have also reported that several patients have asymptomatic brain lesions (Table 7.2). In a French cohort of children with a first attack of CNS inflammatory demyelination, 7% (2/29) with a monofocal ATM at presentation were later diagnosed with multiple sclerosis (Mikaeloff et al. 2004). Another series reported only 2% (1 out of 47) of ATM cases progressing to multiple sclerosis (Pidcock et al. 2007). However, 31% (13 out of 42) of children with polysymptomatic clinical features including transverse myelitis at presentation were later diagnosed with multiple sclerosis (Mikaeloff et al. 2004). This highlights the importance of differentiating isolated ATM from ATM that is part of a polyfocal syndrome.

In adults with multiple sclerosis, spinal lesions are usually fewer than two segments in length and located in the posterolateral aspect of the spinal cord (Campi et al. 1995, Sheerin et al. 2009, Alper et al. 2011). A recent adult study (Young et al. 2009) found that 50% of patients converted to clinically definite multiple sclerosis when they had the combination of ATM and brain lesions (Controlled High-Risk Subjects Avonex Multiple Sclerosis Prevention Study Criteria [Jacobs et al. 2000]; more than one brain lesion greater than 3mm in diameter with at least one periventricular or ovoid). Children with multiple sclerosis have also been shown to tend to have spinal lesions less than three segments (see Fig. 7.4),

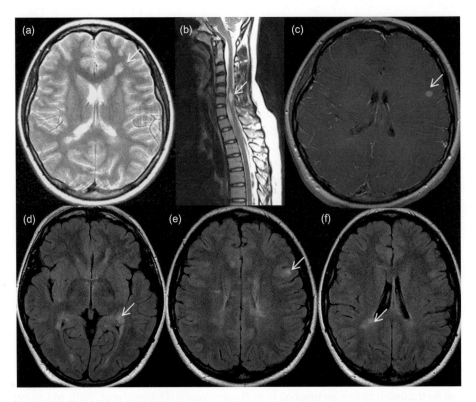

Fig. 7.4. MRI of the brain and spinal cord of a 15-year-old female with clinically relapsing remitting multiple sclerosis (positive oligoclonal bands). There are multiple T_2-weighted and FLAIR lesions: periventricular (a, d, f), juxtacortical (e), gadolinium enhancing on T_1 (c), infratentorial spinal lesion spanning two vertebral cervical segments (b), hence fulfilling McDonald criteria.

although longer segments (longitudinally extensive transverse myelitis) have been reported to progress to multiple sclerosis as well (Verhey et al. 2010). Further prospective studies with longer term follow-up are needed to clarify this.

Radiation myelitis

Radiation myelitis is a white matter injury to the cord and is a consequence of spinal irradiation after a latent period of as early as 2 months to several years (Rampling and Symonds 1998, Okada and Okeda 2001). It involves myelinated fibres and blood vessels. The clinical features of the resulting myelopathy are variable, with onset being acute or with a more insidious chronic presentation. Severity is varied, with the most serious consequences arising with complete transection of the cord at the irradiated level. The condition is regarded as irreversible with no proven treatment. Several factors, such as radiation dose, modify its occurrence and severity. Radiation myelitis has rarely been reported in children. In a case report (Antunes et al. 2002) where a 5-year-old received craniospinal radiation after chemotherapy for a CNS relapse of leukaemia, myelitis developed 2 months after completion of radiation. The child developed a progressive quadriparesis, and MRI revealed an enhancing lesion involving the medulla and upper cervical cord. A high index of suspicion is needed, accompanied by typical MRI findings (low signal intensity on T_1- and high signal intensity on T_2-weighted images respectively, usually with gadolinium enhancement and cord swelling) (Wang et al. 1992) to make the diagnosis.

Tropical spastic paraparesis and HTLV-1-associated myelopathy

HTLV-1 is a human RNA retrovirus and the aetiological agent of tropical spastic paraparesis. Infection by HTLV-I is known to occur in many parts of the world, including southwest Japan, the Caribbean islands, Central and West Africa, the southeast USA, and South America (Bittencourt et al. 2006). HTLV-associated myelopathy/tropical spastic paraparesis is a chronic and disabling demyelinating myelopathy of adults. It occurs rarely in children, with few cases reported in the literature (usually with a preceding history of infective dermatitis caused by HTLV-I and always involving the scalp). In contrast to the adult form of the disease, the paediatric form appears to have a more rapid and progressive clinical course, typically over 1 to 2 years (Primo et al. 2005).

Serological screening for HTLV-1 should hence be performed in children presenting with myelopathy preceded by recurrent or chronic forms of eczema in endemic areas. Additionally, HTLV-1 may be transmitted vertically, with breastfeeding being the primary source.

A recent paediatric case report described a patient presenting with progressive cognitive impairment over a few years in association with a more protracted course of myelopathic motor symptoms as the clinical manifestation of HTLV-I infection (Zorzi et al. 2010). HTLV-I infection may therefore be associated with a wider spectrum of neurological syndromes, requiring a high index of suspicion.

There are no clinical trials for HTLV-associated myelopathy/tropical spastic paraparesis, and its treatment usually includes high dose intravenous methylprednisolone, followed by a few weeks to 3 months of oral prednisolone (1mg/kg/d) with minimal improvement in motor and sphincter function reported (Primo et al. 2005). Other treatment options include interferon-α and immunoglobulins.

Human immunodeficiency virus and myelopathy

Neurological complications related to infection with HIV in children are well-recognized (Lobato et al. 1995, Cooper et al. 1998). HIV encephalopathy predominates. Most children with HIV have congenitally or perinatally acquired infection. Vertical transmission of HIV from mother to child can occur during pregnancy, at the time of delivery, or postnatally through breast-feeding. HIV-infected infants are usually normal at birth.

Symptoms usually start in the first few years of life and include developmental delay or cognitive regression, progressive corticospinal tract dysfunction, and an acquired micro-cephaly. HIV-1 infection of the nervous system in children involves the brain more often than the spinal cord (George et al. 2009). Neurological complications of HIV result from multiple mechanisms; HIV may be neurotoxic; it may cause autoimmune disease due to immune deregulation; or it may lead to opportunistic infections due to immune suppression.

Spinal cord involvement in HIV infection can be categorized as direct (vacuolar myelopathy) and indirect or secondary due to opportunistic processes (Table 7.5). In children, pathology is mainly due to direct HIV infection. Opportunistic infections due to reactivation of dormant organisms are uncommon, as children have not usually been exposed to the responsible organisms.

Vacuolar myelopathy is the most common chronic myelopathy associated with HIV infection in adults. Rarely diagnosed clinically, on autopsy the prevalence in adults is approximately 15% (Petito et al. 1985). In childhood the prevalence is unknown, but is thought to be rare (Dickson et al. 1989).

Clinical signs include a symmetric spastic paraparesis, with lower extremity hyperre-flexia, and impaired proprioception. Sensory ataxia and bladder dysfunction may be present. There is usually no sensory level. Upper extremity dysfunction is less common, although hyperreflexia may be present in the arms. Progression usually occurs slowly over a few months. This myelopathy usually occurs during the late stages of HIV infection, when CD4 lymphocyte counts are low. MRI may occasionally reveal cord atrophy, but neuroimaging is often unremarkable. CSF is non-specific or shows a mild increase in protein levels. Occasionally co-infection with reactivated measles, cytomegalovirus, tuberculosis, herpes zoster, and schistosomiasis has been reported. Pathological examination demonstrates vacu-olization in the posterior and lateral columns of the spinal cord (Dal Pan et al. 1994). Despite

---

TABLE 7.5

Myelopathy and human immunodeficiency virus

Direct: primary human immunodeficiency virus
• Human immunodeficiency virus seroconversion myelopathy
• Vacuolar myelopathy
Indirect: neurological opportunistic processes
• Herpes viruses: varicella zoster virus, cytomegalovirus, herpes
  simplex virus
• Bacterial: tuberculosis
• Neoplasm: lymphoma

---

a clinical and pathological similarity to sub-acute combined degeneration of the spinal cord, vitamin B_{12} levels are normal. Vacuolar myelopathy is very rarely symptomatic or diagnosed in young children with HIV infection (Wilmshurst et al. 2006), although pathological abnormalities of the spinal cord are frequently seen at autopsy (Dickson et al. 1989).

Infectious and neoplastic disorders may cause myelopathy in patients with HIV infection and must be considered in the differential diagnosis of vacuolar myelopathy. Compared with vacuolar myelopathy, other aetiologies may progress more rapidly or are associated with back or radicular pain. Causes of infective myelitis include cytomegalovirus, varicella zoster virus, cryptococcus, and herpes simplex virus (see differential diagnosis of ATM). Children with myelitis associated with cytomegalovirus retinitis have been reported (Gungor et al. 1993, Marriage et al. 1996). Other rarer causes may include *Mycobacterium tuberculosis* and *Toxoplasma gondii* (Bhigjee et al. 2001). The CSF should be tested for the presence of HIV and other pathogens; viral cultures should be done with specific emphasis on cytomegalovirus and herpes simplex virus type 1 and 2, as well as bacterial and fungal cultures and cryptococcal antigen. An acute myelopathy of uncertain pathogenesis can occur at the time of seroconversion to HIV (Denning et al. 1987).

Primary CNS lymphoma is the most common malignancy associated with HIV in childhood (Esptein et al. 1988). There is evidence that nuclear material from polyomavirus, Epstein–Barr virus, cytomegalovirus, herpes virus, and HIV can integrate with the host genome and change the microenvironment, increasing the risk of malignant transformation (Agius 2004).

Clinical and immunological events can be slowed or arrested by antiretroviral therapies, hence influencing the natural course of HIV. However, it remains uncertain whether the incidence of myelopathy has been altered by the use of antiretroviral treatment. Currently there is no specific treatment for vacuolar myelopathy, but supportive and symptomatic treatment of the spasticity and sphincter dysfunction are important management goals.

Spinal cord ischaemia

Spinal cord infarction in children is a rare yet clinically important condition. There are only a few case reports and series in the paediatric literature. Many questions remain unanswered about its incidence, diagnosis, and best management. There is no comprehensive epidemiological review of ischaemic spinal cord infarction in children or adults. Autopsy series have estimated that 5 to 8% of all acute myelopathies in adults are associated with ischaemia (Sandson and Friedman 1989).

Clinical features of spinal cord infarction typically start with sudden-onset sensory symptoms, especially pain followed by weakness within minutes or hours. Urine retention and loss of control of bladder and bowel usually occur. Depending on the vascular supply involved, different spinal cord syndromes have been described (Table 7.6).

The spinal cord is supplied by an anterior spinal artery (arising from the vertebral arteries) and two posterior spinal arteries (arising from the vertebral or posterior inferior cerebellar arteries) and the spinal radicular arteries. The anterior spinal artery supplies the anterior two-thirds of the spinal cord. The anterior and posterior arteries form a plexus surrounding

TABLE 7.6
Summary of the clinical features of spinal cord ischaemic syndromes

Spinal cord stroke syndrome	Clinical features
Anterior spinal artery infarct	Back pain: severe diffuse, radicular or girdle-like
	Corticospinal tract deficit: bilateral weakness
	Spinothalamic deficit: pain and sensory deficit below the cord level
	Sparing of dorsal column: vibration and position sense intact
	Autonomic system deficit: sphincter (bladder/bowel) disturbance
	Depending on cord level: respiratory failure, hypotension
Posterior spinal artery infarct	Dorsal column deficit: loss of proprioception, vibration and position sense
	With or without corticospinal tracts deficit: bilateral weakness

the spinal cord. From the aorta, six to ten spinal radicular arteries arise and supply the spinal cord. The great radicular artery of Adamkiewicz arises from the left between T5 and L3 and is the major blood supply to the lumbar and sacral cord. The mid-thoracic region (T4–T8) is an area of relatively decreased perfusion and is susceptible to infarction.

Occasionally a partial syndrome is seen, and symptoms may also be unilateral and present as a Brown–Sequard syndrome. If grey matter of the cord is mainly affected, the deficit may spare sphincter control and sensory function. A central infarct gives bilateral spinothalamic sensory deficit, but motor control is preserved. A transverse infarct results in bilateral motor deficit and complete sensory deficit (Novy et al. 2006).

Ischaemic spinal cord infarction may be difficult to distinguish from other myelopathies. In contrast to acute cerebral stroke, MRI has been less useful for spinal cord ischemia. The most common MRI abnormality is a swollen spinal cord that is hyper-intense on T_2-weighted images with a 'pencil like' shape which may enhance with gadolinium on T_1-weighted images (Shimizu et al. 1996, Weidauer et al. 2002). A central medullary T_2 hyper-intensity involving multiple levels is the classical feature observed. Sensitivity and specificity of diffusion-weighted imaging in acute spinal cord ischemia is unknown (Thurnher and Bammer 2006). Diffusion-weighted imaging restriction was confirmatory in four children with anterior spinal artery infarcts (Beslow et al. 2008). Ischaemic abnormalities in the vertical bodies producing T_2 hyper-intensity, if present, may help confirm the diagnosis of spinal cord infarct (Suzuki et al. 2003, Parazzini et al. 2006). Spinal angiography can identify an arterio-venous malformation, which is one of the rare causes of spinal cord ischaemia. CT angiography could be an alternative to selective angiography (Ou et al. 2007). Even where urgent imaging fails to provide a definite diagnosis, it is vital in excluding cord compression.

In many children the aetiology of spinal cord infarction remains unclear, even after extensive work-up, or is found to be multi-factorial with no clear single cause (Table 7.7). Paediatric spinal trauma can cause indirect cord injury from an associated vascular injury, such as arterial disruption or thrombosis. Other causes include hypotension, intravascular injury, cerebellar herniation, thrombotic or embolic disease (e.g. vasculitis in CNS infections or other thrombotic disorders, and fibro-cartilaginous embolism), vasculitis, atlanto-axial instability, microcirculatory compromise, and venous congestion due to arteriovenous

172

TABLE 7.7
Aetiology of spinal infarct in children

Probable mechanism	Aetiology of spinal infarct in children
Hypotension (systemic)	Cardiac arrest
	Blood loss
	Perinatal hypoxic ischaemia in newborn (Sladky and Rorke 1986, Clancy et al. 1989)
	Trauma
	Blood loss
Intravascular injury	Umbilical catheters
Instrumentation	Thoracic neuroblastoma surgery
Minor trauma	Aortic coarctation repair
Major trauma	Spinal cord injury without radiological abnormality
Cerebellar herniation	Metabolic encephalopathy with or without lumbar puncture
	Meningitis with lumbar puncture
Thrombotic disease	Thrombotic vasculitis in central nervous system infections
	Thrombotic disorders
Vasculitis	Systemic lupus erythematosus
	Antiphospholipid syndrome (Hasegawa et al. 1993)
	Meningitis
Embolic	Fibrocartilaginous embolism (Tan et al. 2009)
	Sclerotherapy of oesophageal varices
Microcirculatory compromise	Arteriovenous malformations
	Hirayama disease (Elsheikh et al. 2009)
	Tumour infiltration of leptomeninges (Martinez-Lage et al. 2009)
Atlanto-axial instability	Achondrodysplasia
	I-cell disease
	Down syndrome (Sohal et al. 2009)
Venous congestive due to arteriovenous shunting	Scoliosis surgery (Dapunt et al. 2009)
Multifactorial	
Unknown	

shunting. Most of these risk factors are derived from case reports or small series reported in the literature (Nance and Golomb 2007). Causes to consider, although not yet reported in children, include cocaine abuse (Weidauer et al. 2002) and diving-related barotrauma/ decompression sickness (Warren et al. 1988). Indirect damage can also be caused by hyper-extension injury; a distinct subgroup of transverse myelopathy (up to 10% of cases) is recognized and termed spinal cord injury without neuroimaging abnormality (Trigylidas et al. 2010).

The prognosis of spinal cord infarction is thought to be poor; however, there are no good long-term outcome studies in children. Besides the inability to walk, morbidity may include ventilator dependence, loss of bowel and bladder function, recurrent respiratory and urinary tract infections, chronic pain, and spasticity. Several reviews in adults have reported outcomes (Salvador de la Barrera et al. 2001, De Seze et al. 2003). A review of outcomes reported in 199 adult patients reported that 22% died, 24% did not improve, 35% showed some improvement, and 19% improved markedly (Cheshire et al. 1996) This review included only two patients younger than 20 years old. A risk factor for poor outcome is significant motor deficit at presentation (Cheshire et al. 1996, Nedeltchev et al. 2004). A study of 19 children with meningitis and spinal cord infarction reported outcomes of death in five, mild improvement in 12, and normal function in two (Moffett and Berkowitz 1997). In another review of 20 previously reported cases of spinal cord infarction of various types, two children died in the acute stage, and of the remainder, only seven were mobile. Of these seven children, all had neurological sequelae and required assistance to walk (Sohal et al. 2009).

Treatment is primarily based on the underlying aetiology, such as anti-coagulation for thrombotic disorders, and steroid therapy for vasculitis. Supportive care, physiotherapy, occupational therapy, and rehabilitation are important in the management of children with spinal cord infarction.

Neurodegenerative, metabolic, and nutritional disorders affecting the spinal cord
NEURODEGENERATIVE DISORDERS
Childhood neurodegenerative disorders comprise of a large and diverse group of heterogeneous conditions that are often categorized into (1) disorders involving subcellular organelles like the lysosomes, (2) disorders of intermediary metabolism, (3) disorders of metal, especially copper, metabolism, (4) leukodystrophies, and (5) a heredodegenerative group of disorders such as hereditary spastic paraplegia (Aicardi and Hanefeld 2009, Ogier et al. 2009). Clinical manifestations of spinal cord pathology are less prominent than brain involvement, occurring only in a handful of these, although it is likely that subclinical involvement is present more often with spinal cord symptoms and signs masked by the severe brain pathology. Spinal cord pathology may also arise in some disorders as a result of compression from bony involvement in, for example, the mucolipidoses and mucopolysaccharidoses (Wraith 2004). X-linked adrenoleukodystrophy and Krabbe disease are two leukodystrophies that may present with a predominant myelopathy.

X-linked adrenoleukodystrophy
X-linked adrenoleukodystrophy (Online Mendelian Inheritance in Man [OMIM] 300100), results from alteration to the *ABCD1* gene, resulting in a defect in peroxisomal beta oxidation and the accumulation of the saturated very long-chain fatty acids in all tissues of the body (Moser et al. 2007). The disorder primarily affects the adrenal cortex and the nervous system. The phenotypes can be subdivided into four main categories: cerebral inflammatory, adrenomyeloneuropathy (AMN), Addison-only, and asymptomatic (Moser et al. 2007), although different phenotypes may manifest in a patient. In adulthood, for example, the inflammatory phenotype is most commonly superimposed on pre-existing AMN.

In childhood, the most common neurological presentation is the cerebral inflammatory phenotype. The early manifestations (age 4–8y) often resemble attention-deficit–hyperactivity disorder or other learning issues. A progressive behavioural, intellectual, and neurological decline ensues, often leading to total disability within 3 years of presentation. This clinical deterioration is accompanied by neuroradiological and neuropathological features of an inflammatory demyelinating process (Moser et al. 2007). The classic posterior pattern involvement of white matter is observed in the neuroimaging of 80% of male children with this childhood cerebral phenotype (Kumar et al. 1987), with the percentage being somewhat lower in older patients (see Loes et al. 2003). AMN is the most common phenotype to present in adulthood. The principal abnormality in AMN is a non-inflammatory distal axonopathy, which involves the dorsal column and corticospinal tract in the lower thoracic and lumbar regions. Paraparesis can, however, begin in early adolescence although most commonly present after the second decade and is slowly progressive through to adulthood (Fenichel 2005).

Lorenzo's oil, combined with moderate reduction of dietary fat, normalizes or significantly lowers the levels of very long-chain fatty acids in the plasma of patients with X-linked adrenoleukodystrophy. However, this striking biochemical effect did not significantly alter the rate of progression in individuals who were already symptomatic, but may provide a preventive effect in asymptomatic male children whose brain MRI is normal (Moser et al. 2007). An open study of the effects of Lorenzo's oil on neurological progression in 45 adult males with pure AMN demonstrated significantly slower neurological progression compared with the pre-treatment period (Moser et al. 2007). Bone marrow or umbilical cord haemopoietic stem-cell transplantation appears favourable in patients in whom transplantation was performed at the early stage of the illness (Peters et al. 2004). However, the use of transplantation is significantly limited in adulthood, and the potential benefits in patients with AMN remains unclear.

Krabbe disease

Krabbe disease is caused by a deficiency of the enzyme galactocerebrosidase, which results in the accumulation of a toxic intermediate psychosine (Wenger 2000). Severe demyelination of both the CNS and the peripheral nervous system ensues. Most cases are an early infantile form, with onset between 3 and 6 months of life. In this infantile form, or classic Krabbe disease, the disorder is aggressive and rapidly progressive (Korn-Lubetski et al. 2003). The characteristic clinical finding of opisthotonic posturing and absent reflexes alerts the clinician to a central and peripheral nervous system involvement (Korn-Lubetski et al. 2003). Hyperpyrexia, irritability, and inconsolable crying (often described as 'crabby') are also typical. Death usually follows the onset of loss of bulbar function at around the second year of life. Nerve conduction velocities are delayed owing to demyelination of the peripheral nervous system, and the protein content of CSF is always elevated (Ogier et al. 2009). Brain MRI shows signs of leukodystrophy, with symmetric signal abnormalities usually noted in the periventricular region of the posterior cerebral hemispheres.

In the less prevalent late-onset forms, the clinical presentation can be very variable. Intellectual deterioration is not inevitable, where optic atrophy and tremor are more common. Patients may also present with a slowly progressive paraplegia often accompanied by visual failure (Kolodny et al. 1991).

Transplantation of umbilical-cord blood from unrelated donors in asymptomatic infants with infantile Krabbe disease favourably altered the natural history of the disease (Escolar et al. 2005). Allogeneic hematopoietic stem-cell transplantation has been previously reported to be beneficial in patients with early stages of juvenile Krabbe disease (see Krivit et al.

1998), although this remains unevaluated in the primary slow progressive paraparesis phenotype.

Hereditary spastic paraplegias

Hereditary spastic paraplegias (HSPs) are a clinically and genetically heterogeneous group of conditions that are characterized by the presence of lower limb spasticity and weakness (Harding 1993). The onset of HSP is often subtle, with the development of leg stiffness or abnormal wear of the shoes. Compared with other causes of spastic paraplegia, such as multiple sclerosis and spinal injury, there is relative preservation of power despite dramatically increased tone in the legs, particularly in patients with early-onset disease. The key diagnostic clinical findings are of lower limb spasticity and pyramidal weakness, with hyper-reflexia and extensor plantar responses. The common pathological feature of these conditions is retrograde degeneration of the longest nerve fibres in the corticospinal tracts and posterior columns (Harding1993).

HSP can be inherited as an autosomal dominant, recessive, or X-linked recessive trait, and at least 41 spastic paraplegia gene (*SPG*) loci have been mapped and up to 17 genes identified so far (Salinas et al. 2008). For practical purposes, HSP is divided according to mode of inheritance and presence or absence of complicating features. Most cases of pure HSP are autosomal dominant, whereas complicated (other extra spinal features) forms tend to be autosomal recessive.

Autosomal dominant HSP is the most prevalent form and represents around 70% of cases. *SPAST*-gene-associated HSP-associated HSP (OMIM 603277) is the most common type of pure autosomal dominant HSP, accounting for 40 to 45% of such cases (Hazan et al. 1999), and is the form that has been clinically studied in the most detail. This type of HSP typically has onset from childhood through to late adult life (McDermott et al. 2006). More than half of mutation carriers will not develop symptoms under the age of 30 years. In most cases, the phenotype is of a slowly progressive spasticity in the lower limbs with loss of mobility around two decades after the onset of symptoms (McDermott et al. 2006). *SPG3A*-associated HSP (OMIM 606439) is the second most common cause of autosomal dominant HSP, accounting for approximately 10% of cases. It usually has a pure phenotype, presenting earlier (often before the age of 10y), although there is relatively slow progression of symptoms (Namekawa et al. 2006). Mutations in *REEP1* (formerly *SPG31*; OMIM 609139*)* lead to a pure form of autosomal dominant HSP that has a variable age at onset. Mutations in the *REEP1* gene have been identified in 3% of a sample of unrelated patients with HSP, which increased to 8.2% in pure HSP if those with *SPG3A* and *SPAST* mutations were excluded (Beetz et al. 2008).

The most common autosomal recessive HSP with a childhood presentation is *SPG11*-associated HSP (OMIM 610844), which is characterized by a thin corpus callosum, cognitive impairment and severe axonal neuropathy (Stevanin et al. 2008). Most of the other 16 forms of autosomal recessive HSP are rare, with only up to one to 20 families being affected (Salinas et al. 2008). X-linked HSP caused by mutations in *L1CAM* (formerly *SPG1*; OMIM 308840) is characterized by hydrocephalus, intellectual disability, spasticity of the legs, and adducted thumbs (Jouet et al. 1994). The phenotypic spectrum of *L1CAM* syndrome is

X-linked hydrocephalus with aqueduct stenosis, MASA syndrome (intellectual disability, aphasia, spastic paraplegia, and adducted thumbs), and X-linked agenesis of the corpus callosum. Mutations in the proteolipoprotein gene (*PLP1*, formerly *SPG2*; OMIM 300401) at Xq21–q22 have been found in families with mainly complicated HSP in which there may be an associated peripheral neuropathy and white matter changes on brain MRI. Mutations (usually duplications) of this gene also give rise to the dysmyelinating condition Pelizaeus–Merzbacher disease, which is characterized by congenital hypotonia, an eye movement disorder, psychomotor deterioration, and progressive pyramidal, dystonic, and cerebellar signs (Inoue 2005). The variation in phenotype between Pelizaeus–Merzbacher disease and *PLP1*-linked HSP is thought to arise from the differential effect that mutations can have on the two isoforms of the protein product, proteolipoprotein 1 (PLP1) and DM20 (Inoue 2005).

METABOLIC AND NUTRITIONAL DISORDERS
Arginase deficiency
Arginase catalyses the metabolism of arginine to ornithine and urea in the urea cycle. Patients present with motor and cognitive decline in early childhood with ensuing neurological regression. Progressive spastic diplegia, recurrent vomiting, and seizures are invariably present. The diagnosis is suspected on the basis of elevated plasma arginine and ammonia levels, and can subsequently be confirmed either by measuring the enzyme level in erythrocytes (usually <1% of normal) or by genetic testing of *ARG1*, the only gene known to be associated with arginase deficiency. Some patients have been shown to have cognitive and motor improvement after dietary intervention (Prasad et al. 1997).

Vitamin B$_{12}$ (cobalamin) deficiency
Vitamin B$_{12}$ deficiency may cause haematological (pernicious anaemia), gastrointestinal, neurological, and psychiatric involvement (Healton et al. 1991). However, neurological disease can occur in the absence of anaemia or macrocytosis (Green and Kinsella 1995). The neurological features of vitamin B$_{12}$ deficiency in patients include peripheral neuropathy, posterior and lateral column degeneration of the spinal cord termed 'subacute combined degeneration of the cord' (SCD), autonomic dysfunction, optic atrophy, mood and behaviour changes, psychosis, memory impairment, and cognitive decline (Reynolds 2006). Neurological manifestations are caused by predominantly white matter degenerative lesions in the brain, spinal cord, and peripheral nerve. Patients may present with paraesthesia of the feet and fingers, disturbed vibratory and proprioceptive senses, and spasticity.

Although less common in childhood, symptomatic vitamin B$_{12}$ deficiency causing SCD can occur as a consequence of inadequate dietary intake (Cornejo et al. 2001, Licht et al. 2001). SCD has been reported in a 15-year-old male child with early-onset cobalamin C (cblC) disorder, an inborn error of metabolism in which formation of the two coenzymatically active derivatives of vitamin B$_{12}$ (deoxyadenosylcobalamin and methylcobalamin) is impaired (Smith et al. 2006). Deficiency in transcobalamin II, a serum transport protein for vitamin B$_{12}$, has also been reported to cause SCD in childhood (Teplitsky et al. 2003). Congenital (Zittoun et al. 1988) or acquired (Frank and Ashwal 2006) intrinsic factor deficiency, malabsorptive states resulting from surgical resection (Banerji and Hurwitz 1971), inherited disease of the specific ileal receptor (Matthews and Linnell 1982), removal of the vitamin from the intestine by bacteria or parasites, and malnutrition arising from chronic illnesses are other conditions where neurological manifestations including a myelopathy have been reported (Frank and Ashwal 2006).

Intramuscular injection of 1 to 5µg of cobalamin results in prompt haematological improvement and serves as a confirmatory test for deficiency. Oral administration of 1000µg at monthly intervals prevents recurrent deficiency, and 1000µg given at weekly intervals is suggested for the treatment of neurological deficits (Frank and Ashwal 2006). B_{12} deficiency is usually treated with intramuscular dosing and less commonly with high-dose oral vitamin B_{12}, as the oral form generally has low bioavailability, especially in patients with malabsorption. However, more recently, newer proprietary formulations are proving to be as effective and less costly than intramuscular injections (Castelli et al. 2011).

Published experience in adults suggests that sensory symptoms begin to improve more quickly than motor symptoms, usually within the first 6 weeks (Reynolds 2006). No improvement within 3 months should raise doubts about the significance of a low serum vitamin B_{12} concentration in relation to the neurological disorder. In adults, the duration and degree of neurological recovery is correlated with the duration of preceding symptoms and the severity of disability before treatment. In a large series, just fewer than 50% of patients made a complete recovery. About 90% of patients can expect at least 50% improvement in disability and up to 10% may be left with moderate to severe disability (Healton et al. 1991). Although such data are not available for children, an approach of early diagnosis and aggressive treatment is imperative.

Folate deficiency

Folate deficiency also causes a megaloblastic anaemia, with patients demonstrating spinal cord, peripheral nerve, and mental health disorder (Reynolds 2006). Compared with patients with vitamin B_{12} deficiency, patients with folate deficiency appear to have a higher incidence of neuropsychiatric disorders, but a lower incidence of peripheral neuropathy and SCD. In keeping with this, folate deficiency causing SCD has only been reported in a child with 5,10-methylenetetrahydrofolate reductase deficiency, an inborn error of folate metabolism (Clayton et al. 1986), and not in any acquired form of dietary deficiency.

Treatment with 2 to 5mg folic acid for up to a month is sufficient to reverse the non-CNS manifestations of folate deficiency (Frank and Ashwal 2006). As with Vitamin B_{12}, the reversal of neurological deficits in response to folate treatment is slow over many months, at least in part because of the poor CNS penetration (Reynolds 2002). Treatment should be for at least 6 months, but some improvement should be detected within 3 months. Again, the response and the degree of residual disability will be related to the duration and severity of nervous system complications before treatment (Reynolds 2006).

Inadequate maternal folate intake and status is one of several well-established factors that can increase the risk of neural-tube defects, especially spina bifida and anencephaly (Eichholzer et al. 2006). Interestingly, impaired vitamin B_{12} status (Ray and Blom 2003) and high plasma homocysteine (Rosenquist et al. 1996) are also suspected to be additional or related risk factors. Preconception preventive treatment with 400μg folic acid significantly reduces the risk of such defects but at least a third of neural-tube defects are not preventable (MRC Vitamin Study Research Group 1991).

Copper deficiency

Acquired copper deficiency has been recognized as a rare cause of anaemia and neutropenia for over half a century. Copper deficiency myelopathy was only described within the past decade, and represents a treatable cause of non-compressive myelopathy that closely mimics subacute degeneration of the cord due to vitamin B_{12} deficiency (Schleper and Stuerenburg 2001). Patients typically present with gait difficulties, which arise through sensory ataxia due to dorsal column dysfunction and spasticity. Clinical examination usually reveals a spastic paraparesis or tetraparesis with a truncal sensory level for dorsal column modalities. A sensori-motor neuropathy frequently coexists and manifests as depression of distal reflexes and superimposed sensory impairment in a glove-and-stocking distribution (Jaiser and Winston 2010). Of the 55 cases reported in the literature, this myelopathy most frequently presented in the fifth and sixth decades, with only one case presenting in the 20s (Jaiser and Winston 2010). Risk factors included previous upper gastrointestinal surgery, zinc overload, and malabsorption syndromes, all of which impair copper absorption in the upper gastrointestinal tract.

The effects of copper deficiency on the developing brain appears complex, and children born to mothers with copper deficiency have impaired cognitive and behavioural function (Gambling and McArdle 2004). In Menkes disease (OMIM 309400), the basolateral membrane by a P-type ATPase (ATP7A) is deficient, causing impaired copper absorption that occurs predominantly in the duodenum and potentially also in the stomach (Jaiser and Winston 2010). The integral role of many copper-dependent enzymes in human biology is reflected in the multisystem and severe presentation of this condition, which includes a relentless neurodegenerative process with an arteriopathy (Kodama et al. 1999). CNS demyelination secondary to hypocupraemia has been reported in a patient with Wilson disease who was over-treated (Narayan and Kaveer 2006), but as yet a pure myelopathy has not been reported in childhood. Given the increased awareness of copper deficiency in the past few years, it is likely that reports of childhood presentation will emerge.

Abetalipoproteinaemia and vitamin E deficiency

Studies in patients with abetalipoproteinaemia, other chronic and severe fat malabsorptive states, and a selective defect in vitamin E absorption, together with neuropathological studies, indicate that vitamin E is important for normal neurological function (Muller 2010). Abetalipoproteinemia is a rare, autosomal recessive disorder caused by mutations in the gene encoding the large subunit of microsomal triglyceride transfer protein (MTP; OMIM 157147). It is characterized by fat malabsorption, acanthocytosis, and hypocholesterolemia in infancy. Its longer-term effects are mediated by the deficiency of fat-soluble vitamins causing atypical retinitis pigmentosa, coagulopathy, spinal pathology, and myopathy (Zamel et al. 2008). In particular, the long-term sequelae on the CNS result from vitamin E deficiency. Other causes of vitamin E deficiency include malabsorption due to disorders of fat metabolism, and mutations in *TTPA* gene (OMIM 277460), which encodes for a soluble protein that binds α-tocopherol (causing ataxia and vitamin E deficiency).

Treatment with high oral doses of fat-soluble vitamins, including vitamin E (2400–1200IU) appears to have been associated with arrest of the CNS symptoms and other complications in some patients (see Muller et al. 1977, Zamel et al. 2008). Neuropathological studies in patients and animals deficient in vitamin E reveal degeneration of the axons of the posterior columns and a selective loss of large calibre myelinated sensory axons in the spinal cord and peripheral nerves, which is particularly severe in the posterior columns (Nelson et al. 1981). Concordant with that finding, patients who have either primary or secondary vitamin E deficiency all appear to demonstrate the characteristic phenotype of an ataxic myeloneuropathy.

Biotinidase deficiency
Biotinidase deficiency is an autosomal recessive disorder due to alteration in the *BTD* gene (OMIM 609019), which affects the endogenous recycling of biotin, resulting in multiple carboxylase deficiency, often manifesting during childhood with various cutaneous and neurological symptoms. Neurological symptoms commonly include seizures, ataxia, hearing loss, optic atrophy, and developmental delay (Wolf 2001). Spinal cord involvement is less frequently reported (Wiznitzer and Bangert 2003), but can occur in the absence of the more characteristic neurological manifestation (Chedrawi et al. 2008). Importantly, biotin replacement may modify or reverse the neurological features including myelopathy.

REFERENCES

Absoud M, Cummins C, Desai N, et al. Childhood optic neuritis clinical features and outcome. *Arch Dis Child* 2011; **96**: 860–862.

Agius LM. Viral participation in cellular and microenvironmental transformation and amplification towards malignancy in AIDS patients. *Med Hypotheses* 2004; **62**: 593–599.

Aicardi J, Hanefeld F. In Aicardi J, editor. Diseases of the Nervous System in Children (3rd edition). London: Mac Keith Press, 2009: 327–380.

Alper G, Petropoulou KA, Fitz CR, Kim Y. Idiopathic acute transverse myelitis in children: an analysis and discussion of MRI findings. *Mult Scler* 2011; **17**: 74–80.

Antunes NL, Wolden S, Souweidane MM, Lis E, Rosenblum M, Steinherz PG. Radiation myelitis in a 5-year-old girl. *J Child Neurol* 2002; **17**: 217–219.

Bailey SL, Carpentier PA, McMahon EJ, Begolka WS, Miller SD. Innate and adaptive immune responses of the central nervous system. *Crit Rev Immunol* 2006; **26**: 149–188.

Banerji NK, Hurwitz, LJ. Nervous system manifestations after gastric surgery. *Acta Neurol Scand* 1971; **47**: 485–513.

Banwell BL. The long (-itudinally extensive) and the short of it: transverse myelitis in children. *Neurology* 2007; **68**: 1447–1449.

Banwell B, Ghezzi A, Bar-Or A, Mikaeloff Y, Tardieu M. Multiple sclerosis in children: clinical diagnosis, therapeutic strategies, and future directions. *Lancet Neurol* 2007; **6**: 887–902.

Banwell B, Kennedy J, Sadovnick D, et al. Incidence of acquired demyelination of the CNS in Canadian children. *Neurology* 2009; **72**: 232–239.

Banwell B, Tenembaum S, Lennon et al. Neuromyelitis optica-IgG in childhood inflammatory demyelinating CNS disorders. *Neurology* 2008; **70**: 344–352.

Becher B, Bechmann I, Greter M. Antigen presentation in autoimmunity and CNS inflammation: how T lymphocytes recognize the brain. *J Mol Med* 2006; **84**: 532–43.

Beetz C, Schule R, Deconinck T, et al. REEP1 mutation spectrum and genotype/phenotype correlation in hereditary spastic paraplegia type 31. *Brain* 2008; **131**: 1078–1086.

Belman AL, Chitnis T, Renoux C, Waubant E. Challenges in the classification of pediatric multiple sclerosis and future directions. *Neurology* 2007; **68**: S70–S74.

Beslow LA, Ichord RN, Zimmerman RA, Smith SE, Licht DJ. Role of diffusion MRI in diagnosis of spinal cord infarction in children. *Neuropediatrics* 2008; **39**: 188–191.

Bhat A, Naguwa S, Cheema G, Gershwin ME. The epidemiology of transverse myelitis. *Autoimmun Rev* 2010; **9**: A395–A399.

Bhigjee AI, Madurai S, Bill PL, et al. Spectrum of myelopathies in HIV seropositive South African patients. *Neurology* 2001; **57**: 348–351.

Bittencourt AL, Primo J, Oliveira MF. Manifestations of the human T-cell lymphotropic virus type I infection in childhood and adolescence. *Jornal de Pediatria* 2006; **82**: 411–420.

Brabb T, Von Dassow P, Ordonez N, Schnabel B, Duke B, Goverman J. In situ tolerance within the central nervous system as a mechanism for preventing autoimmunity. *J Exp Med* 2000; **192**: 871–880.

Campi A, Filippi M, Comi G, et al. Acute transverse myelopathy: spinal and cranial MR study with clinical follow-up. *AJNR Am J Neuroradiol* 1995; **16**: 115–123.

Carrithers MD, Visintin I, Viret C, Janeway CS Jr. Role of genetic background in P selectin-dependent immune surveillance of the central nervous system. *J Neuroimmunol* 2002; **129**: 51–57.

Castelli MC, Friedman K, Sherry J, et al. G Comparing the efficacy and tolerability of a new daily oral vitamin B12 formulation and intermittent intramuscular vitamin B12 in normalizing low cobalamin levels: a randomized, open-label, parallel-group study. *Clin Ther* 2011; **33**: 358–371 e2.

Chedrawi AK, Ali A, Al Hassnan ZN, Faiyaz-Ul-Haque M, Wolf B. Profound biotinidase deficiency in a child with predominantly spinal cord disease. *J Child Neurol* 2008; **23**: 1043–8.

Cheshire WP, Santos CC, Massey EW, Howard JF Jr. Spinal cord infarction: etiology and outcome. *Neurology* 1996; **47**: 321–330.

Clancy RR, Sladky JT, Rorke LB. Hypoxic-ischemic spinal cord injury following perinatal asphyxia. *Ann Neurol* 1989; **25**: 185–189.

Clayton PT, Smith I, Harding B, Hyland K, Leonard JV, Leeming RJ. Subacute combined degeneration of the cord, dementia and parkinsonism due to an inborn error of folate metabolism. *J Neurol Neurosurg Psychiatry* 1986; **49**: 920–927.

Collongues N, Marignier R, Zephir H, et al. Neuromyelitis optica in France: a multicenter study of 125 patients. *Neurology* 2010a; **74**: 736–742.

Collongues N, Marignier R, Zephir H, et al. Long-term follow-up of neuromyelitis optica with a pediatric onset. *Neurology* 2010b; **75**: 1084–1048.

Cooper ER, Hanson C, Diaz C, et al. Encephalopathy and progression of human immunodeficiency virus disease in a cohort of children with perinatally acquired human immunodeficiency virus infection. Women and Infants Transmission Study Group. *J Pediatr* 1998; **132**: 808–812.

Cornejo W, Gonzalez F, Toro ME, Cabrera D. [Subacute combined degeneration. A description of the case of a strictly vegetarian child.] (In Spanish.) *Rev Neurol* 2001; **33**: 1154–1157.

Dajusta DG, Wosnitzer MS, Barone JG. Persistent motor deficits predict long-term bladder dysfunction in children following acute transverse myelitis. *J Urol* 2008; **180**: 1774–1777.

Dal Pan GJ, Glass JD, McArthur JC. Clinicopathologic correlations of HIV-1-associated vacuolar myelopathy: an autopsy-based case-control study. *Neurology* 1994; **44**: 2159–2164.

Daput UA, Mok JM, Sharkey MS, Davis AA, Foster-Barber A, Diab M. Delayed presentation of tetraparesis following posterior thoracolumbar spinal fusion and instrumentation for adolescent idiopathic scoliosis. *Spine* 2009; **34**: E936–E941.

De Goede CG, Holmes EM, Pike MG. Acquired transverse myelopathy in children in the United Kingdom—a 2 year prospective study. *Eur J Paediatr Neurol* 2010; **14**: 479–487.

De Seze M, Joseph PA, Wiart L, Nguyen PV, Barat M. [Functional prognosis of paraplegia due to cord ischemia: a retrospective study of 23 patients.] (In French.) *Rev Neurol (Paris)* 2003; **159**: 1038–1045.

Defresne P, Hollenberg H. Husson B, et al. Acute transverse myelitis in children: clinical course and prognostic factors. *J Child Neurol* 2003; **18**: 401–6.

Defresne P, Meyer L, Tardieu M, et al. Efficacy of high dose steroid therapy in children with severe acute transverse myelitis. *J Neurol Neurosurg Psychiatry* 2001; **71**: 272–274.

Denning DW, Anderson J, Rudge P, Smith H. Acute myelopathy associated with primary infection with human immunodeficiency virus. *BMJ* 1987; **294**: 143–144.

Dickson DW, Belman AL, Kim TS, Horoupian DS, Rubinstein A. Spinal cord pathology in pediatric acquired immunodeficiency syndrome. *Neurology* 1989; **39**: 227–235.

Dunne K, Hopkins IJ, Shield LK. Acute transverse myelopathy in childhood. *Dev Med Child Neurol* 1986; **28**: 198–204.

Eichholzer M, Tonz O, Zimmermann R. Folic acid: a public-health challenge. *Lancet* 2006; **367**: 1352–1361.

Elsheikh B, Kissel JT, Christoforidis G, et al. Spinal angiography and epidural venography in juvenile muscular atrophy of the distal arm "Hirayama disease". *Muscle Nerve* 2009; **40**: 206–212.

Escolar ML, Poe MD, Provenzale JM, et al. Transplantation of umbilical-cord blood in babies with infantile Krabbe's disease. *N Engl J Med* 2005; **352**: 2069–2081.

Esptein, LG, Dicarlo, FJ, Jr, Joshi, VV, et al. Primary lymphoma of the central nervous system in children with acquired immunodeficiency syndrome. *Pediatrics* 1988; **82**: 355–363.

Fenichel GM. In: Fenichel GM, editor. Clinical Paediatric Neurology (5th edition). Philadelphia, PA: Elsevier Saunders, 2005: 255–272.

Frank Y, Ashwal S. In: Swaiman KF, Ashwal S, Ferriero DM, editors. Pediatric Neurology: Principles & Practice. Philadelphia, PA: Mosby Elsevier, 2006: 2285–2352.

Frohman EM, Wingerchuk DM. Clinical practice transverse myelitis. *N Engl J Med* 2010; **363**: 564–572.

Gambling L, McArdle HJ. Iron, copper and fetal development. *Proc Nutr Soc* 2004; **63**: 553–562.

George R, Andronikou S, Du Plessis J, Du Plessis AM, Van Toorn R, Maydell A. Central nervous system manifestations of HIV infection in children. *Pediatr Radiol* 2009; **39**: 575–85.

Goverman J. Autoimmune T cell responses in the central nervous system. *Nat Rev Immunol* 2009; **9**: 393–407.

Green R, Kinsella LJ. Current concepts in the diagnosis of cobalamin deficiency. *Neurology* 1995; **45**: 1435–1440.

Greenberg BM, Thomas KP, Krishnan C, Kaplin AI, Calabresi PA, Kerr DA. Idiopathic transverse myelitis: corticosteroids, plasma exchange, or cyclophosphamide. *Neurology* 2007; **68**: 1614–1617.

Gungor T, Funk M, Linde R, Jacobi G, Horn M, Kreuz W. Cytomegalovirus myelitis in perinatally acquired HIV. *Arch Dis Child* 1993; **68**: 399–401.

Harding AE. Hereditary spastic paraplegias. *Semin Neurol* 1993; **13**: 333–336.

Hasegawa M, Yamashita J, Yamashima T, Ikeda K, Fujishima Y, Yamazaki M. Spinal cord infarction associated with primary antiphospholipid syndrome in a young child. Case report. *J Neurosurg* 1993; **79**: 446–450.

Hazan J, Fonknechten N, Mavel D, et al. Spastin, a new AAA protein, is altered in the most frequent form of autosomal dominant spastic paraplegia. *Nat Genet* 1999; **23**: 296–303.

Healton EB, Savage DG, Brust JC, Garrett TJ, Lindenbaum J. Neurologic aspects of cobalamin deficiency. *Medicine* 1991; **70**: 229–245.

Hickey WF. Basic principles of immunological surveillance of the normal central nervous system. *Glia* 2001; **36**: 118–124.

Huppke P, Bluthner M, Bauer O, et al. Neuromyelitis optica and NMO-IgG in European pediatric patients. *Neurology* 2010; **75**: 1740–1744.

Inoue K. PLP1-related inherited dysmyelinating disorders: Pelizaeus-Merzbacher disease and spastic paraplegia type 2. *Neurogenetics* 2005; **6**: 1–16.

Jacobs LD, Beck RW, Simon JH, et al. Intramuscular interferon beta-1a therapy initiated during a first demyelinating event in multiple sclerosis. CHAMPS Study Group. *N Engl J Med* 2000; **343**: 898–904.

Jaiser SR, Winston GP. Copper deficiency myelopathy. *J Neurol* 2010; **257**: 869–881.

Jouet M, Rosenthal A, Armstrong G, et al. X-linked spastic paraplegia (SPG1), MASA syndrome and X-linked hydrocephalus result from mutations in the L1 gene. *Nat Genet* 1994; **7**: 402–407.

Kalra V, Sharma S, Sahu J, et al. Childhood acute transverse myelitis: clinical Profile, Outcome, and association with antiganglioside antibodies. *J Child Neurol* 2009; **24**: 466–471.

Kodama H, Murata Y, Kobayashi M. Clinical manifestations and treatment of Menkes disease and its variants. *Pediatr Int* 1999; **41**: 423–429.

Kolodny EH, Raghavan S, Krivit W. Late-onset Krabbe disease (globoid cell leukodystrophy): clinical and biochemical features of 15 cases. *Dev Neurosci* 1991; **13**: 232–239.

Korn-Lubetzki I, Dor-Wollman T, Soffer D, Raas-Rothschild A, Hurvitz H, Nevo, Y Early peripheral nervous system manifestations of infantile Krabbe disease. *Pediatr Neurol* 2003; **28**: 115–118.

Krishnan C, Kerr DA. Idiopathic transverse myelitis. *Arch Neurol* 2005; **62**: 1011–1013.

Krivit W, Shapiro EG, Peters C, et al. Hematopoietic stem-cell transplantation in globoid-cell leukodystrophy. *N Engl J Med* 1998; **338**: 1119–1126.

Krupp LB, Banwell B, Tenembaum S. Consensus definitions proposed for pediatric multiple sclerosis and related disorders. *Neurology* 2007; **68**: S7–S12.

Kumar AJ, Rosenbaum AE, Naidu S, et al. Adrenoleukodystrophy: correlating MR imaging with CT. *Radiology* 1987; **165**: 497–504.

Lennon VA, Wingerchuk DM, Kryzer TJ, et al. A serum autoantibody marker of neuromyelitis optica: distinction from multiple sclerosis. *Lancet* 2004; **364**: 2106–2112.

Licht DJ, Berry GT, Brooks DG, Younkin DP. 2001 Reversible subacute combined degeneration of the spinal cord in a 14-year-old due to a strict vegan diet. *Clin Pediatr (Phila)* 2001; **40**: 413–415.

Lobato MN, Caldwell MB, Ng P, Oxtoby MJ. Encephalopathy in children with perinatally acquired human immunodeficiency virus infection. Pediatric Spectrum of Disease Clinical Consortium. *J Pediatr* 1995; **126**: 710–715.

Loes DJ, Fatemi A, Melhem ER, et al. Analysis of MRI patterns aids prediction of progression in X-linked adrenoleukodystrophy. *Neurology* 2003; **61**: 369–374.

Lotze TE, Northrop JL, Hutton GJ, Ross B, Schiffman JS, Hunter JV. Spectrum of pediatric neuromyelitis optica. *Pediatrics* 2008; **122**: e1039–e1047.

Marriage SC, Booy R, Hermione Lyall EG, et al. Cytomegalovirus myelitis in a child infected with human immunodeficiency virus type 1. *Pediatr Infect Dis J* 1996; **15**: 549–551.

Martinez-Lage JF, Almagro MJ, Izura V, Serrano C, Ruiz-Espejo AM, Sanchez-Del-Rincon, I. Cervical spinal cord infarction after posterior fossa surgery: a case-based update. *Childs Nerv Syst* 2009; **25**: 1541–1546.

Matthews DM, Linnell JC. Cobalamin deficiency and related disorders in infancy and childhood. *Eur J Pediatr* 1982; **138**: 6–16.

McDermott CJ, Burness CE, Kirby J, et al. Clinical features of hereditary spastic paraplegia due to spastin mutation. *Neurology* 2006; **67**: 45–51.

McKeon A, Lennon VA, Lotze T, et al. CNS aquaporin-4 autoimmunity in children. *Neurology* 2008; **71**: 93–100.

Mikaeloff Y, Suissa S, Vallee L, et al. First episode of acute CNS inflammatory demyelination in childhood: prognostic factors for multiple sclerosis and disability. *J Pediatr* 2004; **144**: 246–252.

Miller DH, Weinshenker BG, Filippi M, et al. Differential diagnosis of suspected multiple sclerosis: a consensus approach. *Mult Scler* 2008; **14**: 1157–1174.

Miyazawa R, Ikeuchi Y, Tomomasa T, Ushiku H, Ogawa T, Morikawa A. Determinants of prognosis of acute transverse myelitis in children *Pediatr Int* 2003; **45**: 512–516.

Moffett KS, Berkowitz FE. Quadriplegia complicating *Escherichia coli* meningitis in a newborn infant: case report and review of 22 cases of spinal cord dysfunction in patients with acute bacterial meningitis. *Clin Infect Dis* 1997; **25**: 211–214.

Moser HW, Mahmood A, Raymond GV. X-linked adrenoleukodystrophy. *Nat Clin Pract Neurol* 2007; **3**: 140–151.

MRC Vitamin Study Research Group. Prevention of neural tube defects: results of the Medical Research Council Vitamin Study. *Lancet* 1991; **338**: 131–137.

Muller DP. Vitamin E and neurological function. *Mol Nutr Food Res* 2010; **54**: 710–718.

Muller DP, Lloyd JK, Bird AC. Long-term management of abetalipoproteinaemia. Possible role for vitamin E. *Arch Dis Child* 1977; **52**: 209–214.

Namekawa M, Ribai P, Nelson I, et al. SPG3A is the most frequent cause of hereditary spastic paraplegia with onset before age 10 years. *Neurology* 2006; **66**: 112–114.

Nance JR, Golomb MR. Ischemic spinal cord infarction in children without vertebral fracture. *Pediatr Neurol* 2007; **36**: 209–216.

Narayan SK, Kaveer N. CNS demyelination due to hypocupremia in Wilson's disease from overzealous treatment. *Neurol India* 2006; **54**: 110–111.

Nedeltchev K, Loher TJ, Stepper F, et al. Long-term outcome of acute spinal cord ischemia syndrome. *Stroke* 2004; **35**: 560–565.

Nelson JS, Fitch CD, Fischer VW, Broun GO Jr, Chou AC. Progressive neuropathologic lesions in vitamin E-deficient rhesus monkeys. *J Neuropathol Exp Neurol* 1981; **40**: 166–186.

Novy J, Carruzzo A, Maeder P, Bogousslavsky J. Spinal cord ischemia: clinical and imaging Patterns, pathogenesis, and outcomes in 27 patients. *Arch Neurol* 2006; **63**: 1113–1120.

Ogier H, Hanefeld F, Aicardi J. In Aicardi J, editor. Diseases of the Nervous System in Childhood (3rd edition). London: Mac Keith Press, 2009: 247–326.

Okada S, Okeda R. Pathology of radiation myelopathy. *Neuropathology* 2001; **21**: 247–265.

Oliveri RL, Valentino P, Russo C, et al. Randomized trial comparing two different high doses of methyl-prednisolone in MS: a clinical and MRI study. *Neurology* 1998; **50**: 1833–1836.

Ou P, Schmit P, Layouss W, Sidi D, Bonnet D, Brunelle F. CT angiography of the artery of Adamkiewicz with 64-section technology: first experience in children. *AJNR Am J Neuroradiol* 2007; **28**: 216–219.

Palace J, Leite MI, Nairne A, Vincent, A. Interferon beta treatment in neuromyelitis optica: increase in relapses and aquaporin 4 antibody titers. *Arch Neurol* 2010; **67**: 1016–1017.

Parazzini C, Rossi L, Righini A, et al. Spinal cord and vertebral stroke: a paediatric case. *Neuropediatrics* 2006; **37**: 107–109.

Peters C, Charnas LR, Tan Y, et al. Cerebral X-linked adrenoleukodystrophy: the international hematopoietic cell transplantation experience from 1982 to 1999. *Blood* 2004; **104**: 881–888.

Petito CK, Navia BA, Cho ES, Jordan BD, George DC, Price RW. Vacuolar myelopathy pathologically resembling subacute combined degeneration in patients with the acquired immunodeficiency syndrome. *N Engl J Med* 1985; **312**: 874–879.

Pidcock FS, Krishnan C, Crawford TO, Salorio CF, Trovato M, Kerr DA. Acute transverse myelitis in childhood: center-based analysis of 47 cases. *Neurology* 2007; **68**: 1474–1480.

Polman CH, Reingold SC, Edan G, et al. Diagnostic criteria for multiple sclerosis: 2005 revisions to the "McDonald Criteria". *Ann Neurol* 2005; **58**: 840–846.

Prasad AN, Breen JC, Ampola MG, Rosman NP. Argininemia: a treatable genetic cause of progressive spastic diplegia simulating cerebral palsy: case reports and literature review. *J Child Neurol* 1997; **12**: 301–309.

Primo JR, Brites C, Oliveira Mde F, Moreno-Carvalho O, Machado M, Bittencourt AL. Infective dermatitis and human T cell lymphotropic virus type 1–associated myelopathy/tropical spastic paraparesis in childhood and adolescence. *Clin Infect Dis* 2005; **41**: 535–541.

Quain R. A Dictionary of Medicine: including General Pathology, General Therapeutics, Hygiene, and the Diseases Peculiar to Women and Children. Longmans, Green, 1882.

Rampling R, Symonds P. Radiation myelopathy. *Curr Opin Neurol* 1998; **11**: 627–632.

Ray JG, Blom HJ. Vitamin B12 insufficiency and the risk of fetal neural tube defects. *QJM* 2003; **96**: 289–295.

Reynolds E. Vitamin B12, folic acid, and the nervous system. *Lancet Neurol* 2006; **5**: 949–960.

Reynolds EH. Benefits and risks of folic acid to the nervous system. *J Neurol Neurosurg Psychiatry* 2002; **72**: 567–571.

Rosenquist TH, Ratashak SA, Selhub J. Homocysteine induces congenital defects of the heart and neural tube: effect of folic acid. *Proc Natl Acad Sci U S A* 1996; **93**: 15227–15232.

Salinas S, Proukakis C, Crosby A, Warner TT. Hereditary spastic paraplegia: clinical features and pathogenetic mechanisms. *Lancet Neurol* 2008; **7**: 1127–1138.

Salvador de la Barrera S, Barca-Buyo A, Montoto-Marques A, Ferreiro-Velasco ME, Cidoncha-Dans M, Rodriguez-Sotillo A. Spinal cord infarction: prognosis and recovery in a series of 36 patients. *Spinal Cord* 2001; **39**: 520–525.

Sandson TA, Friedman JH. Spinal cord infarction. Report of 8 cases and review of the literature. *Medicine* 1989; **68**: 282–292.

Schleper B, Stuerenburg HJ. Copper deficiency-associated myelopathy in a 46-year-old woman. *J Neurol* 2001; **248**: 705–706.

Scott TF, Frohman EM, De Seze J, Gronseth GS, Weinshenker BG. Evidence-based guideline: clinical evaluation and treatment of transverse myelitis: report of the Therapeutics and Technology Assessment Subcommittee of the American Academy of Neurology. *Neurology* 2011; **77**: 2128–2134.

Sellner J, Boggild M, Clanet M, et al. EFNS guidelines on diagnosis and management of neuromyelitis optica. *Eur J Neurol* 2010; **17**: 1019–1032.

Sheerin F, Collison K, Quaghebeur G. Magnetic resonance imaging of acute intramedullary myelopathy: radiological differential diagnosis for the on-call radiologist. *Clin Radiol* 2009; **64**: 84–94.

Shimizu M, Hamano S, Nara T, Eto Y, Maekawa K. [MRI findings of anterior spinal artery syndrome in childhood.] (In Japanese.) *No To Hattatsu* 1996; **28**: 438–442.

Sladky JT, Rorke LB. Perinatal hypoxic/ischemic spinal cord injury. *Pediatr Pathol* 1986; **6**: 87–101.

Smith SE, Kinney HC, Swoboda KJ, Levy HL. Subacute combined degeneration of the spinal cord in cblC disorder despite treatment with B12. *Mol Genet Metab* 2006; **88**: 138–145.

Sohal AS, Sundaram M, Mallewa M, Tawil M, Kneen, R. Anterior spinal artery syndrome in a girl with Down syndrome: case report and literature review. *J Spinal Cord Med* 2009; **32**: 349–354.

Stevanin G, Azzedine H, Denora P, et al. Mutations in SPG11 are frequent in autosomal recessive spastic paraplegia with thin corpus callosum, cognitive decline and lower motor neuron degeneration. *Brain* 2008; **131**: 772–784.

Suzuki T, Kawaguchi S, Takebayashi T, Yokogushi K, Takada J, Yamashita T. Vertebral body ischemia in the posterior spinal artery syndrome: case report and review of the literature. *Spine* 2003; **28**: E260–E264.

Tan K, Hammond ER, Kerr D, Nath A. Fibrocartilaginous embolism: a cause of acute ischemic myelopathy. *Spinal Cord* 2009; **47**: 643–645.

Teplitsky V, Huminer D, Zoldan J, Pitlik S, Shohat M, Mittelman M. Hereditary partial transcobalamin II deficiency with neurologic, mental and hematologic abnormalities in children and adults. *Isr Med Assoc J* 2003; **5**: 868–872.

Thurnher MM, Bammer R. Diffusion-weighted MR imaging (DWI) in spinal cord ischemia. *Neuroradiology* 2006; **48**: 795–801.

Transverse Myelitis Consortium Working Group. Proposed diagnostic criteria and nosology of acute transverse myelitis. *Neurology* 2002; **59**: 499–505.

Trigylidas T, Yuh SJ, Vassilyadi M, Matzinger MA, Mikrogianakis A. Spinal cord injuries without radiographic abnormality at two pediatric trauma centers in Ontario. *Pediatr Neurosurg* 2010; **46**: 283–289.

Verhey LH, Branson HM, Makhija M, Shroff M, Banwell B. Magnetic resonance imaging features of the spinal cord in pediatric multiple sclerosis: a preliminary study. *Neuroradiology* 2010; **52**:1153–1162.

Wang PY, Shen, WC, Jan JS. MR imaging in radiation myelopathy. *AJNR Am J Neuroradiol* 1992; **13**: 1049–1055.

Warren LP Jr, Djang WT, Moon RE, et al. Neuroimaging of scuba diving injuries to the CNS. *AJR Am J Roentgenol* 1988; **151**: 1003–1008.

Weidauer S, Nichtweiss M, Lanfermann H, Zanella FE. Spinal cord infarction: MR imaging and clinical features in 16 cases. *Neuroradiology* 2002; **44**: 851–857.

Weinshenker BG, O'Brien PC, Petterson TM, et al. A randomized trial of plasma exchange in acute central nervous system inflammatory demyelinating disease. *Ann Neurol* 1999; **46**: 878–886.

Wenger, DA. Murine, canine and non-human primate models of Krabbe disease. *Mol Med Today* 2000; **6**: 449–451.

Wilmshurst JM, Burgess J, Hartley P, Eley B. Specific neurologic complications of human immunodeficiency virus type 1 (HIV-1) infection in children. *J Child Neurol* 2006; **21**: 788–794.

Wingerchuk DM, Lennon VA, Pittock SJ, Lucchinetti CF, Weinshenker BG. Revised diagnostic criteria for neuromyelitis optica. *Neurology* 2006; **66**: 1485–1489.

Wiznitzer M, Bangert BA. Biotinidase deficiency: clinical and MRI findings consistent with myelopathy. *Pediatr Neurol* 2003; **29**: 56–58.

Wolf B. In Scriver CR, Beaudet AL, Sly WS, Valle D, editors. The Metabolic and Molecular Bases of Inherited Disease (8th edition). New York, NY: McGraw Hill, 2001: 3935–3962.

Wraith JE. In Platt FM, Walkley SU, editors. Lysosomal Storage Disorders of the Brain. Oxford: Oxford University Press, 2004: 50–80.

Yiu EM, Kornberg AJ, Ryan MM, Coleman LT, Mackay, MT. Acute transverse myelitis and acute disseminated encephalomyelitis in childhood: spectrum or separate entities? *J Child Neurol* 2009; **24**: 287–296.

Young J, Quinn S, Hurrell M, Taylor B. Clinically isolated acute transverse myelitis: prognostic features and incidence. *Mult Scler* 2009; **15**: 1295–1302.

Zamel R, Khan R, Pollex RL, Hegele RA. Abetalipoproteinemia: two case reports and literature review. *Orphanet J Rare Dis* 2008; **3**: 19.

Zittoun J, Leger J, Marquet J, Carmel R. Combined congenital deficiencies of intrinsic factor and R binder. *Blood* 1988; **72**: 940–943.

Zorzi G, Mancuso R, Nardocci N, Farina L, Guerini FR, Ferrante P. Childhood-onset HAM/TSP with progressive cognitive impairment. *Neurol Sci* 2010; **31**: 209–212.

185

8
SPECIFIC ISSUES IN MANAGEMENT AND REHABILITATION

Lawrence Vogel and Allison Graham

Unique issues in the management and rehabilitation of children and adolescents with spinal cord dysfunction are related to the dynamic nature of growth and development interacting with the manifestations and complications of the dysfunction in the paediatric population (Betz and Mulcahey 1996, Vogel et al. 1997, Sarwark and Lubicky 2002, Vogel and Anderson 2003). This chapter will primarily focus on the management and rehabilitation of acquired spinal cord injuries (SCIs); however, as appropriate, issues unique to myelomeningocele will be highlighted. Both SCIs and myelomeningocele share many of the same manifestations related to spinal cord dysfunction, namely paralysis, sensory loss, and autonomic nervous system, bladder, bowel, and sexual dysfunction. Children with both disorders also experience similar complications consequent to growth, such as scoliosis and hip dysplasia. In contrast, myelomeningocele has several distinctive manifestations because of its prenatal onset and associated brain abnormalities, resulting in congenital malformations, such as congenital talipes equinovarus, cognitive and behavioural abnormalities, respectively (Sarwark and Lubicky 2002, Vogel and Sturm 2008). Hydrocephalus is present in 80 to 90% of children with myelomeningoceles, and a Chiari II malformation occurs in virtually all affected individuals (Rauzzino and Oakes 1995, Urui and Oi 1995).

Rehabilitation: general paediatric and adolescent issues
Rehabilitation and habilitation of children with spinal cord dysfunction is a dynamic process with developmentally based goals that are constantly changing (Betz and Mulcahey 1994). At each developmental phase, goals must focus on independence and full participation comparable to the adolescent's uninjured peers. The ultimate goal in caring for children with spinal cord dysfunction is that they become adults who fully participate in their communities with a high quality of life. From the time of injury (or birth, in the case of myelomeningocele) rehabilitation goals across the child's lifespan need to be delineated. The expectation that the child with spinal cord dysfunction will become an independent adult participating fully in their community must be established early and reinforced subsequently. In addition to the child and their parents, these expectations must be endorsed by others who are involved with the child with spinal cord dysfunction, including teachers,

healthcare providers, and extended family members. Transition from adolescence to adulthood requires a comprehensive plan that facilitates this important progression into becoming an independent and productive adult. Transition is a continuous process that begins during childhood and intensifies during adolescence. It encompasses a variety of areas including health care and finances, psychosocial and sexual function, independent living and employment (Anderson et al. 1998, Zebracki et al. 2010).

Rehabilitation of children with spinal cord dysfunction requires an interdisciplinary team that focuses on a broad spectrum of issues, including spinal cord dysfunction-specific education, skin, bladder and bowel management, recreation and leisure time activities, mobility, self-care activities, social services, psychological and vocational counselling, and prevention and management of complications. Management must be family centred and sensitive to educational, psychosocial, cultural, and spiritual aspects of the patient and family. Children and their parents need to be an integral part of the rehabilitation team, and actively participate in decision-making activities throughout their lives.

As children with spinal cord dysfunction move into adolescence, they need to assume an increasing role in the decision-making process to transition into adulthood successfully. At all ages, a major goal should be independence and increased knowledge and skills about their SCI. Parents are normally responsible for all aspects of care for infants and toddlers. Over the years, the child will progressively take on more of the responsibilities for their care with the goal that they transition into adulthood with the expectation that they are fully capable of managing their own care (Anderson et al. 1998, Zebracki et al. 2010). This process of gradually transferring responsibility to the young person is complicated because the consequences of poor compliance may be serious or even life-threatening.

Two examples of this include skin care and bladder management. Because pressure ulcers are associated with significant morbidity, the performance of regular pressure reliefs and skin inspections are crucial. To prevent urinary tract infections, incontinence, and long-term urological complications, such as renal failure or stones, strict adherence to a catheterization programme is essential. Although an 8-year-old child with an SCI may be able to self-catheterize and perform pressure relief and skin inspections, they may forget or simply decide not to do it. At the same time, parents can appreciate the importance of these issues for their child's health but may be reluctant to turn responsibility over to the child. It is difficult to attain the right balance, and parents often need to be vigilant and provide a safety net as the child gradually takes on the responsibility for their care.

The SCI team should provide supervision and encouragement for both the child and their parents during this dynamic process. To encourage transition, adolescents should be seen alone without their parents for increasing periods during outpatient visits.

Motor rehabilitation
MOBILITY: GENERAL ASPECTS
Mobility is an important aspect of the rehabilitation of children with spinal cord dysfunction. The concept of mobility should be viewed in a comprehensive manner that goes beyond ambulation to include effective mobility in all spheres of an individual's life, including home, school, community, and the world at large. Depending upon the individual's age and

degree of neurological impairment, the nature of mobility may vary. However, the broad categories of mobility ranging from bed mobility and transfers to movement at home, and in the wider community apply to all ages and all degrees of neurological severity.

As children age, mobility significantly affects activity and participation specific to each developmental stage that is critical to successful progression and outcomes throughout childhood and adolescence (Rosen et al. 2009). At one extreme is the child born with a myelomeningocele or a child diagnosed with an SCI at birth; mobility impairment affects the infant and toddler's exploration of their environment, which is critical to their development. Similarly, because of mobility limitations, adolescents with SCIs may not have the opportunities to access community activities spontaneously that non-injured peers experience, such as 'hanging out'.

STANDING AND AMBULATION

There are numerous options for ambulation and upright mobility for children and adolescents with SCIs. The types of orthotics and assistive devices used and the degree and duration of ambulation is dependent upon several factors, including age, body size, compliance, cognitive function, preferences, musculoskeletal complications (such as contractures or spasticity), and the degree of the neurological deficit (Hussey and Stauffer 1973, Vogel and Lubicky 1995, Kelly and Stokes 1996, Vogel et al. 2007).

For those with SCIs, the extent of the neurological deficit is defined by the neurological level and injury severity as measured by the American Spinal Injury Association Impairment Scale (AIS) score (Table 8.1) (American Spinal Injury Association 2011). Younger age and less neurological severity are associated with greater degrees of ambulation. Individuals with upper thoracic paraplegia (T1–T6) may ambulate primarily in a therapeutic setting, and those with lower thoracic and upper lumbar lesions (T7–L2) may be household ambulators. In contrast, those with functional motor incomplete SCIs (AIS D) or those with

TABLE 8.1
American Spinal Injury Association Impairment Scale (AIS) score

A, complete. No sensory or motor function is preserved in the sacral segments S4–S5.

B, sensory incomplete. Sensory but not motor function is preserved below the neurological level and includes the sacral segments S4–S5, *and* no motor function is preserved more than three levels below the motor level on either side of the body.

C, motor incomplete. Motor function is preserved below the neurological level,[a] and more than half of key muscle functions below the single neurological level of injury have a muscle grade less than 3 (grades 0–2).

D, motor incomplete. Motor function is preserved below the neurological level[a], and at least half (half or more) of key muscle functions below the neurological level of injury have a muscle grade greater or equal to 3.

E, normal. If sensation and motor function as tested with the International Standards for Neurological Classification of Spinal Cord Injury are graded as normal in all segments, and the patient had previous deficits, the AIS grade is E.

[a]For an individual to receive a grade C or D, i.e. motor incomplete, they must have either (1) voluntary anal sphincter contraction or (2) sacral sparing (at S4/5 or deep anal pressure) with sparing of motor functions more than three levels below the motor level for that side of the body.

L3 and lower lesions are capable of being community ambulators, although they generally require wheelchairs for long distances (Hussey and Stauffer 1973, Vogel et al. 2007, Schottler 2012). For children with spina bifida, prediction of ambulation is similarly based on specific patterns of lower extremity muscle strength (McDonald et al. 1991a, b).

For children with spina bifida, the presence of perineal sensation has also been shown to predict the ability to ambulate (Oakeshott et al. 2007).

Children are more likely to be active ambulators than adolescents and adults, because of their smaller size, increased energy level, and less awareness of appearance (Vogel and Lubicky 1995, Vogel et al. 2007). By 9 to 15 months of age, infants can begin standing in a variety of standers or parapodia, which are dynamic standers that allow mobility. Toddlers and young children with paraplegia can ambulate using a variety of orthotics and assistive devices, whereas those with tetraplegia may continue using standing devices or parapodia. As children grow older, especially during adolescence, they tend to ambulate less and use their wheelchairs as their primary mode of mobility. This change from ambulation to wheeled mobility should be viewed as a transition and not as a failure, and reflects the need for efficient mobility as individuals progress through childhood into adolescence and young adulthood.

As children and adolescents grow, new equipment is required both because of increasing size and changing needs. As an example, infants and young toddlers may crawl, progress to parapodia for standing and minimal mobility, and use pushchairs (strollers or buggies) for wheeled mobility. Older children should avoid crawling because of the risk of inadvertent trauma to insensate areas of the body that individuals beyond toddlers may be susceptible to because of their larger body size. Preschool and early school-aged children may crawl at home, but use a variety of orthotics and assistive devices for ambulation or standing in school. They should also be independent in appropriate types of wheelchair. Except for children with less severe neurological impairments that allow for community ambulation, older children and adolescents would primarily, if not exclusively, use wheelchairs for all their mobility.

Parapodia allow children with SCIs to stand without the need for upper extremity weight bearing, so that they can perform activities with both hands (Fig. 8.1) (Vogel and Lubicky 1995, 1997). Patients who use parapodia are either therapeutic or household ambulators; nonetheless, parapodia facilitate independent mobility and provide an opportunity to be upright and face their peers at eye level. Requirements for using parapodia include head control and the absence of significant lower extremity contractures. Parapodia can be initiated in children as young as 9 to 12 months of age, which is a developmentally appropriate time to stand. Parapodia provide the young child the opportunity to be upright, before the use of other orthotics. Parapodia have the advantage of not requiring intensive therapy.

Although parapodia are accepted by preschool and early school-aged children, most children stop using them by 7 to 10 years of age for a variety of reasons including the relative bulk of the parapodia, awareness of appearance and inefficiency of this mode of mobility. The child can ambulate by swivelling (by twisting their upper trunk and swinging their arms), or they can perform a swing-to or a swing-through gait using walkers or forearm crutches (Fig. 8.1).

189

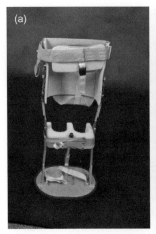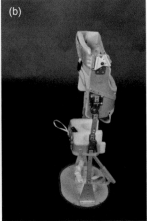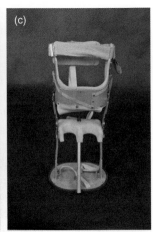

Fig. 8.1. Parapodium; (a) front, (b) side, and (c) rear views.

In addition to parapodia, there are a variety of static and mobile standing devices that are suitable for children and adolescents, including standing wheelchairs, standing frames and mobile standing devices (Fig. 8.2) (Fitzsimmons 1996, Vogel and Lubicky 1997). Standing devices are primarily used for household, school, or vocational activities, such as food preparation at a counter top or classroom work at the chalk board. Parapodia encourage the development of stance, weight shifting, and trunk rotation which are necessary antecedents for ambulation; whereas, static or wheeled standers do not engender the development of balance and trunk shifting (McDonald 1995).

Reciprocating gait orthoses (RGOs) are orthotics that extend from the thoracic region to the feet and allow for flexion in one hip with the extension of the opposite hip as a result of either a cable system or stainless steel rocker bar mounted on a moulded pelvic bar (Fig. 8.3). RGOs can be prescribed for individuals with paraplegia with L2 or higher-level lesions (see Vogel and Lubicky 1995, 1997, Vogel et al. 2007). RGOs may be initiated in children as young as 15 to 18 months old. Children who are most likely to be community ambulators with RGOs are those with active hip flexors, those who are young and well motivated, and those who are able to ambulate with forearm crutches. Compared with other orthotics, such as hip–knee–ankle–foot orthoses (HKAFOs) or knee–ankle–foot orthoses (KAFOs), RGOs provide a reciprocating gait and are more energy efficient.

Children with thoracic or upper lumbar paraplegia (T1–L2) can ambulate with HKAFOs with a swing-to or swing-through gait using a walker or forearm crutches (Fig. 8.4). However, the use of HKAFOs is limited by the relatively slow and energy inefficient gait pattern. Young people with lower thoracic or upper lumbar paraplegia (T7–L2) may also be able to ambulate with KAFOs. Children with L2 level injuries with strong hip flexors may be able to ambulate with a reciprocating gait. However, similar to HKAFO users, most KAFO users ambulate with a swing-to or swing-through gait. Using assistive devices such as forearm crutches or a walker, a swing-to gait is accomplished by swinging both legs in

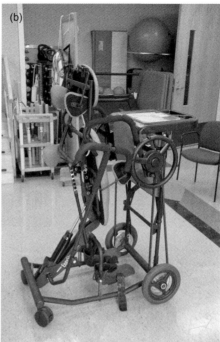

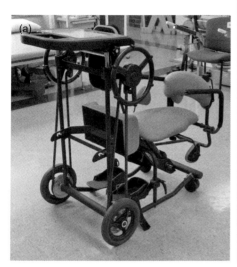

Fig. 8.2. Mobile standing device; (a) front and (b) side views.

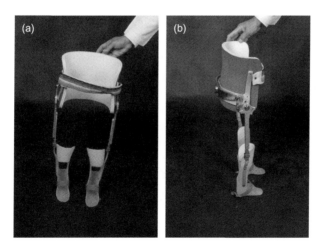

Fig. 8.3. Reciprocating gait orthosis; (a) front and (b) side views.

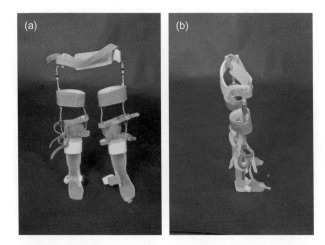

Fig. 8.4. Hip knee ankle–foot orthosis; (a) front and (b) side views.

parallel forward so that the body lands at the position of the assistive device. In contrast, in a swing-through gait using crutches, both legs are swung in parallel forward so that the body lands past the crutches with every step. Similar to the HKAFOs, the use of KAFOs is limited by the relatively slow and energy-inefficient gait pattern and the need to support most of one's body weight through the upper extremities.

Children with L3 neurological levels who exhibit strong iliopsoas and quadriceps strength (of 4–5/5) can be community ambulators. They may use floor-reaction ankle–foot orthoses (AFOs) or KAFOs with an unlocked knee joint to protect the medial longitudinal ligament. Floor- (or ground-) reaction AFOs place the extension force closer to the knee to accentuate knee-extension at midstance (Fig. 8.5). In younger children with spina bifida who frequently have significant internal tibial torsion, twister cables may be necessary to provide better leg alignment and foot progression in a neutral position.

Young people with low lumbar to high sacral levels have strong iliopsoas, quadriceps and medial hamstrings (4–5 muscle strength), relatively strong anterior tibialis and glutei (3–5), and weaker gastrocnemius (0–3). This group of patients will be community ambulators, and those with strong hip extensors may seldom require a wheelchair. Standard or floor-reaction AFOs are usually needed because of weak plantar flexors and a mildly crouched gait.

Young people with sacral-level lesions demonstrate partial weakness of the gluteus maximus, gastrocnemius, soleus, and foot intrinsic muscles, and are usually community ambulators. They rarely need assistive devices or orthotics or at most they may need supra-malleolar AFOs to maintain the foot in a neutral position (Fig. 8.6). They frequently exhibit cavus and intrinsic foot deformities and are prone to pressure ulcers of their feet; therefore they need to pay close attention to footwear, the amount of standing and walking, and avoidance of adverse local factors such as moisture and extremes of temperature.

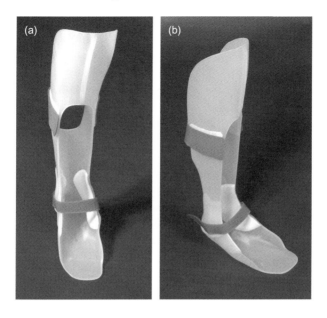

Fig. 8.5. Floor-reaction ankle–foot orthosis; (a) front and (b) side views.

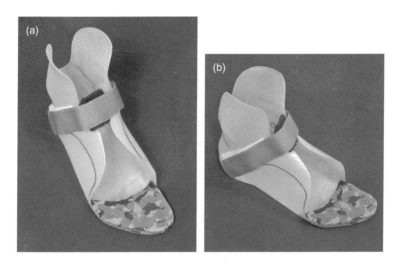

Fig. 8.6. Supramalleolar ankle–foot orthosis; (a) front and (b) side views.

Another potential ambulation option for children with SCIs is functional electrical stimulation (FES) in which electrical stimulation is applied to a peripheral nerve to cause contraction of the corresponding muscle. FES systems have been demonstrated to be feasible and practical (Johnston et al. 2003). Using implanted FES systems, adolescents are able to stand at home, allowing them to perform common activities while standing such as reaching high places (Johnston et al. 2003).

Compared with KAFOs, implanted FES systems were more effective in promoting independence and were preferred for most activities (Bonaroti et al. 1999). Contraindications for lower extremity implanted FES systems include hip dislocation, contractures, severe scoliosis, and myocutaneous flaps performed for pressure ulcers (Triolo et al. 1994). Therefore, it is important to prevent these complications in children and adolescents with SCIs, who may benefit in the future from innovative treatments such as FES. Although implanted FES systems are not currently available, the Parastep System®, a system approved by the United States Food and Drug Administration, is commercially available and uses surface electrical stimulation of the quadriceps, hamstring, and gluteus muscles for ambulation (Chaplin 1996).

Regardless of the type of upright mobility device used, particular attention to and careful monitoring of the shoulder, elbow, and wrist must occur to prevent overuse syndromes and pain. Children, particularly as they get older, should engage in a routine upper limb exercise programme to maintain strength and range of motion, and prevent upper extremity pain and overuse syndromes.

WHEELCHAIRS AND SEATING

Most individuals with SCIs will require a wheelchair for most of their community mobility; therefore, custom-fitted wheelchairs should be introduced as early as 15 months of age to maximize independence at all ages (Krey and Calhoun 2004). Wheelchairs must be sized correctly throughout the growing years, with annual evaluations to ensure the wheelchair fits appropriately and is properly maintained. Ideally wheelchairs that are prescribed for children before completing their growth during adolescence should have growth potential that includes adjustment for seat depth and width, and foot plate height.

The ability of the young person to operate the wheelchair independently should determine whether a manual or power chair is prescribed. In general, the use of traditional pushchairs (strollers/buggies) should be reserved for children less than 15 months of age. Children as young as 15 months of age should be able to operate either a manual or power wheelchair independently, depending upon their neurological impairment and their cognitive functioning. Children with paraplegia and those with lower level tetraplegia (C7–C8) will generally use a manual wheelchair. Children with C6-level tetraplegia may use manual wheelchairs but may require power wheelchairs for longer distances. In contrast, power wheelchairs would be appropriate for those with higher levels of tetraplegia (C5 and higher) and some with lower levels of tetraplegia. Pushrim-activated, power-assisted wheelchairs are an option for children with lower level tetraplegia or higher-level paraplegia. Power-assisted wheelchairs have an add-on powered motor on each of the rear wheels that augments the force applied to the pushrim with additional rear-wheel torque (Fig. 8.7).

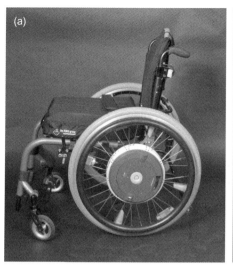 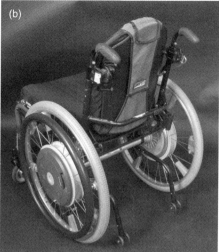

Fig. 8.7. Power-assisted wheelchair; (a) side and (b) rear views.

Major factors associated with readiness to use a power wheelchair include cognition and problem solving skills, sensorimotor integration skills, and temperament (attentiveness, persistence, and motivation) (Krey and Calhoun 2004). Manual wheelchairs for preschool children can be equipped with handles so that a caregiver can assist in pushing the child for longer distances. An important factor that must be considered when prescribing a wheelchair is long-term upper extremity overuse syndromes associated with manual chairs.

Therefore, children who use a manual wheelchair should have their wheelchair propulsion characteristics evaluated every 1 to 2 years. During these periodic evaluations, proper wheelchair propulsion mechanics that must be emphasized include decreased number of strokes as well as long, smooth, wheelchair-propulsive strokes (Fig. 8.8) (Consortium for Spinal Cord Medicine 2005). The rear wheel should be positioned as far forward as possible to decrease rolling resistance and improve propulsion efficiency. Additionally, the seat should be positioned so that when the hand is placed at the top dead-centre position on the pushrim, the angle between the upper arm and forearm is between 100 and 120° (Fig. 8.9). Ideally for those who use manual wheelchairs, an ultralight chair, weighing less than 9 kg, should be prescribed because lighter wheelchairs require less force to propel, are more adjustable, are made with better components, and cost less to operate (Cooper et al. 1997, Beekman et al. 1999, Fitzgerald et al. 2001).

The most appropriate interface for operating a power wheelchair is dependent upon the degree of neurological impairment. Children with C5 or lower neurological levels can usually operate a power chair with a joystick, which may need to be modified with a T-piece for those with C5 or weak C6 lesions. Children with C4 or higher lesions will use either a sip and puff interface or a head array system. Power wheelchairs should be equipped with a tilt or recline function to allow for pressure relief. Power wheelchairs can also be

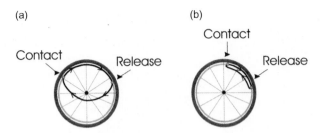

Fig. 8.8. The recommended propulsion pattern is shown in (a). An example of poor propulsion pattern is shown in (b) (arc pattern). The thick line on the wheel is the path followed by the hand. Reprinted with permission from the Paralyzed Veterans of America 2005.

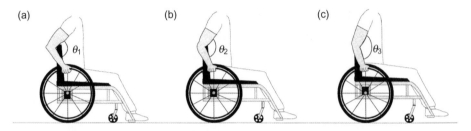

Fig. 8.9. (a–c) Differences in the elbow flexion angle (θ) from adjusting the height of the axle. (b) The recommended elbow angle ($\theta_2 = 100–120°$). (a) Angle θ_1 is smaller because the seat is too low (axle too high). (c) Angle θ_3 is larger because the seat is too high (axle too low). Reprinted with permission from the Paralyzed Veterans of America 2005.

configured with power seat elevators or a stand feature. For those with high cervical lesions and poor neck control, proper head support should be provided.

Irrespective of the type of wheelchair, children and adolescents of all ages should have a customized pressure-reducing seating system prescribed based on pressure mapping. A wheelchair cushion should redistribute the child's body weight in an even fashion over their entire seating surface to avoid excess weight on bony prominences, especially the ischial tuberosities. There are a wide variety of wheelchair cushions, including foam, gel, air, polyurethane honeycomb, and hybrid cushions that combine two or more materials. Pressure mapping systems measure the pressure distribution of a seated individual using a pressure sensing mat (Fig. 8.10). Evaluation of pressure-reducing seating systems should be performed at least annually. These sessions are also important for biofeedback to allow the child to see the areas of high pressure and how they can influence changes in pressure by using the appropriate weight shifting manoeuvres.

Ready access to one's community is important at all ages, but becomes most critical in adolescence. Whether public or private, motorized transportation must be accessible and enhance an adolescent's independence. Individuals with lesions as high as C5 are capable of driving an appropriately adapted motor vehicle, so it is imperative that they receive proper driver's evaluations and prescriptions for motor vehicle adaptations. The age when

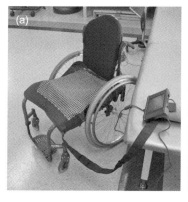 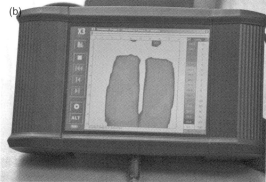

Fig. 8.10. (a) Pressure mapping system and (b) an example of a printout demonstrating excessive areas of pressure.

adolescents can obtain a drivers permit and eventually a driving licence varies between countries as well as regions or states but generally is 16 to 18 years of age.

Adolescents with paraplegia should be able to be transfer independently from an ultra-lightweight manual chair to the driver's seat of a motor vehicle and then transfer the wheelchair into the car. Most adolescents with tetraplegia, especially those who use power wheelchairs, will need an adapted van with a wheelchair lift and an automatic locking system for their wheelchair, either in the driver's position or as a passenger. Using an adapted van with a wheelchair lift, adolescents with tetraplegia or paraplegia who use a manual wheelchair would generally transfer themselves into the driver's seat. If the adolescent transfers onto the motor vehicle seat, their pressure-reducing seating system should be used.

Individuals of all ages with spinal cord dysfunction should be properly restrained in motor vehicles ranging from car seats for infants and toddlers, boosters for older children, specialized restraint systems for children with poor trunk or neck control, three-point restraints for appropriately sized older children and adolescents, to approved restraint systems for those who remain in their wheelchairs that are properly locked down.

Home modifications

As age-appropriate, children and adolescents with spinal cord dysfunction should be able to enter, exit, and manoeuvre independently throughout their living space, which should incorporate a barrier-free design. Barrier-free design with a one-floor plan not only facilitates independence but must also support safety. Ideally, access into and throughout the living space should be level and the surface should be firm and stable. If a ramp is needed for access into the house, its slope should be no more than 1:12, its width at least 42 inches wide, and it should have a non-slip surface. Each segment of the ramp should not exceed 30 feet. A ramp should incorporate a platform for rest, which should measure 5 feet × 5 feet (approximately 1.52 m × 1.52 m), and the entrance to the house should be covered to protect the child from inclement weather. For safety reasons, there should be two accessible exits out of the child's living quarters. At a minimum, doorways should be 32 inches (1 inch = 2.54cm) and hallways 36 inches wide, and preferably doorways should be 36 inches and hallways 42 inches wide. Interior and exterior doors should be equipped with lever-type door handles.

Within the living quarters, flooring should be a solid material such as wood or tile, rather than carpeting, to minimize the energy required to propel a manual wheelchair. Light switches should not be higher than 36 inches from the floor. Depending upon the neurological severity, the child's home should be equipped with appropriate environmental control units so that the child can access lighting, audiovisual equipment, computer, and communication equipment including a phone and an intercom.

The most challenging rooms are the kitchen and bathroom. The design of the kitchen should facilitate independent access and use of appliances, counter- and tabletops, sink, and cabinets. Side-by-side refrigerator–freezers or refrigerators with freezers at the bottom improve accessibility. Countertops should be 30 to 35 inches above the floor rather than the standard 36 inches. Access to countertops or the sink requires that there is no base cabinet below the countertop or sink. Pull-out work surfaces that can accommodate the child seated in a wheelchair are also useful. The sink height should be 30 to 31 inches and shallow enough to gain knee space below; the drain and water supply must be located in the rear and insulated to prevent thermal injury. The taps should be a single-lever design and placed to the side of the sink to facilitate usage. The cooker should have controls on the front or the side and the oven should be located low enough for easy access from a wheelchair (Fig. 8.11).

Bathroom design should allow for the use of a padded wheeled shower/commode chair that can easily fit over a commode and into a roll-in shower (Fig. 8.12). A roll-in shower should be two or three sided, it should be at least 5 by 5 feet and have no entrance threshold.

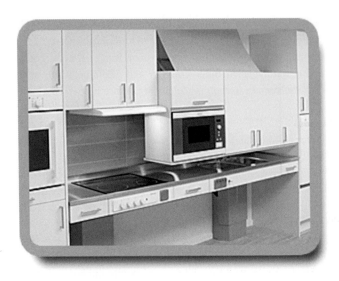

Fig. 8.11. Wheelchair-accessible stove top.

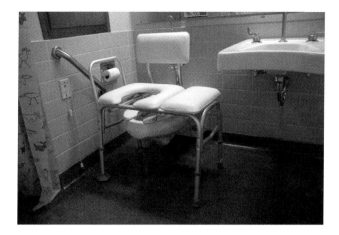

Fig. 8.12. Padded wheeled shower/commode chair.

If a roll-in shower is not possible, then a padded bath seat is essential. The bathroom sink should be mounted from the wall and allow the child in a wheelchair or a shower/commode chair to fit under the sink so that the sink should be no higher than 34 inches from the floor. The drain and water supply must be located in the rear and be insulated to prevent thermal injury. Water-mixing valves should be used for both the sink and shower, and a hand-held shower head with an on/off switch on its handle is essential. The bathroom should be connected to the child's bedroom and afford appropriate privacy.

Sensation

SKIN

Sensory loss places children with spinal cord dysfunction at risk of pressure ulcers or thermal skin injuries from the extremes of heat or cold (Hickey et al. 2000). In addition to pressure, risk factors for developing pressure ulcers include moisture, friction, and shearing.

Urinary incontinence places the adolescent at greater risk of pressure ulcers as a result of moisture; therefore, avoiding incontinence and nappies is important. Poorly performed transfers can create shearing and friction, and can be avoided by proper transfer techniques and the use of sliding boards.

As discussed in the wheelchairs and seating section, children and adolescents of all ages should have a customized pressure-reducing seating system prescribed based on pressure mapping. Other important measures in preventing pressure ulcers include regular pressure reliefs every 15 to 20 minutes while sitting, skin inspections at least twice daily, and repositioning every 2 to 4 hours while in bed.

Obesity may contribute to the development of pressure ulcers if being overweight interferes with transfers or the performance of pressure reliefs. Other contributing factors to the development of pressure ulcers include scoliosis, hip dysplasia, and heterotopic ossification. To prevent pressure ulcers of the foot it is important that properly fitted footwear be used. Although management of pressure ulcers is beyond the scope of this chapter, the basic principles of pressure ulcer management include prevention, correction of underlying factors, debridement, and moist wound healing (Priebe et al. 2010). More detailed information on the prevention and management of pressure ulcers can be found in Consortium for Spinal Cord Medicine (2000).

Burns including full-thickness skin loss can occur from relatively minor contact with warm or hot objects such as hair curling irons, laptop computers, or radiators. Lastly, inadvertent trauma can cause pathological fractures as well as soft-tissue trauma including abrasions and intramuscular or subcutaneous hematomas.

PAIN

Pain is a common complication after sustaining an SCI, and can be classified in several ways (Siddall et al. 1997, Bryce and Ragnarsson 2000). Musculoskeletal pain can be caused by overuse of muscle groups such as the shoulder muscles, related to transfers, wheelchair use, and overhead activities. In addition, musculoskeletal pain can be exacerbated by muscle imbalance around a joint.

Pain at the zone of injury (the neurological level) may be caused by nerve root compression at the level of injury or from mechanical instability. Dysaesthesia, or central pain, may be located at the zone of injury or below the zone of injury. Self-abusive behaviour, or self-mutilation, is occasionally seen in children and adolescents with SCIs with normal cognitive function and may be a manifestation of dysaesthesia (Vogel and Anderson 2002). Self-abusive behaviour most commonly involves biting of fingertips, which can result in finger amputations.

Irrespective of the cause, pain interferes with the rehabilitation of children with SCIs and significantly impacts their lives, including activities of daily living, participation, and their psychosocial well-being. Pain management should be performed by an interdisciplinary team, combining pharmacological, physical, and psychological modalities (Lau and McCormack 1996). Physical modalities may include physical therapy, hydrotherapy, or transcutaneous electrical neural stimulation. Medications commonly used for dysesthesia in the paediatric population with SCIs include anticonvulsants (gabapentin, pregabalin, carbamazepine, phenytoin), antidepressants (amitriptyline), or clonidine.

Respiratory complications

Pulmonary complications are major problems during both the acute and chronic phase of SCIs (DeVivo 1999, Massagli 2000). All children with SCIs should receive pneumococcal vaccine and annual influenza vaccines. Pulmonary function and an effective cough are impaired in children with tetraplegia and thoracic paraplegia because of respiratory and abdominal muscle paralysis and restrictive lung disease in those with associated scoliosis. Management of these impairments may include chest physiotherapy, inspiratory muscle training and assisted cough techniques. Non-invasive systems such as biphasic positive airway pressure and airway secretion management, such as mechanical insufflation/exsufflation or external vibration systems, may be used in the paediatric population with SCIs (Tromans et al. 1998, Nelson 2000).

Children with high cervical injuries will usually require lifelong ventilatory support. Phrenic nerve or diaphragmatic pacing may allow children to be independent of their ventilator for part or all of the day (Weese-Mayer et al. 1992, Onders et al. 2007). A phrenic nerve stimulator can be placed in the neck/supraclavicular region, which avoids the need for thorascopic surgery as required for diaphragmatic pacing. Bilateral phrenic nerve stimulation generally must be performed to avoid excessive mediastinal shifts. Tracheostomies are needed because of the upper airway obstruction that occurs in young children during phrenic nerve pacing. Some children may experience failure to thrive if they are entirely dependent upon phrenic nerve pacing, which may necessitate supplemental night-time positive pressure ventilation through a tracheostomy (Weese-Mayer et al. 1992).

Young people with tetraplegic SCIs, especially those who were injured at an early age, may be at risk of incipient respiratory failure, manifested by sleep-disordered breathing with sleep apnoea, snoring, morning confusion, headache, daytime somnolence, and lethargy and poor school performance (Flavell et al. 1992). Because the symptoms of sleep-disordered breathing may be subtle, a high index of suspicion must be maintained and sleep studies should be considered. Risk factors for sleep-disordered breathing include obesity and medications such as baclofen or diazepam (Bonekat et al. 1990). Management of sleep-disordered breathing may include nocturnal non-invasive ventilation with biphasic positive airway pressure, tonsillectomy, and adenoidectomy in selected cases.

Autonomic disturbances

Autonomic disturbances associated with spinal cord dysfunction include cardiovascular, thermoregulatory, bladder, bowel, and sexual dysfunction. Cardiovascular abnormalities include autonomic dysreflexia, bradycardia and orthostatic hypotension.

Autonomic dysreflexia is a result of sympathetic over-reactivity in individuals with T6 and higher-level lesions. It results from a noxious stimulus below the zone of injury, most commonly bladder distension (Consortium for Spinal Cord Medicine, 2002). Autonomic dysreflexia is manifested by hypertension, headache, facial flushing, sweating, and heart rate changes, most notably bradycardia.

Because of the varying cognitive and verbal abilities of children, autonomic dysreflexia may present in younger children with vague symptoms rather than complaints of a pounding headache, and infants and toddlers may only manifest irritability (Hickey et al. 2004, McGinnis et al. 2004, Schottler et al. 2009). Because of the potential life-threatening nature of the hypertension, prompt and accurate diagnosis and management are essential (Krassioukov et al. 2009).

Symptomatic measures, such as the relief of bladder distention by intermittent catheterization, are generally successful in managing most episodes of autonomic dysreflexia. For episodes that are not responsive to conservative measures, treatment includes either the application of nitropaste or nifedipine administered by chew and swallow for those who can follow directions or sublingually for younger children and infants.

Children who experience recurrent episodes of autonomic dysreflexia should be studied to exclude underlying inciting factors such as urinary stones or hip dysplasia. Recurrent autonomic dysreflexia can be managed with alpha-1 blockers, such as prazosin, doxazosin, or terazosin. It is important for children to have blood pressure checks as part of annual review and be aware of their 'normal' blood pressure to help assess the effect of elevation due to autonomic dysreflexia. All schools should be informed how to assist the child if autonomic dysreflexia develops.

Hyperhidrosis is seen primarily in those with tetraplegia or upper thoracic paraplegia. It is related to sympathetic overactivity of the spinal cord immediately below the zone of injury as a response to a noxious stimulus (Staas et al. 1989, Anderson et al. 1992). The sympathetic innervation of the sweat glands of the face and neck originates from T1–7, those for the trunk from T4–12, and those for the legs from T9–L2 (Staas et al. 1989). The primary focus of management should include avoidance or alleviation of precipitating factors; medications that may be beneficial include propantheline (Canaday and Stanford 1995) or transdermal scopolamine (Staas et al. 1989).

Bradycardia is primarily a problem during the first 4 to 6 weeks after injury for those with tetraplegia (Teasell et al. 2000). It is a result of increased vagal tone, unopposed by sympathetic activity, and may be precipitated by manoeuvres that precipitate increased vagal tone, such as tracheal suctioning or belching. If bradycardia is symptomatic, management could include avoidance of precipitating factors or vagolytic drugs such as atropine, particularly before tracheal suctioning. If bradycardia is associated with symptomatic hypotension and is unresponsive to anticholinergic therapy, transcutaneous pacing may be necessary.

Orthostatic hypotension primarily occurs in those with tetraplegia and upper thoracic paraplegia. It is manifested by light-headedness, headache, and occasionally syncope when a patient moves from a supine to sitting or standing position (Teasell et al. 2000, Claydon et al. 2006). Orthostatic hypotension results from inadequate vascular tone, poor venous return from the lower extremities due to muscle paralysis, and inadequate sympathetic control below the zone of injury. Management should include conservative measures such as abdominal binders, graduated elastic stockings, adequate fluid intake, use of a tilt table, and gradual change to the upright or sitting posture. For those who are unresponsive to conservative measures, options include alpha-agonists (pseudoephedrine, ephedrine, or midodrine) or mineralocorticoids (fludrocortisone).

THERMOREGULATORY DISTURBANCE

Spinal cord injuries at T6 or above may result in a poikilothermic state because the spinal cord damage interferes with central control of the thoracolumbar sympathetics and voluntary muscles of the lower body (Formal 1992). The child is unable to increase their core temperature by vasoconstriction and shivering below the zone of injury, and is unable to decrease core body temperature by vasodilatation and sweating below the zone of injury. This places these children at risk of hypothermia or hyperthermia as a result of environmental temperatures or exercise (Petrofsky 1992). Younger children are particularly vulnerable to environmental temperature extremes because of their relatively large surface area and their limited cognitive and verbal abilities. In contrast, adolescents with SCIs may be susceptible to hypothermia or hyperthermia because of their unpredictable behaviour and judgement.

BLADDER AND BOWEL DYSFUNCTION

Bladder and bowel dysfunction after an SCI result from the partial or total loss of bladder and bowel sensation with the inability to control the initiation or postponement of urination or defecation, respectively. Consequences of bladder and bowel dysfunction may include urinary or faecal incontinence, urinary tract infections, and constipation (Merenda and Brown 2007). In the absence of urological complications, the use of nappies is the primary mode of bladder and bowel management in infants and children younger than 2 to 3 years of age. Fears about possible bladder or bowel incontinence may lead, despite the associated embarrassment, to the wearing of nappies and may inhibit a young person's participation in activities with their peer group. Therefore, a major goal of bladder and bowel management is that nappy-like undergarments should not be worn after 3 years of age. Because bladder or bowel incontinence is a feared event for all children with a neurogenic bowel or bladder, appropriate contingency plans, including a change of clothing, are necessary.

Bladder management

Clean intermittent catheterization is the standard for bladder management of children and adolescents with SCIs (Lapides et al. 1972, Fernandes et al. 1994, McLaughlin et al. 1996, Vogel and Pontari 1997). The catheterization programme is generally initiated at approximately 3 years of age, or earlier if the child has recurrent urinary tract infections or renal impairment. For children with adequate hand function, self-catheterization is begun when they are developmentally 5 to 7 years of age (McLaughlin et al. 1996).

Children should be afforded appropriate privacy during catheterization, which may be difficult for children attending school because of the lack of accessible toileting facilities and adequate privacy. For children who are unable to perform their own catheterization, properly trained personnel need to be available to perform the catheterization in a private and professional manner and with minimal disruption to the school schedule.

Prophylactic antibiotics should be limited to children with recurrent or severe urinary tract infections and those with compromised renal function or obstructive uropathy, such as vesico-ureteric reflux or hydronephrosis (National Institute on Disability and Rehabilitation Research Consensus Statement 1992). Patients with asymptomatic bacteriuria are generally not treated unless they have compromised renal function. Treatment of urinary tract infections should be limited to symptomatic infections associated with systemic toxicity (fever, chills, autonomic dysreflexia, or exacerbation of spasticity), incontinence, or cloudy and foul-smelling urine. Because of the potential adverse effects of fluoroquinolones on articular cartilage and tendons, fluoroquinolones should be used sparingly in children younger than 18 years of age (Schaad 1999).

Continence and independence are important goals of bladder management for children with SCIs. Management of incontinence may include anticholinergics (antimuscarinics), modification of fluid intake and catheterization schedule, and treatment of urological complications, such as urolithiasis and urinary tract infections. Children with incontinence associated with neurogenic detrusor overactivity are most likely to benefit from the use of antimuscarinic medications, such as oxybutynin, tolterodine, solifenacin, and trospium. For children with limited bladder capacity unresponsive to a antimuscarinic medications, options include botulinum toxin injections into the detrusor (Giannantoni et al. 2009) or bladder augmentation (Kass and Koff 1983, Gray and Yang 2000).

Continent catheterizable conduits may be a beneficial alternative for children who are unable or have difficulty performing intermittent catheterization (Gray and Yang 2000). A continent catheterizable conduit (the Mitrofanoff procedure) involves creating a catheterizable conduit using the appendix or a segment of small bowel connecting the bladder to a stoma in either the umbilicus or on the lower abdominal wall (Mitrofanoff 1980). Young people with C6 or C7 lesions with limited hand function are usually able to catheterize themselves using a continent catheterizable stoma (Chaviano et al. 2000, Pontari et al. 2000, Chulamorkodt et al. 2004, Merenda et al. 2007). Continent catheterizable conduits are also good alternatives for young people who have difficulty accessing their urethra, such as females who cannot actively abduct their legs, or those who have difficulty transferring to a commode or toilet.

Urological evaluation of children with SCIs should include baseline urodynamics, renal ultrasound, and voiding cystourethrogram (Pannek et al. 1997). Routine follow-up generally includes annual renal ultrasounds, whereas urodynamics should be repeated in those with persistent incontinence and renal scans performed in those with renal compromise.

Bowel management

Important elements of bowel management include complete and regular emptying, a quick rather than time-consuming bowel programme, continence, aesthetics, privacy, and the prevention of constipation or diarrhoea (Gleeson 1990, Goetz et al. 1998, Merenda and Brown 2007). Regularity in performing bowel programmes is frequently in conflict with the non-conformity of childhood and adolescent lifestyles. However, anxiety about fecal incontinence is a strong incentive for compliance with a bowel programme. Bowel programmes should be initiated when children are 2 to 3 years of age, which is a developmentally appropriate age. A regular pattern of bowel emptying through use of laxatives and suppositories should be established. Parents often choose an evening routine to ensure the procedure is less rushed than before the school run.

Children with adequate hand function should be taught to perform their own bowel programmes when they are 5 to 7 years old. Ideally, bowel programmes should be performed on a toilet or a commode both for hygienic reasons and because the sitting position facilitates defaecation. The child should be taught and encouraged to grunt or blow bubbles by increasing intra-abdominal pressure. Laxatives (such as senna or polyethylene glycol), stool softeners (docusate or lactulose), and suppositories (such as glycerine, enemeez/docusate mini-enemas, or magic bullet/water-soluble bisacodyl) are frequently helpful in establishing and maintaining a successful bowel programme.

Other alternative bowel programmes include retrograde irrigation systems (such as the Peristeen) (Puet et al. 1997) or the Malone antegrade continence enema procedure (Mace procedure) (Herndon et al. 2004). Candidates for either the retrograde irrigation systems or antegrade continence enemas include young people with myelomeningocele and poorly controlled bowel movements or those with SCIs and limited upper extremity function that inhibits their ability to transfer independently to a commode and perform bowel programme manoeuvres such as the insertion of suppositories or manual extraction. These programmes should ideally be performed while the child is sitting safely and well supported on a toilet so that appropriate training with qualified staff is needed to assist in the best compliance with these methods. Using the Malone antegrade continence enema procedure (Mace procedure), antegrade evacuation of the bowel is accomplished by administering an enema directly into the caecum through a surgically created conduit, commonly using the appendix, which is accessible through an abdominal wall stoma.

SEXUALITY

Sexuality should be addressed from a developmental perspective from the time of initial rehabilitation and should be continued during regular follow-up encounters (Yarkony and Anderson 1996, Anderson 1997a, Sawyer and Roberts 1999, Sipski Alexander and Alexander 2007). The topic of sexuality should be initiated at the time of injury, regardless of the age of the child, so that parents have accurate information about future sexuality issues for their child. For those with SCIs without an associated traumatic brain injury, sexual development and puberty, including the onset of menses, should not be affected (Anderson et al. 1997). Females who had menarche before their injury will usually have resumption of menstruation within 6 months of sustaining their SCI. The characteristics of menstruation in individuals with SCIs will not differ from those without an SCI. Young people with myelomeningocele may experience an early onset of puberty, so it is important that they and their parents be prepared for precocious puberty (Trollman et al. 1998).

Sexuality issues should be addressed during infancy and early childhood and include educating caregivers about their child's future sexuality and fertility. Parents should be aware that their children will be able to engage in sexual activity and have children when they grow up; these are concerns that parents may have shortly after their child sustains an SCI but are afraid to ask. School-aged children and adolescents need to be provided with developmentally appropriate sexuality information, which should include fertility, sexual functioning, the progression of sexual development, and onset or resumption of menses. When children are 9 to12 years of age and sexuality programmes are initiated in school, they may have questions about how their spinal cord dysfunction impacts on sexual function and menstruation. Adolescents may have more specific questions about erection, ejaculation, sexual intercourse, fertility, birth control, and pregnancy. Both females and males with myelomeningocele should be counselled about their increased risk of having a child with myelomeningocele (Toriello and Higgins 1983).

Females with SCIs are as capable of becoming pregnant as those without SCIs. Those with T6 and higher neurological levels need to be aware of the potential of autonomic dysreflexia during labour and delivery, which presents with hypertension and must be distinguished from pre-eclampsia (Consortium for Spinal Cord Medicine 2002, Jackson 2010). Menstruation in females with SCIs is frequently complicated by bladder spasms, worsening of muscle spasticity, and autonomic symptoms such as sweating, flushing, or headaches (Jackson and Wadley 1999). These peri-menstrual problems may be alleviated by anti-inflammatory medication (Jackson 2010). Managing menstrual flow is a matter of personal choice for the female and may require the input of carers.

The extent and specifics of sexual dysfunction depend upon the level of the SCI, its severity (AIS), and whether it is an upper or lower motoneuron lesion (Elliott 2010a, b). For those with complete upper motoneuron lesions, the sacral reflexes remain intact so that males will have reflex erections and females may experience reflex vaginal lubrication. Those with complete lower motoneuron lesions, or flaccid paralysis, do not have intact sacral reflexes, but they usually have central control of the thoracolumbar sympathetics. As a result, they may not experience reflex erections or vaginal lubrication but may experience psychogenic erections or vaginal lubrication as well as ejaculation in males. Individuals with incomplete lesions generally possess a greater degree of sexual functioning, including the ability to experience orgasm, than those with complete lesions.

Males with spinal cord dysfunction frequently have problems with fertility, including erection and ejaculation. Therefore, they need to be aware of the availability of fertility clinics that have expertise with individuals with spinal cord dysfunction and the myriad of available procedures to assist in fertility. Potential management of erectile dysfunction includes vacuum pump with constriction rings; intracavernous injections of papaverine, phentolamine, or prostaglandins (PGE1, alprostadil); or phosphodiesterase type 5 inhibitors (sildenafil, tadalafil, or vardenafil). Use of penile implants is limited because of the high rate of infection and erosion. Lastly, erections may be obtained in males by the insertion of sacral anterior root stimulator implants (The Brindley Finetech SARSI®); however, this requires the surgical implantation of an electrical stimulation device and division of the sacral posterior roots.

The two main methods of managing ejaculatory dysfunction include vibrostimulation or electroejaculation (Elliot 2010a). The first line of management of ejaculatory dysfunction is vibrostimulation, which involves the application of a high-amplitude vibration to the glans penis using a hand-held vibrator. Ejaculation occurs as a result of intact sacral ejaculatory reflex. Electroejaculation is performed using commercially available electroejaculation stimulation equipment in which direct electrical current is applied through a rectal probe. Ejaculation most probably results from direct sympathetic stimulation to the prostate and seminal vesicles.

Female patients should be counselled to enhance their experience of sexuality. This may include use of vibrator therapy or lubrication gels, but for specific information referral to sexuality specialists is necessary.

Orthopaedic complications
Scoliosis is common in children who sustain an SCI before skeletal maturity, with 98% developing scoliosis and 67% requiring surgery; whereas, for those injured after skeletal maturity, scoliosis occurs in 20%, with 5% requiring surgical correction (Dearolf et al. 1990). These spine deformities result from muscle weakness, residual deformity, or may be iatrogenic, such as after laminectomy, and may be associated with pelvic obliquity, poor sitting balance, pressure ulcers, pain, or cardiopulmonary and gastrointestinal problems (Betz 1997). Thoracolumbosacral spine radiographs should be performed every 6 months before skeletal maturity and every 12 months thereafter. In certain centres, long spine radiograph are obtained with physical traction applied by a trained physiotherapist.

Additionally, some centres perform photography with anthropometric monitoring to reduce the radiation.

The role of prophylactic bracing with thoracolumbosacral orthoses is unclear. In a retrospective review of 123 children with SCIs, surgical fusion was reduced to 50% in those who were braced when their curve was 20° or less compared with 86% in those not wearing a brace (Mehta et al. 2004). In addition, the time to surgical correction was delayed 4 years in those braced compared with those not braced, which is significant in reference to spinal growth before a fusion is performed. In contrast, for those who were braced when their curve was 20 to 40°, there was a lesser reduction in those needing surgery from 86 to 60% and only a 1 year delay of surgery compared with those who were not braced. Major disadvantages of bracing include interference with independent function and mobility (Chavetz et al. 2007, Sison-Williamson et al. 2007). Irrespective of the severity of scoliosis, thoracolumbosacral orthoses may improve trunk support, facilitating sitting and upper extremity functioning.

Because of the difficulties and lack of compliance with bracing 24 hours a day, one author will recommend sleep systems or a lycra suit to attempt to manage posture throughout the day and night. It is important to consider the night-time as a possible treatment time for stretching and enabling the child to lie in a non-chair-shaped position.

When a curve progresses beyond 40° in children older than 10 years old, spine surgery is generally performed (Betz and Mulcahey 1994). For younger children, curves up to 80° are tolerated if they are flexible and decrease while in thoracolumbosacral orthoses; otherwise, a growing spinal system is recommended while waiting for enough spinal growth to perform a fusion. For adolescents who have completed their growth, the decision to correct the scoliosis surgically must take into account the loss of spine flexibility after a spine fusion versus the relatively slow progression of the spine deformity in skeletally mature individuals.

Scoliosis is also a very common complication of myelomeningocele, and is a result of a variety of factors, including congenital vertebral anomalies, neuromuscular weakness, pelvic obliquity, and hip contractures (Piggott 1980). Progression of scoliosis may be caused by uncompensated hydrocephalus, syringomyelia, or a re-tethered spinal cord (Tomlinson et al. 1994). Correction of hydrocephalus, syringomyelia, or a re-tethered spinal cord may slow curve progression in patients with less severe curvatures (less than 40°), but generally do not affect more severe curves.

Hip subluxation, dislocation, and contractures are frequent complications in children who sustain an SCI at younger ages (Betz and Mulcahey 1994, Miller and Betz 1996, Betz 1997, McCarthy and Betz 2006). In one series, hip dysplasia occurred in 100% of children who were injured when they were less than 5 years of age and in 93% of those injured less than 10 years of age (Betz and Mulcahey 1994, Miller and Betz 1996). Hip dysplasia occurs in patients regardless of their neurological level, presence or absence of spasticity, or their sex. Prevention and management of hip dysplasia in children with SCIs are not clear-cut. On the one hand, an aggressive approach to managing hip instability could be entertained in view of the future applications of the FES systems for upright mobility and the future possibility for spinal cord regeneration (Betz and Mulcahey 1994, Betz et al. 2001). The use of various types of orthoses to prevent hip dysplasia is without supporting evidence.

Radiology of the pelvis to assess hip location every 6 to 12 months before skeletal maturity is recommended.

As a result of post-traumatic immobilization, osteopenia begins shortly after sustaining an SCI with continued bone mineral loss for several years after injury (Giangregorio and McCartney 2006, Maimoun et al. 2006). In one study, children and adolescents with SCIs were found to have bone densities of approximately 60% of healthy age- and sex-matched comparisons (see Betz et al. 1991). Because of the role of vitamin D in bone metabolism, several studies have looked at the incidence of vitamin D deficiency in populations with SCIs. In one study of adults with SCIs, vitamin D deficiency was found in 34.5 to 53.8% of acutely injured adults, and 61.5 to 78.6% of those with chronic SCIs (see Oleson et al. 2010). In a pilot study at one of the authors' institutions, 39% of 82 children and adolescents with SCIs had vitamin D deficiency (Zebracki et al. 2013). Because of the high incidence of vitamin D deficiency, 25-hydroxy-vitamin D levels should be routinely monitored in individuals with SCIs and those with vitamin D deficiency should be treated with oral vitamin D to attain a 25-hydroxy-vitamin D level greater than 30 ng/ml (Bauman et al. 2011). The role of standing, walking, vibration, and FES on preventing or reversing bone loss in individuals with SCIs is unclear and requires further study (Giangregorio and McCartney 2006, Clark et al. 2007, Rauch 2009).

Spasticity
Approximately 50% of children with SCIs have spasticity. The management of spasticity should include a thorough history and physical examination with attention directed to potential exacerbating factors, such as hip dysplasia which is common in the paediatric population with SCIs. Goals should be to improve function, prevent complications, and alleviate pain (Vogel 1996). Advantages as well as disadvantages of spasticity must be considered when managing it. Potential advantages of spasticity include assistance in standing, sit-to-stand transfers, and maintenance of muscle bulk. Disadvantages of spasticity may include causing pain, interference with activities of daily living, disturbance of sleep, or development of contractures. The mainstay of management includes avoidance of precipitating factors, maintenance of good skin, bowel and bladder programmes, and mechanical-stretching, range-of-motion exercises and positioning.

Baclofen is the drug of choice for managing spasticity that interferes with function and is not responsive to conservative management. Use of baclofen must be closely monitored to ensure excessive daytime drowsiness and problems with school participation are avoided. Other medications that may be beneficial in the management of spasticity include diazepam, tizanidine, dantrolene, gabapentin, and clonidine. The use of diazepam is limited because of its sedative and abuse potential. Children treated with tizanidine or dantrolene must have liver function studies performed periodically because of potential hepatotoxicity.

For spasticity unresponsive to standard management, the primary options are intrathecal baclofen and localized injection of botulinum toxin (Penn 1989, Jankovic 1991). Intrathecal baclofen is beneficial in managing severe spasticity in children with SCIs; however, it is expensive and occasionally associated with serious adverse reactions (Armstrong et al. 1992).

Wellness/fitness

Because of the relatively long lifespan of children with SCIs, it is important to prevent complications, such as cardiovascular complications, that affect the quality and longevity of their lives. Exercise is critical in preventing cardiovascular complications, but is challenging in children with SCIs because of motor limitations and compliance that vary with age. Children and adolescents with tetraplegia and upper thoracic SCIs demonstrate decreased cardiovascular adaptations to exercise, including decreased cardiac output, reduced aerobic capacity, hyperthermia, and exertional hypotension (King et al. 1992, Petrofsky 1992, Hopman et al. 1993, Widman et al. 2007). The use of FES machines with cycling has yet to be evaluated for improving fitness.

Children with spinal cord dysfunction should participate in adapted physical education and therapeutic recreational activities, with goals of cardiovascular fitness, increased aerobic capacity, muscle strengthening, and endurance (Johnson and Klaas 2000, Liusuwan et al. 2007). Fitness programmes must be developmentally based, consistent with pre-injury interests, facilitate independence, be incorporated into family and community activities and, most importantly, be fun.

Children with spinal cord dysfunction should be assessed for their cardiovascular risks, including obesity, sedentary lifestyle, smoking, hypertension, hyperlipidemia, and family history, and screening for lipid abnormalities should be performed in those at high risk.

Psychosocial issues

Most SCIs in children or adolescents occur abruptly in individuals who have been developing normally and participating fully in their lives. This abrupt and severe change in function is devastating for the affected young people and their families (Warshausky et al. 1996, Anderson 1997b).

Although preschool children may not fully understand the implications of an SCI, they may be adversely affected by hospital procedures, therapy sessions, unfamiliar environments, and limitations to their functioning (Johnson et al. 1991). Preschool children may also be affected by the stress and grief that their parents experience (Aitken et al. 2005).

Older children and parents may have some familiarity with the concept of an SCI and paralysis, but few will be aware of all of the ramifications and intrusion on daily life such as catheterization, bowel programmes, pressure reliefs, and multiple medications. In addition to dealing with the initial shock of the diagnosis of SCI, young people and their parents must also adjust to the considerable burden of care that is lifelong, including the need to learn an extensive amount of new information about the care required for an SCI and how to perform the care.

At one time, it was thought that most individuals who sustained an SCI would go through a series of stages of emotional adjustment, including denial, anger, and depression. Empirically that theory was not supported and it did not take into account variations among individuals, styles of coping, and support available (Trieschmann 1998, Fitchtenbaum and Kirshblum 2002).

For young people and their parents, the initial adjustment to injury is further complicated by childhood developmental issues. Infants and preschool children tend to focus on the present and are most comforted by family. Because of the central role of play in the lives of younger children, rehabilitation should incorporate play activities. Along with other rehabilitation specialists, child life specialists (play specialists) are important in assisting these endeavours, including the use of adapted toys, electronically controlled devices, and large push buttons. School-age children, who were independent in toileting, dressing, feeding, and bathing before their SCI, may feel frustrated after injury by their dependency and the need for help from others. Many will verbalize that they want to walk and return to their pre-morbid activities such as bicycle riding or playing sports.

Because school-aged children are often very social, they will fear being left out of neighbourhood and school activities. Even younger school-aged children may grasp the concept that their disability is permanent, although they may continue to make statements about being able to walk when they 'get better'. Other concerns for children are fears that others will make fun of them, stare, ask what is wrong, and refuse to include them in play activities.

Adolescence is the most common age for paediatric-onset SCIs and may be the most difficult age at which to sustain an injury (Kennedy et al. 1995, Bloom and Joseph 2003). Adolescents are at a stage of establishing independence from parents and relating more with peers than family. Adolescents face a myriad of challenges including psychosocial issues, sexuality, and participation in school and community activities. Appearance, popularity, fitting-in, and self-esteem are particularly important (Mulcahey 1992). Older adolescents are in the process of transitioning into adulthood, which encompasses increasing independence, vocational planning, and assumption of an adult identity; an SCI significantly disrupts this process. Adolescents who sustain an SCI become more dependent on their parents and generally spend more time with them than with their peers during initial rehabilitation.

Adolescents may react to their loss of independence by showing anger towards staff and parents (Augutis et al. 2007). Adolescents may exhibit avoidance behaviours such as excessive sleeping, placing blankets over their heads so they cannot see or be seen, and refusing therapy or community expeditions (Augutis et al. 2007). During a developmental stage when privacy and sexuality are particularly relevant, bowel and bladder programmes, and bathing performed by staff or parents, may be particularly humiliating to an adolescent. The turbulent nature of adolescence makes them more vulnerable to SCI-related complications such as pressure ulcers, urinary tract infections, and depression.

Symptoms of post-traumatic stress disorder are commonly experienced by individuals after sustaining an SCI, with 25% of children and adults aged 11 to 24 years experiencing them (Boyer et al. 2000). Common symptoms include flashbacks or re-experiencing of the event, such as a car crash that caused the injury, and avoidance of discussions, images, or individuals that might be associated with the traumatic event.

In addition to the psychosocial issues that young people with spinal cord dysfunction face, the needs of their parents and other family members must also be addressed. Parents may experience guilt for a variety of reasons, including that they were involved to varying degrees in causing the injury or that they were unable to prevent it. During the acute hospitalization and initial rehabilitation, parents are under immense stresses related to absence from work, financial worries, and the needs of the rest of their family. Interventions to help parents to regain control of their situation include individual and family counselling as well as education, advice, for example on home modifications, and assistance with resources.

Many families fear that their child, regardless of age at injury, may not be able to live independently, have a job, become financially independent, or have a family of their own. Therefore, it is important to allay those fears by providing realistic expectations for future functioning and independence so that they continue to raise their child with appropriate expectations and goals in mind. Parents benefit from specific information about their child and general education about SCIs and the opportunity to meet with other parents and successful individuals with SCIs. Siblings are also an important part of the young person's family and need to be supported in the process and enabled to express their views and fears.

Throughout development, it is important that young people with spinal cord dysfunction keep up with peers in all aspects of community participation as they grow. As an example, it is common for school-aged children to attend birthday parties of classmates; however, children with spinal cord dysfunction may not be invited because parents of uninjured children are nervous or their houses are inaccessible. As a result the child with spinal cord dysfunction may experience social isolation and develop poor self-esteem. Similar issues arise for most of the activities of childhood and adolescence, whether it is scouting, sport, school outings, musical and theatrical activity. At each clinical review, community participation must be assessed so that appropriate guidance and suggestions, including integration strategies and resources for specialized recreation programmes, are provided. It is also important to make sure parents are aware that participation is important for all children and adolescents regardless of their injury.

SCHOOL

School is a major aspect of the lives of all children and adolescents, and is critical to their psychosocial development. Furthermore, education is important in preparation for future employment, which in turn is critical for independent living and life-satisfaction as an adult (Massagli et al. 1996, Anderson and Vogel 2002). Therefore, it is important that children with spinal cord dysfunction receive a well-rounded education in the least restrictive environment. Young people who have a concomitant traumatic brain injury and SCI, and children with myelomeningocele with associated cognitive impairments, may require additional educational interventions, but this should be provided in an inclusive fashion. In addition to the primary educational objective of school, children with spinal cord dysfunction should also participate as fully as possible in extracurricular activities with their peers. Schooling should recommence as early as possible during the rehabilitation hospitalization. Using internet technology, the child may be able to keep in touch with current activities in their own school.

One of the important objectives of discharge planning for young people with SCIs is to facilitate their return to school (Anderson 1997b). Ideally, the young person should return to the school they previously attended. The young person and their parents are frequently reluctant for the child to return to school for a variety of reasons, such as the need for a wheelchair and adaptive equipment, or the need to catheterize, and anxieties about social exclusion. Compared with the relative ease of the young person's previous experiences at school, it can be overwhelming to think of returning after an SCI. Parents may be concerned that their child will not receive adequate attention for their medical needs in school; this is addressed in discharge planning with the community team including the school health service. In addition, adolescents with a new SCI may worry about how their teachers and classmates will react.

Although schools may have experience with educating children with physical disabilities, they may not be familiar with the life-threatening medical complications related to spinal cord dysfunction, such as autonomic dysreflexia or hyperthermia. School personnel need to be educated about a variety of complications related to loss of sensation for young people with spinal cord dysfunction. Prevention of pressure ulcers requires frequent pressure reliefs, proper pressure-reducing seating systems, skin inspections, and avoidance of thermal injuries such as sun burns or burns from contact with a radiator. Most young people with spinal cord dysfunction are able to perform pressure relief independently by repositioning themselves in their wheelchair or altering the recline angle in power chairs. School staff need to be familiar with preventive measures and may need to remind some of the less compliant young people to sit on their cushions or perform pressure relief. Those with higher neurological levels may require assistance in feeding, toileting, writing, and participating in activities.

Privacy during catheterization is imperative, appropriately trained staff must be available for those who require assistance, and all efforts must be made to expedite the process to minimize disruption in the participation in the school schedule. Although older school-age children and adolescents can be responsible for remembering to catheterize, younger and less mature children may need assistance.

A learning support assistant may be employed to allow the child to keep up in the classroom. They need to be sensitive to the needs of the child and be aware of affecting how the child interacts with other children. This is particular important when children who may be ventilated are always surrounded by adults; those adults should be able to withdraw safely to allow the child private time with friends.

To avoid the inconvenience of adapting the school to the needs of the young person with an SCI, the school may take the position that the child does not have to return to school for the rest of the year because 'we will pass them anyway'. This approach can be detrimental to a young person with SCI because it limits the full spectrum of educational, recreational, and psychosocial elements of attending school, which are critical for development and transition into adulthood. If returning to school is delayed, it becomes increasingly difficult for the young person with an SCI to transition back into school. Additionally, returning to school shortly after discharge facilitates the child's return to their pre-injury lifestyle, resulting in a healthier, and a more satisfied social individual.

For elementary (junior) schoolchildren, three additional issues commonly arise about school. The first is the activity of the child on the playground and during break-time. Although teachers may be tempted to encourage the child to stay in the classroom and play games or read books, the best solution from a psychosocial and fitness perspective is to have accessible playgrounds and encourage activities that the child can participate in with their classmates.

A second problem area for many children with spinal cord dysfunction is physical education and the best solution is innovative programming that will include the child with an SCI in all activities. Finally, children must participate fully in extracurricular activities, such as field trips. Because much of the fun of field trips is socializing on the bus, having all of the children together on an accessible bus is the ideal solution. Similarly, high- (senior-)school students with spinal cord dysfunction should be included in all of the typical activities, such as dances or sporting events, with special efforts made to assure accessibility.

Vocational planning is an integral component of caring for adolescents with spinal cord dysfunction, with objectives changing throughout their developmental. For children of all ages, chores are the foundation for future employment, so that parents need to establish appropriate expectations that their children can participate in chores commensurate with their developmental age and physical abilities. In addition to household chores, young people should be encouraged to obtain neighbourhood jobs such as cutting lawns or baby-sitting and eventually part-time jobs as adolescents. Because parents of young people with spinal cord dysfunction may be overwhelmed with spinal cord dysfunction-related care and therapy issues, expectations that their children participate in chores or jobs assume a relatively low priority. It may be difficult to identify jobs that are suitable for young people with spinal cord dysfunction, especially those with more severe neurological impairments. As a consequence, adolescents with spinal cord dysfunction generally have less work experience than their peers and hence are at a disadvantage as they transition into adulthood (Anderson and Vogel 2000). Therefore, this is an area that deserves additional attention during regular follow-up visits to prepare adolescents gradually for transition to adulthood; it is also an area in which the spinal team must be proactive in allowing the parents to promote their children to be involved, and in allowing parents to discipline their children and set boundaries appropriately as they did before.

Scenario 1

This was a previously healthy male who at the age of 6½ years sustained a complete (AIS A) T3 SCI in a motor vehicle crash in March 1988, in which he was a rear-seated, restrained passenger. He exhibited a T2 to T3 interspinous ligamentous disruption with a non-displaced fracture of T3 and bilateral facet dislocation (Fig. 8.13) for which he underwent a posterior reduction and internal fixation. His only other associated injuries were free intraperitoneal air without obvious cause and a brief period of unconsciousness after the crash.

He was started on an intermittent catheterization programme and a daily bowel programme for his neurogenic bladder and bowel, respectively. Within 3 months of his injury, he exhibited severe lower extremity spasticity that was managed with oral baclofen.

Within 7 months he demonstrated a 45° thoracolumbar curve (Fig. 8.14). Because of rapidly progressive scoliosis despite use of a thoracolumbosacral orthosis, he underwent a posterior spine fusion with instrumentation from T5 to the sacrum 15 months after the injury when he was 7 years 11 months of age (Fig. 8.15).

One month later at 8 years of age, he underwent bilateral hip flexion contracture releases, a left femoral shortening and derotational osteotomy, and a left acetabular shelf

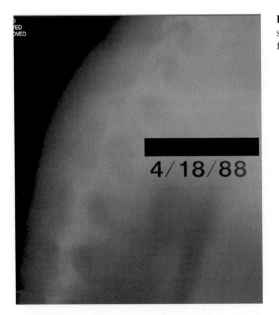

4/18/88

Fig. 8.13. Lateral tomogram of thoracic spine demonstrating perched T2–T3 facets.

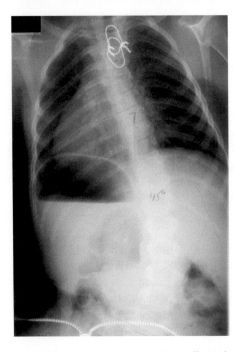

Fig. 8.14. Anterior–posterior spine radiograph demonstrating a 45° thoracolumbar scoliosis 7 months after injury.

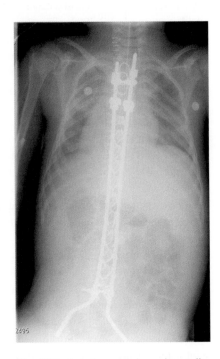

Fig. 8.15. Anterior–posterior spine radiograph after spine fusion performed 15 months after injury.

214

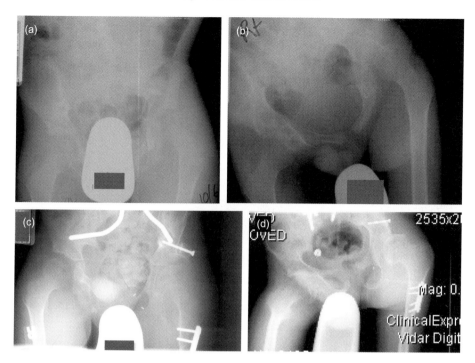

Fig. 8.16. (a) Anterior–posterior pelvic radiographs 7 months after injury; (b) 1 year after injury; (c) 3 months after bilateral hip flexion contracture releases, left femoral shortening and derotational osteotomy and left acetabular shelf procedure; and (d) 2½ years later.

procedure because of bilateral hip flexion contractures of 45° and a subluxed left hip (Fig. 8.16). Postoperatively, he was placed in a hip spica cast, but he developed a stage 2 sacral pressure ulcer which necessitated that a window be placed in the cast. The cast was removed 3 months later, but 3 days later he was diagnosed with a left distal femoral fracture that was managed with a knee immobilizer (Fig. 8.17). Within 6 months his hip flexion contractures had recurred (70° on the right and 30° on the left).

At 10 years of age, an intrathecal baclofen pump was inserted which significantly improved his spasticity; however, it was removed 1 year later because of skin erosion over the pump and subsequent infection.

At 12 years of age, he underwent an anterior spine fusion and revision of the posterior spine fusion because of hardware failure and a pseudoarthrosis (Fig. 8.18). Because of recurrence of the pseudoarthrosis, he underwent a second revision of his posterior spine fusion when he was 13½ years of age.

At his last clinic visit at 21 years of age, he continued to have significant hip and knee contractures. Currently he is 30 years of age, lives and drives independently, is unmarried, states that he is retired and lives on a large trust fund. He rates his life as extremely satisfying.

215

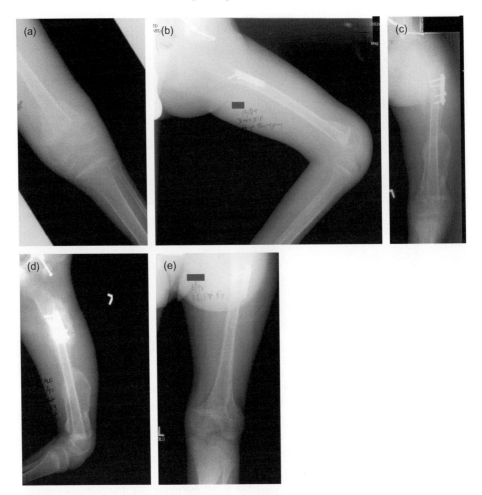

Fig. 8.17. (a) Anterior–posterior and (b) lateral radiographs of left femur 3 months after hip surgery demonstrating supracondylar femoral fracture. (c) Anterior–posterior and (d) lateral radiographs of left femur 6 weeks after femoral fracture demonstrating exuberant callus formation. (e) Anterior–posterior radiographs of left femur 2½ years after femoral fracture demonstrating remodelling of left femur.

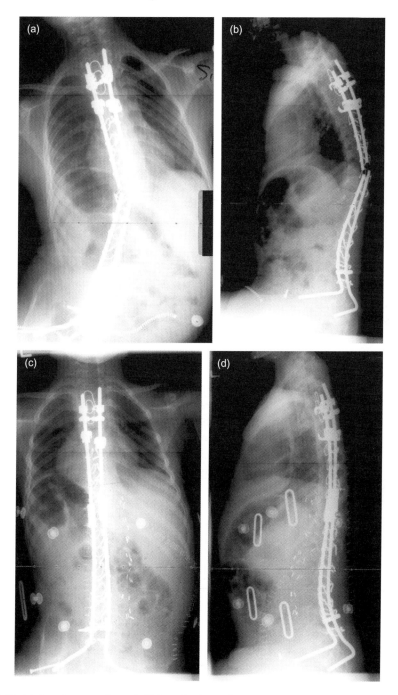

Fig. 8.18. (a) Anterior–posterior and (b) lateral spine radiographs 3 years after spine fusion demonstrating pseudoarthrosis and hardware failure. (c) Anterior–posterior and (d) lateral spine radiographs after anterior spine fusion and revision of posterior spine fusion.

Illustrative points include the following:

1. His severe spasticity and rapid progression of scoliosis, hip contractures, and subluxation
2. The development of pseudoarthrosis with failure of the posterior fusion was most probably related to his severe spasticity and spine fusion in a skeletally immature child. Contemporary practice would use surgical techniques that avoid fusion such as growing rods
3. The recurrence of the hip contractures after surgical release is not uncommon in children and adolescents. Therefore, releases of hip contractures should probably be limited to children or adolescents who are community ambulators
4. The development of a pathological fracture of the distal femur is not an uncommon occurrence in individuals with SCIs because of osteoporosis. The preceding use of a hip spica cast also contributed to the development of this fracture
5. Despite his SCI and multiple musculoskeletal complications including chronic back pain, he lives and drives independently and is extremely satisfied with his life. However, he does not work because he has a large trust fund.

Scenario 2

This was a 16½-year-old female who sustained a complete C6 SCI in a motor vehicle crash in January 1996 as the restrained driver. There were no associated injuries, other than a C6 burst fracture for which she underwent a C6 corpectomy and fusion.

At 18 years of age, she underwent a continent catheterizable conduit (an appendicovesicostomy or Mitrofanoff procedure). Four months and 8 months later she underwent bilateral deltoid to triceps transfers and staged House procedures on her left hand to reconstruct palmar grasp and key pinch. The upper extremity surgery allowed her to perform intermittent catheterization independently through her appendicovesicostomy and increase the efficiency and spontaneity with activity of daily living tasks, thereby increasing her independence (Fig. 8.19).

She is currently 31 years old, lives and drives independently, has a 10-year-old daughter, is divorced and rates her life as satisfying.

Illustrative points include the following:

1. This highlights the need for proper drivers' education and attention to automotive safety, including distracted driving, which in the 21st century includes use of mobile telephones and texting
2. The use of surgical interventions, such as the Mitrofanoff procedure and upper extremity tendon transfers, to increase independence and life satisfaction in individuals with SCIs
3. In individuals with C6 SCIs, the benefits of surgical procedures to reconstruct elbow extension include improved overhead reach, improved bed mobility, and transfers. An alternative to deltoid to triceps transfer is a biceps to triceps transfer, which may be preferable if there are pre-existing elbow flexion contractures.

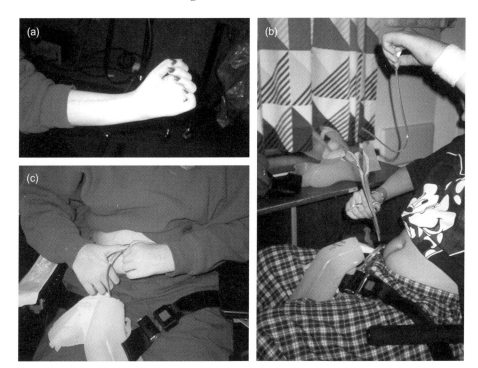

Fig. 8.19. (a) Key pinch after upper extremity surgery allowing her (b) to grasp catheter, and (c) perform catheterization through her appendicovesicostomy.

Summary

This chapter has provided an overview of unique issues in the management and rehabilitation of children and adolescents with spinal cord dysfunction. The two case scenarios demonstrate many of the complications that these individuals face throughout their lifespan. These also highlight the resiliency of these individuals and their ability to have full and satisfying lives, emphasizing the importance of developmentally appropriate care throughout their lifespan.

REFERENCES

Aitken ME, Korchbandi P, Parnell D, et al. Experience from the development of a comprehensive family support program for pediatric trauma and rehabilitation patients. *Arch Phys Med Rehabil* 2005; **86**: 175–179.

American Spinal Injury Association. International Standards for Neurological Classification of Spinal Cord Injury, Revised 2011. Atlanta, GA: American Spinal Injury Association, 2011.

Anderson CJ. Psychosocial and sexuality issues in pediatric spinal cord injury. *Top Spinal Cord Inj Rehabil* 1997a; **3**: 70–78.

Anderson CJ. Unique Management needs of pediatric spinal cord injury patients: Psychological issues. *J Spinal Cord Med* 1997b; **20**: 21–24.

Anderson CJ, Johnson KA, Klaas SJ, Vogel LC. Pediatric spinal cord injury: transition to adulthood. *J Voc Rehabil* 1998; **10**: 103–113.

Anderson CJ, Mulcahey MJ, Vogel LC. Menstruation and pediatric spinal cord injury. *J Spinal Cord Med* 1997; **20**: 56–59.

Anderson CJ, Vogel LC. Employment outcomes of adults who sustained spinal cord injuries as children or adolescents. *Arch Phys Med Rehabil* 2002; **83**: 791–801.

Anderson CJ, Vogel LC. Work experience in adolescents with spinal cord injuries. *Dev Med Child Neurol* 2000; **42**: 515–517.

Anderson LS, Biering-Sorensen F, Muller PG, et al. The prevalence of hyperhidrosis in patients with spinal cord injuries and an evaluation of the effect of dextropropoxyphene hydrochloride in therapy. *Paraplegia* 1992; **30**: 184–191.

Armstrong RW, Steinbok P, Farrell K, et al. Continuous intrathecal baclofen treatment of severe spasms in two children with spinal cord injury. *Dev Med Child Neurol* 1992; **34**: 731–738.

Augutis M, Levi R, Asplund K, Berg-Kelly K. Psychosocial aspects of traumatic spinal cord injury with onset during adolescence: a qualitative study. *J Spinal Cord Med* 2007; **30**: S55–S64.

Bauman WA, Emmons RR, Cirnigliaro CM, Kirshblum SC, Spungen AM. An effective oral vitamin D replacement therapy in persons with spinal cord injury. *J Spinal Cord Med* 2011; **34**: 455–460.

Beekman CE, Miller-Porter L, Schoneberger M. Energy cost of propulsion in standard and ultralight wheel-chairs in people with spinal cord injuries. *Phys Ther* 1999; **79**: 146–158.

Betz RR, Triolo RJ, Hermida VM, et al. The effects of functional neuromuscular stimulation on the bone mineral content in the lower limbs of spinal cord injured children. *J Am Paraplegia Soc* 1991; **14**: 65–66.

Betz RR, Mulcahey MJ. In Weinstein SL, editor. The Pediatric Spine: Principles and Practice. New York, NY: Raven Press, 1994: 781–810.

Betz RR, Mulcahey MJ, editors. The Child with a Spinal Cord Injury. Rosemont, IL: American Academy of Orthopaedic Surgeons, 1996.

Betz RR. Orthopaedic problems in the child with spinal cord injury. *Top Spinal Cord Inj Rehabil* 1997; **3**: 9–19.

Betz RR, Mulcahey MJ, Smith BT, et al. Implications of hip subluxation for FES-assisted mobility in patients with spinal cord injury. *Orthopedics* 2001; **24**: 181–184.

Bloom L, Joseph M. The effect of spinal cord injury in adolescence. *SCI Psychosoc Process* 2003; **16**: 237–243.

Bonaroti D, Akers J, Smith BT, et al. Comparison of functional electrical stimulation to long leg braces for upright mobility in children with complete thoracic level spinal injuries. *Arch Phys Med Rehabil* 1999; **80**: 1047–1053.

Bonekat HW, Anderesen G, Squires J. Obstructive disordered breathing during sleep in patients with spinal cord injury. *Paraplegia* 1990; **28**: 392–398.

Boyer BA, Knolls ML, Kafkalas CM, Tollen LG. Prevalence of posttraumatic stress disorder in patients with pediatric spinal cord injury: relationship to functional independence. *Top Spinal Cord Inj Rehabil* 2000; **6**: S125–133.

Bryce TN, Ragnarsson KT. Pain after spinal cord injury. *Phys Med Rehabil Clin N Am* 2000; **11**: 157–168.

Canaday BR, Stanford RH. Propantheline bromide in the management of hyperhidrosis association with spinal cord injury. *Ann Pharmcother* 1995; **29**: 489–492.

Chavetz RS, Mulcahey MJ, Betz RR, et al. Impact of prophylactic thoracolumbosacral orthosis bracing on functional activities and activities of daily living in the pediatric spinal cord injury population. *J Spinal Cord Med* 2007; **30**: S178–S183.

Chaviano AH, Matkov TG, Anderson CJ, McGovern PA, Vogel LC. Mitrofanoff continent catheterizable stoma for pediatric patients with spinal cord injury. *Top Spinal Cord Inj Rehabil* 2000; **6**: S30–35.

Chaplin E. Functional neuromuscular stimulation for mobility in people with spinal cord injuries. The Parastep®I System. *J Spinal Cord Med* 1996; **19**: 99–105.

Chulamorkodt NN, Estrada CR, Chaviano AH. Continent urinary diversion: 10-year experience of Shriners Hospitals for Children in Chicago. *J Spinal Cord Med* 2004; **27**: S84–S87.

Clark JM, Jelbart M, Rischbieth H, et al. Physiological effects of lower extremity functional electrical stimulation in early spinal cord injury: lack of efficacy to prevent bone loss. *Spinal Cord* 2007; **45**: 78–85.

Claydon VE, Steeves JD, Krassioukov A. Orthostatic hypotension following spinal cord injury understanding clinical pathophysiology. *Spinal Cord* 2006; **44**: 341–351.

Consortium for Spinal Cord Medicine. Acute management of autonomic dysreflexia: individuals with spinal cord injury presenting to health-care facilities. *J Spinal Cord Med* 2000; **24**: S39–101.

Consortium for Spinal Cord Medicine. Acute management of autonomic dysreflexia: individuals with spinal cord injury presenting to health-care facilities (2nd edition). *J Spinal Cord Med* 2002; **25**: S67–88.

Consortium for Spinal Cord Medicine. Preservation of upper limb function following spinal cord injury: a clinical practice guideline for health-care providers. *J Spinal Cord Med* 2005; **28**: 433–470.

Cooper RA, Gonzalez J, Lawrence B, Renschler A, Bonniger ML, VanSickle DP. Performance of selected lightweight wheelchairs on ANSI/RESNA tests. American National Standards Institute-Rehabilitation Engineering and Assistive Technology Society of North America. *Arch Phys Med Rehabil* 1997; **78**: 1138–1144.

Dearolf WW III, Betz RR, Vogel LC, et al. Scoliosis in pediatric spinal cord-injured patients. *J Pediatr Orthop* 1990; **10**: 214–218.

DeVivo MJ, Krause JS. Lammertse DP. Recent trends in mortality and causes of death among persons with spinal cord injury. *Arch Phys Med Rehabil* 1999; **80**: 1411–1419.

Elliott S. In Lin V, editor. Spinal Cord Medicine: Principles and Practice (2nd edition). New York, NY: Demos, 2010a: 409–428.

Elliott S. In Lin V, editor. Spinal Cord Medicine: Principles and Practice (2nd edition). New York, NY: Demos, 2010b: 429–437.

Fernandes ET, Reinberg Y, Vernier R, et al. Neurogenic bladder dysfunction in children: review of pathophysiology and current management. *J Pediatr* 1994; **124**: 1–7.

Fitchtenbaum J, Kirshblum S. Psychologic adaptation to spinal cord injury. In Kirshblum S, Campangnolo DI, DeLisa JA, editors. Spinal Cord Medicine. Philadelphia, PA: Lippincott Williams and Wilkins, 2002: 299–311.

Fitzgerald SG, Cooper RA, Bonninger ML, Renschler A. Comparison of fatigue life for 3 types of manual wheelchairs. *Arch Phys Med Rehabil* 2001; **82**: 1484–1488.

Fitzsimmons AS. In Betz RR, Mulcahey MJ, editors. The Child with a Spinal Cord Injury. Rosemont, IL: American Academy of Orthopaedic Surgeons, 1996: 533–535.

Flavell H, Marshall R, Thornton AT, et al. Hypoxia episodes during sleep in high tetraplegia. *Arch Phys Med Rehabil* 1992; **73**: 623–627.

Formal C. Metabolic and neurologic changes after spinal cord injury. *Phys Med Rehabil Clin N Am* 1992; **3**: 783–796.

Giangregorio L, McCartney N. Bone loss and muscle atrophy in spinal cord injury: epridemiology, fracture prediction, and rehabilitation strategies. *J Spinal Cord Med* 2006; **29**: 489–500.

Giannantoni A, Mearini E, Del Zingaro M Porena M. Six year follow-up of Botulinum Toxin A intradetrusorial injections in patients with refractory neurogenic detrusor overactivity: clinical and urodynamics results. *Eur Urol* 2009; **55**: 705–711.

Gleeson RM. Bowel continence for the child with a neurogenic bowel. *Rehabil Nurs* 1990; **15**: 319–321.

Goetz LL, Hurvitz EA, Nelson VS, et al. Bowel management in children and adolescents with spinal cord injury. *J Spinal Cord Med* 1998; **21**: 335–341.

Gray GJ, Yang C. Surgical procedures of the bladder after spinal cord injury. *Phys Med Rehabil Clin N Am* 2000; **11**: 57–72.

Herndon CDA, Rink RC, Cain MP, et al. In situ Malone antegrade continence enema in 127 patients: a 6-year experience. *J Urol* 2004; **172**: 1689–1691.

Hickey KJ, Anderson CJ, Vogel LC. Pressure ulcers in pediatric spinal cord injury. *Top Spinal Cord Inj Rehabil* 2000; **6**: S85–S90.

Hickey KJ, Vogel LC, Willis KM, Anderson CJ. Prevalence and etiology of autonomic dysreflexia in children with spinal cord injuries. *J Spinal Cord Med* 2004; **27**: S54–S60.

Hopman MT, Oeseburg B, Binkhorst RA. Cardiovascular responses in persons with paraplegia to prolonged arm exercise and thermal stress. *Med Sci Sports Exerc* 1993; **25**: 577–583.

Hussey RW, Stauffer ES. Spinal cord injury: requirements for ambulation. *Arch Phys Med Rehabil* 1973; **54**: 544–547.

Jackson AB, Wadley VA. A multicenter study of women's self-reported reproductive health after spinal cord injury. *Arch Phys Med Rehabil* 1999; **80**: 1420–1428.

Jackson AB. In Lin V, editor. Spinal Cord Medicine: Principles and Practice (2nd edition). New York, NY: Demos, 2010: 438–457.

Jankovic J, Brin MF. Therapeutic uses of botulinum toxin. *N Engl J Med* 1991; **324**: 1186–1194.

Johnson KA, Klaas SJ. Recreation involvement and play in pediatric spinal cord injury. *Top Spinal Cord Inj Rehabil* 2000; **6** (Suppl): 105–109.

Johnson KM, Berry ET, Goldeen RA, Wicker E. Growing up with a spinal cord injury. SCI Nursing 1991; **8**: 11–19.

Johnston TE, Betz RR, Smith BT, Mulcahey MJ. Implanted functional electrical stimulation: an alternative for standing and walking in pediatric spinal cord injury. *Spinal Cord* 2003; **41**: 144–152.

Kass EJ, Koff SA. Bladder augmentation in the pediatric neuropathic bladder. *J Urol* 1983; **129**: 552–555.

Kelly MA, Stokes KS. In Betz RR, Mulcahey MJ, editors. The Child with a Spinal Cord Injury. Rosemont, IL: American Academy of Orthopaedic Surgeons, 1996: 519–532.

Kennedy P, Gorsuch N, Marsh N. Childhood onset of spinal cord injury: sel-esteem and self-perception. *Br J Clin Pyschol* 1995; **34**: 581–588.

King M, Freeman DM, Pellicone JT, et al. Exertional hypotension in thoracic spinal cord injury: case report. *Paraplegia* 1992; **30**: 261–266.

Krassioukov A, Warburton DE, Teasell R, Eng JJ. A systematic review of the management of autonomic dysreflexia after spinal cord injury. *Arch Phys Med Rehabil* 2009; **90**: 682–695.

Krey CH, Calhoun CL. Utilizing research in wheelchair and seating selection and configuration for children with injury/dysfunction of the spinal cord. *J Spinal Cord Med* 2004; **27**: S29–S37.

Lapides J, Diokno AC, Silber SJ, et al. Clean intermittent self-catheterization in the treatment of urinary tract disease. *J Urol* 1972; **107**: 458–461.

Lau C, McCormack G. In Betz RR, Mulcahey MJ, editors. The Child with a Spinal Cord Injury. Rosemont, IL: American Academy of Orthopaedic Surgeons, 1996: 653–670.

Liusuwan RA, Widman LM, Abresch RT, Johnson AJ, McDonald CM. Behavioral intervention, Exercise, and Nutrition Education to improve health and Fitness (BENEfit) in adolescents with mobility impairment due to spinal dysfunction. *J Spinal Cord Med* 2007; **30**: S119–S126.

Maimoun L, Fattal C, Micallef J-P, Peruchon E, Rabischong P. Bone loss in spinal cord-injured patients: from physiopathology to therapy. *Spinal Cord* 2006; **44**: 203–210.

Massagli TL, Dudgeon BJ, Ross BW. Educational performance and vocational participation after spinal cord injury in childhood. *Arch Phys Med Rehabil* 1996; **77**: 995–999.

Massagli TL. Medical and rehabilitation issues in the care of children with spinal cord injury. *Phys Med Rehabil Clin N Am* 2000; **11**: 169–182.

McCarthy JJ, Betz RR. Hip disorders in children who have spinal cord injury. *Orthop Clin N Am* 2006; **37**: 197–202.

McDonald CM. Rehabilitatioin of children with spinal dysraphism. *Neurosurg Clin N Am* 1995; **6**: 393–412.

McDonald CM, Jaffe KM, Mosca VS, Shurtleff DB. Ambulation outcome of children with myelomeningocele: effect of lower-extremity muscle strength. *Dev Med Child Neurol* 1991a; **33**: 482–490.

McDonald CM, Jaffe KM, Shurtleff DB, Menelaus MB. Modifications to the traditional description of neurosegmental innervation in myelomeningocele. *Dev Med Child Neurol* 1991b; **33**: 473–481.

McGinnis KB, Vogel LC, McDonald CM, et al. Recognition and management of autonomic dysreflexia in pediatric spinal cord injury. *J Spinal Cord Med* 2004; **27**: S61–S74.

McLaughlin JF, Murray M, Van Zandt K, et al. Clean intermittent catheterization. *Dev Med Child Neurol* 1996; **38**: 446–454.

Mehta S, Betz RR, Mulcahey MJ, McDonald C, Vogel LC. Effect of bracing on paralytic scoliosis secondary to spinal cord injury. *J Spinal Cord Med* 2004; **27**: S88–S92.

Merenda L, Brown JP. Bladder and bowel management for the child with spinal cord dysfunction. *J Spinal Cord Med* 2007; **27**: S16–S23.

Merenda LA, Duffy T, Betz RR, Mulcahey MJ, Dean G, Pontari M. Outcomes of urinary diversion in children with spinal cord injuries. *J Spinal Cord Med* 2007; **30**: S41–S47.

Miller F, Betz RR. In Betz RR, Mulcahey MJ, editors. The Child with a Spinal Cord Injury. Rosemont, IL: American Academy of Orthopaedic Surgeons, 1996: 353–361.

Mitrofanoff P. Trans-appendicular continent cystotomy in the management of the neurogenic bladder. *Chir Pediatr* 1980; **21**: 297–305.

Mulcahey MJ. Returning to school after a spinal cord injury: perspectives from four adolescents. *Am J Occup Ther* 1992; **46**: 305–332.

National Institute on Disability and Rehabilitation Research Consensus Statement. The prevention and management of urinary tract infections among people with spinal cord injuries. *J Am Paraplegia Soc* 1992; **15**: 194–204.

Nelson VS. Noninvasive mechanical ventilation for children and adolescents with spinal cord injuries. *Top Spinal Cord Inj Rehabil* 2000; **6** (Suppl): 12–15.

Oakeshott P, Hunt GM, Whitaker RH, Kerry S. Perineal sensation: an important predictor of long-term outcome in open spina bifida. *Arch Dis Child* 2007; **92**: 67–70.

Oleson CV, Patel PH, Wuermser L-A. Influence of season, ethnicity, and chronicity on vitamin D deficiency in traumatic spinal cord injury. *J Spinal Cord Med* 2010; **33**: 202–213.

Onders RP, Elmo MJ, Ignagni AR. Diaphragm pacing stimulation system for tetraplegia in individuals injured during childhood or adolescence. *J Spinal Cord Med* 2007; **30**: S25–S29.

Pannek J, Diederichs W, Botel U. Urodynamically controlled management of spinal cord injury in children. *Neurourol Urodyn* 1997; **16**: 285–292.

Paralyzed Veterans of America Consortium for Spinal Cord Medicine. Clinical Practice Guidelines. Preservation of Upper Limb Function Following Spinal Cord Injury: A Clinical Practice Guideline for Health-Care Professionals. Washington, DC: Paralyzed Veterans of America.

Penn RD, Savoy SM, Corcos D, et al. Intrathecal baclofen for severe spinal spasticity. *N Engl J Med* 1989; **320**: 1517–1521.

Petrofsky JS. Thermoregulatory stress during rest and exercise in heat in patients with a spinal cord injury. *Eur J Appl Physiol* 1992; **64**: 503–507.

Piggott H. The natural history of scoliosis in myelodysplasia. *J Bone Joint Surg* 1980; **62B**: 54–58.

Pontari MA, Weibel B, Morales V, Dean G, Gaughan J, Betz RR. Improved quality of life after continent urinary diversion in pediatric patients with tetraplegia after spinal cord injury. *Top Spinal Cord Inj Rehabil* 2000; **6**: 25–29.

Priebe M, Wuermser L-A, McCormack. In Ed Lin VW. Spinal Cord Medicine. Principles and Practice, second edition. New York, NY: Demos, 2010: 659–672.

Puet TA, Jackson H, Amy S. Use of pulsed irrigation evacuation in the management of the neuropathic bowel. *Spinal Cord* 1997; **35**: 694–699.

Rauch F. Vibration therapy. *Dev Med Child Neurol* 2009; **51** (Suppl 4): 166–168.

Rauzzino M, Oakes WJ. Chiari II malformation and syringomyelia. *Neurosurg Clin N Am* 1995; **6**: 293–309.

Rosen L, Arva J, Furumasu J, et al. RESNA position on the application of power wheelchairs for pediatric users. *Assit Technol* 2009; **21**: 218–226.

Sarwark JF, Lubicky JP, editors. Caring for the Child with Spina Bifida. Rosemont, IL: American Academy of Orthopaedic Surgeons, 2002.

Sawyer SM, Roberts KV. Sexual and reproductive health in young people with spina bifida. *Dev Med Child Neurol* 1999; **41**: 671–675.

Schaad UB. Pediatric use of quinolones. *Pediatr Infect Dis J* 1999; **18**: 469–470.

Schottler J, Vogel L, Chafetz R, Mulcahey MJ. Patient and caregiver knowledge of autonomic dysreflexia among youth with spinal cord injury. *Spinal Cord* 2009; **47**: 681–686.

Siddall PJ, Taylor DA, Cousins MJ. Classification of pain following spinal cord injury. *Spinal Cord* 1997; **35**: 69–75.

Sipski Alexander M, Alexander CJ. Recommendations for discussing sexuality after spinal cord injury/dysfunction in children, adolescents and adults. *J Spinal Cord Med* 2007; **30**: S65–S70.

Sison-Williamson MM, Bagley A, Hongo A, et al. Effect of thoracolumbosacral orthoses on reachable workspace volumes in children with spinal cord injury. *J Spinal Cord Med* 2007; **30**: S184–191.

Staas WE, Nemunaitis G. Management of reflex sweating in spinal cord injured patients. *Arch Phys Med Rehabil* 1989; **70**: 544–546.

Teasell R, Arnold AP, Krassioukov AV, Delaney GA. Cardiovascular consequences of loss of supraspinal control of the sympathetic nervous system following spinal cord injuries. *Arch Phys Med Rehabil* 2000; **81**: 506–516.

Tomlinson RJ, Wolfe MW, Nadall JM, et al. Syringomyelia and developmental scoliosis. *J Pediatr Orthop* 1994; **14**: 580–585.

Toriello HV, Higgins JV. Occurrence of neural tube defects among first-, second-, and third-degree relatives of probands: results of a United States study. *Am J Med Genet* 1983; **15**: 601–606.

Trieschmann RB. Spinal Cord Injuries: Psychological, Social, and Vocational Rehabilitation. New York, NY: Demos, 1998.

Triolo RJ, Betz RR, Mulcahey et al. Application of functional neuromuscular stimulation to children with spinal cord injuries: candidate selection for upper and lower extremity research. *Paraplegia* 1994; **32**: 824–843.

Trollman R, Strehl E, Dorr HG. Precocious puberty in children with myelomeningocele. Treatment with gonadotropin-releasing hormone analogues. *Dev Med Child Neurol* 1998; **40**: 38–43.

Tromans AM, Mecci M, Barrett FH, et al. The use of the BiPAP biphasic positive airway pressure system in acute spinal cord injury. *Spinal Cord* 1998; **36**: 481–484.

Urui S, Oi S. Experimental study of the embryogenesis of open spinal dysraphism. *Neurosurg Clin N Am* 1995; **6**: 195–202.

Vogel LC. In Betz RR, Mulcahey MJ, editors. The Child with a Spinal Cord Injury. Rosemont, IL: American Academy of Orthopaedic Surgeons, 1996: 261–268.

Vogel LC, Lubicky JP. Ambulation in children and adolescents with spinal cord injuries. *J Pediatr Orthop* 1995; **15**: 510–516.

Vogel LC, Lubicky JP. Pediatric spinal cord injury issues: ambulation. *Top Spinal Cord Inj Rehabil* 1997; **3** (2): 37–47.

Vogel LC, Mulcahey MJ, Betz RR. The child with a spinal cord injury. *Dev Med Child Neurol* 1997; **39**: 202–207.

Vogel LC, Pontari M. Pediatric spinal cord injury issues: medical issues. *Top Spinal Cord Inj Rehabil* 1997; **3**: 20–30.

Vogel LC, Anderson CJ. Self-injurious behavior in children and adolescents with spinal cord injuries. *Spinal Cord* 2002; **40**: 666–668.

Vogel LC, Anderson CJ. Spinal cord injuries in children and adolescents: a review. *J Spinal Cord Med* 2003; **26**: 193–203.

Vogel LC, Mendoza MM, Schottler JC, Chlan KM, Anderson CJ. Ambulation in children and youth with spinal cord injuries. *J Spinal Cord Med* 2007; **30**: S158–164.

Vogel LC, Sturm P. Management of Patients with Developmental and Hereditary Spinal Cord Disorders. *Top Spinal Cord Inj Rehabil* 2008; **14** (2): 53–62.

Warschausky S, Engel L, Kewman D, Nelson VS. In Betz RR, Mulcahey MJ, editors. The Child with a Spinal Cord Injury. Rosemont, IL: American Academy of Orthopaedic Surgeons, 1996: 471–478.

Weese-Mayer DE, Hunt CE, Brouillette RT, et al. Diaphragm pacing in infants and children. *J Pediatr* 1992; **120**: 1–8.

Widman LM, Abresch RT, Styne DM, McDonald CM. Aerobic fitness and upper extremity strength in patients aged 11 to 21 years with spinal cord dysfunction as compared to ideal weight and overweight controls. *J Spinal Cord Med* 2007; **30**: S88–S96.

Yarkony GM, Anderson CJ. In Betz RR, Mulcahey MJ, editors. The Child with a Spinal Cord Injury. Rosemont, IL: American Academy of Orthopaedic Surgeons, 1996: 625–637.

Zebracki K, Anderson CJ, Chlan KM, Vogel LC. Outcomes of adults with pediatric-onset spinal cord injury: longitudinal findings and implications on transition to adulthood. *Top Spinal Cord Inj Rehabil* 2010; **16**: 17–25.

Zebracki K, Hwang M, Patt PL, Vogel LC. Cardiovascular dysfunction and vitamin D deficiency in pediatric spinal cord injury. *J Pediatr Rehabil Med* 2013; **6**: 45–52

9
PROSPECTS FOR SPINAL CORD REPAIR

Elizabeth Muir and Roger Keynes

Restoring function after spinal cord injury (SCI) presents a formidable challenge for regenerative medicine. In his seminal studies on nerve regeneration, Ramon y Cajal (Cajal 1928) recognized the root causes of central nervous system (CNS) regenerative failure after injury as '. . . proliferative inability and irreversibility of intra-protoplasmic differentiation'; or, in contemporary language, 'failure of neuronal stem cell renewal and absence of axon regeneration'. Over the past 30 years there has been a tremendous increase in the number of laboratory studies of SCI, and several approaches for its treatment are now in development. These are mostly directed at promoting axon regeneration and/or plasticity, for the difficulties in restoring spinal cord neural circuits by introducing neuronal stem cells, which are not normally present in the mature spinal cord, remain considerable. Accordingly, in this review we discuss recent advances in understanding the molecular basis for regenerative failure of injured spinal cord axons, and possible ways to stimulate functional recovery by axon sprouting and long-distance extension. Our focus is on traumatic injury, which is the most commonly investigated animal model of SCI. However, dysfunction resulting from regenerative failure of the spinal cord also arises when the primary insult is due to other causes such as inflammation, malignancy, and metabolic disease.

SCI triggers many further tissue-damaging processes which, in turn, often cause secondary tissue loss and cavitation. These include inflammatory responses, and release of excitotoxic transmitters, such as glutamate, that lead to excess calcium entry into cells. Neurons may be deprived of neurotrophic support from their target cells. Moreover, the constituent cells of a CNS-protective glial 'scar' – reactive astrocytes, oligodendrocyte precursor cells, and fibroblastic meningeal cells – create a barrier to axon outgrowth by expression of diverse molecules that inhibit axon regeneration (Afshari et al. 2009; see Table 9.1 for summary). Prominent among these are members of the semaphorin family of axon guidance molecules (e.g. Sema3A; Giger et al. 2010), and of the Eph family of tyrosine kinase receptors (e.g. EphA4; Goldshmit et al. 2004, Afshari et al. 2009) and their ephrin ligands (Giger et al. 2010). The scar extracellular matrix also contains other inhibitory molecules, in particular chondroitin sulphate proteoglycans (CSPGs) such as NG2, phosphacan, brevican and neurocan, and tenascin C (Afshari et al. 2009). Myelin proteins (e.g. Nogo, Mag, and OMgp) provide a further barrier to axon regeneration (Giger et al. 2010), and the 'repulsive guidance molecule' (RGM) expressed on neurons, astrocytes, and leukocytes accumulates extracellularly (Mueller et al. 2006).

TABLE 9.1
Extracellular inhibitors of axon outgrowth

Molecules	Produced by	Reference
Sema 3A	Meningeal fibroblasts	Niclou et al. (2003)
Ephs/ephrins	Injured axons	Afshari et al. (2009)
	Astrocytes	Fabes et al. (2007)
Myelin inhibitors	CNS myelin	Filbin (2003)
Nogo, myelin-associated glycoprotein, oligodendrocyte myelin glycoprotein	Oligodendrocytes	Schwab (2010)
Keratan sulphates	Macrophages	Jones and Tuszynski (2002)
	Reactive microglia	
	Oligodendrocyte progenitors	
Tenascins/tenascin R	Oligodendrocytes	Fawcett and Asher (1999)
	Meningeal cells	
	Scar astrocytes	
Chondroitin sulphate proteoglycans		
Neurocan	Scar astrocytes	Fawcett and Asher (1999)
Brevican	Scar astrocytes	Afshari et al. (2009)
NG2[a]	Meningeal cells	
	Scar astrocytes	
	Oligodendrocyte progenitors	
Versican	Oligodendrocyte progenitors	
Phosphacan	Oligodendrocyte progenitors	
Repulsive guidance molecule	Neurons	Mueller et al. (2006)
	Astrocytes	
	Leucocytes	

[a] NG2 (neuron-glial antigen 2), a chondroitin sulphate proteoglycan.

Each process listed above provides a potential target for therapeutic intervention, and it is likely that a combination of therapies will prove most successful. A further point is that complete regeneration and restoration of neural circuits is not necessarily required, for even limited regeneration may prove clinically beneficial.

Targeting the acute injury phase
After SCI there is an initial influx of neutrophils followed by macrophages into the injury site and adjacent parenchyma (Schültke et al. 2010). Activated neutrophils cause oxidative damage to proteins and lipids, and release hydrolytic enzymes into the extracellular matrix, so increasing the extent of secondary damage after primary trauma. Further disturbances include glutamate-induced excitotoxicity, changes in ionic homeostasis, and vascular abnormalities (Baptiste and Fehlings 2006).

Until recently the most common strategy to curb the inflammatory process has been administration of steroids. However, this has only a modest effect at best (Nesathurai 1998), and indeed may be detrimental to the recovery process. Certain components of the immune system are required for protection and repair of the spinal cord after acute or chronic injury

TABLE 9.2
Targeting the acute phase: limitation of secondary damage

Curb inflammatory response	Promote tissue repair / limit further damage
Quercetin	Riluzole
Serine protease inhibitor	Augment blood-derived monocytes
Promote intrinsic ability of axotomized axons to regenerate	*Rescuing vasculature*
Rho inhibitors, e.g. cethrin	Promote endothelial cell survival, e.g. angiopoietin-1 receptor

(Shechter et al. 2009). More recently, attempts to limit damage at this early time point have met with some success. Schültke et al. (2010) have demonstrated that the flavonoid quercetin, which is a potent inhibitor of myeloperoxidase, a key regulator in oxidant production by cellular mediators of inflammation, improves motor function after spinal cord compression injury in the adult rat. However, another trial of antioxidant therapy in humans, albeit for acute stroke, has not proved successful (Lees et al. 2006).

The vascular changes that follow SCI can also influence the severity of primary damage. Endothelial cells and blood vessels begin to degenerate within 30 minutes of injury, increasing ischaemia. Surviving blood vessels are leaky, promoting oedema and leukocyte ingression, in turn contributing to further tissue loss. This process has been manipulated for therapeutic purposes by targeting the angiopoietin-1 receptor, Tie2, and $\alpha_v\beta_3$-integrin to stimulate endothelial cell survival (Han et al. 2010). Tie2 is expressed on endothelial cells and promotes their survival; $\alpha_v\beta_3$-integrin acts similarly, probably by interaction with the matrix glycoprotein laminin, so preventing endothelial cell detachment that normally follows SCI. Han et al. (2010) showed that after contusion SCI in the mouse, daily intravenous injections of an angiopoietin mimetic, combined with an $\alpha_v\beta_3$-binding peptide, promote angiogenesis in the lesion epicentre and rescue white matter; inflammation is reduced and locomotor function significantly improved.

Several other agents are being assessed for their neuroprotective efficacy in animal models of SCI, including riluzole, a sodium channel inhibitor, and erythropoietin (Baptiste and Fehlings 2006). An anti-inflammatory serine protease inhibitor expressed by astrocytes and neutrophils has been shown to exert an early protective effect in a mouse model of spinal cord contusion injury (Ghasemlou et al. 2010). Another strategy targets the wound-healing response in the spinal cord, and attempts to augment the number of monocytes recruited to the injury site (Schwartz 2010). Table 9.2 summarizes these various approaches to limit the extent of secondary damage after SCI.

Targeting post-acute events

CNS trauma can result in permanent neurological deficits due to loss of neurons and/or interruption of ascending and descending axon pathways. Discussion of neuronal replacement strategies, including the use of neuronal stem cells, is beyond the scope of this review. Regarding damaged axons, one important aim is to re-establish functional neuronal

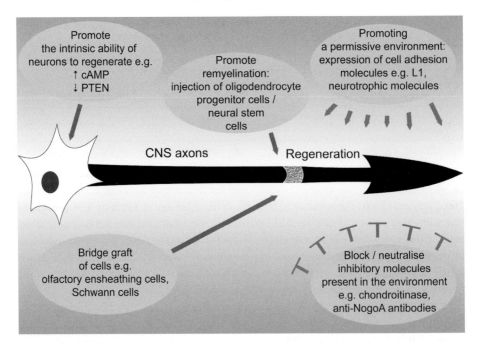

Fig. 9.1. Strategies for treating spinal cord injury based on promoting axon regeneration and remyelination.

pathways, and this could be achieved by axon regeneration and reconnection with original targets, and/or sprouting ('plasticity') of intact spared axons to preserve connectivity (Duan and Giger 2010). However, since Cajal's classic studies (Cajal 1928), it has been clear that CNS axon regrowth is severely compromised after the initial phase of damage. It is now widely accepted that this has two major causes: the regenerative ability of some CNS neuron populations diminishes as they mature (but see David and Aguayo 1981), and, second, the CNS parenchyma provides an inhibitory environment for regenerative axon growth. These will now be discussed in turn, and the related strategies for promoting spinal cord repair are summarized in Figure 9.1.

MODULATION OF THE INTRINSIC CAPACITY OF NEURONS FOR AXON OUTGROWTH: CYCLIC AMP SIGNALLING
Several recent studies have focused on identifying the intrinsic changes that occur as a neuron matures, and that may cause regenerative failure after injury. Such changes are suggested by the observation that although embryonic neurons can be induced to regenerate readily, and can grow extensively when transplanted onto myelinated adult CNS tissue, adult neurons do not extend long neurites on immature CNS tissue (Shewan et al. 1995, Peace and Shewan 2011). Among mature neurons there are also clear differences between populations in their ability to regenerate after injury. For example, the regenerative ability of unmyelinated versus myelinated mature axons is well known (Berry 1982), rubrospinal axons have a

greater potential to regenerate than corticospinal axons in rodents (see Hendriks et al. 2006), and Purkinje cell axons show very limited regeneration (Rossi et al. 2006).

The signalling pathways that may underlie these maturational changes are potential targets for therapeutic intervention. One important contributory factor is a decline in basal levels of neuronal cyclic adenosine monophosphate (cAMP) activity during the later stages of vertebrate development, which coincides with the onset of environmental inhibition of axon outgrowth (Peace and Shewan 2011). It is well established that regeneration of centrally projecting primary sensory neurons through otherwise inhibitory substrates is promoted by raising neuronal cAMP levels, whether by application of neurotrophins (Cai et al. 1999), by performing a conditioning lesion (e.g. sciatic nerve crush, Qiu et al. 2002), or by direct injection of dibutyryl cAMP into the dorsal root ganglion (Neumann et al. 2002, Qiu et al. 2002). It has also been shown that cAMP levels fall after SCI (contusion injury) in the rostral spinal cord, sensorimotor cortex, and brainstem, which is likely to weaken further any regenerative response (Pearse et al. 2004). cAMP levels can be raised artificially by application of rolipram, a phosphodiesterase inhibitor that prevents cAMP breakdown, which has been shown to promote anatomical and functional recovery (Pearse et al. 2004). These findings suggest that manipulating signalling molecules such as cyclic nucleotides, as well as their downstream effectors such as protein kinase A and the guanine nucleotide exchange factor Epac (Peace and Shewan 2010), provides a promising approach to stimulating CNS axon regeneration in a growth-inhibitory microenvironment (Fig. 9.2).

PTEN/MTOR

A significant advance has been made recently in elucidating whether intrinsic molecular mechanisms that might restrain regeneration in mature neurons can be manipulated to promote CNS axon regeneration. Studies of regeneration of both retinal ganglion cell axons and corticospinal axons, anatomical systems that normally show poor regenerative potential, have revealed a key role for the tumour suppressor phosphatase PTEN in restricting axon regeneration. In both systems, conditional PTEN deletion in the mouse results in robust axon sprouting and extension, and this has been shown to be partly mediated through the mTOR signalling pathway controlling the available levels of protein synthesis machinery (Park et al. 2008, Liu et al. 2010). PTEN is a negative regulator of mTOR, and PTEN deletion therefore up-regulates mTOR activity and protein synthesis. In the case of injured corticospinal axons, although Liu et al. (2010) did not examine the degree to which PTEN deletion promotes functional recovery, the degree of anatomical regeneration beyond the lesion was comparable to that seen after manipulating the Nogo system (see below), and the observation that regenerating corticospinal axons make new synapses in spinal segments distal to the injury site is encouraging. A challenge for the future will be to develop PTEN inhibitors that can replicate these effects seen in transgenic animals.

ENVIRONMENTAL INHIBITION OF AXON GROWTH

Studies of environmental influences on mammalian CNS axon regeneration have focused particularly on myelin-associated inhibitors that signal through the Nogo receptor, and on the CSPGs present in the injury-induced glial scar.

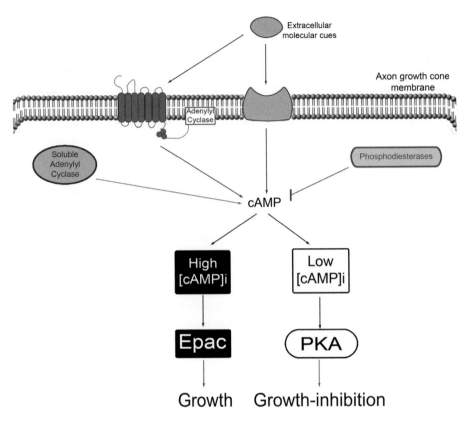

Fig. 9.2. Diagram adapted from Murray et al. (2009) showing distinct pathways mediating cyclic adenosine monophosphate (cAMP)-triggered growth responses in the axon growth cone. Extracellular molecular cues lead to changes in cAMP levels resulting in either forward axon growth or growth-inhibition. Epac, (guanine-nucleotide) exchange protein directly activated by cAMP; PKA, protein kinase A.

MYELIN-ASSOCIATED INHIBITORS OF AXON REGENERATION

The possibility that myelin-derived molecules might inhibit regeneration was first raised by Berry (1982), who pointed out the correlation between CNS regenerative ability and lack of myelination (e.g. cut optic axons in the retina and hypothalamo-hypophyseal tract axons). Schwab's laboratory explored this further in a series of pioneering experiments, culminating in the discovery of the 250kDa myelin protein Nogo, also expressed in oligo-dendrocyte membranes, as a significant inhibitor of CNS axon regeneration (Schwab et al. 1993, Chen et al. 2000, Schwab 2010). Myelin-associated glycoprotein (MAG) and oligo-dendrocyte myelin glycoprotein (OMgp) have also been identified as core myelin compo-nents that block axon growth (Yiu and He 2006). Several co-receptor proteins have been shown to transduce myelin-based growth-inhibition (for review see Giger et al. 2010). A receptor for Nogo, MAG, and OMgp (NgR) is expressed on neurons, and this interacts with two members of the tumour necrosis factor receptor superfamily, p75 and TROY, in concert with a further co-receptor Lingo-1. Another high-affinity receptor for Nogo, MAG, and OMgp has been shown recently to be leukocyte immunoglobulin-like receptor B2 (human LILRB2), whose mouse orthologue, PirB, acts cooperatively with NgR in mediating myelin inhibition of axon growth in vitro (Atwal et al. 2008).

Although in vitro experiments have consistently indicated roles for these proteins in myelin-based axon growth inhibition, it has proved difficult to draw similarly firm conclusions regarding their function in vivo. Genetic ablation studies in the mouse, either of single genes or combinations, have produced variable and often conflicting results between different laboratories. For example, a recent meticulous study of dorsal hemisection SCI in the Nogo/MAG/OMgp triple mutant mouse showed no significant regeneration of corticospinal and serotonergic axons, and only modest promotion of lesion-induced plasticity and behavioural recovery (Lee et al. 2010). On the other hand, in a similar study of triple Nogo/MAG/OMgp knockout mouse, Cafferty et al. (2010) have reported marked anatomical regeneration and significant behavioural recovery. Silver (2010) has argued that such divergent results may result from variations in the degree of experimental axon tract damage, with compensatory sprouting of spared corticospinal and serotonergic axons promoting recovery in the absence of myelin inhibitors. Variations in mouse age or genetic backgound, as well as neuronal labelling artefacts, may provide further confounding factors (Zheng et al. 2003, Steward et al. 2007). On the receptor side, genetic ablation of neither NgR nor PirB promotes corticospinal tract regeneration (Zheng et al. 2005, Omoto et al. 2010) or serotonergic axon regeneration (NgR only (Lee et al. 2010). In the face of these uncertainties the therapeutic potential of humanized neutralizing anti-Nogo antibodies, currently under clinical trial for treating human SCI, is awaited with interest (Zörner and Schwab 2010).

CSPGS AND BACTERIAL CHONDROITINASE

A CSPG comprises a core protein with one or more covalently attached sulphated glycosaminoglycan (GAG) chains, and GAG chains are the major axon growth-inhibitory components of the different CSPG family members (Bradbury and Carter 2011). A promising method to neutralize CSPG-based growth inhibition concerns the use of the bacterial enzyme chondroitinase, which cleaves CSPG GAG chains. Application of bacterial chondroitinase has proven successful as a treatment for acute experimental SCI in many laboratories, in many injury models and in three mammalian species (rat, mouse, and cat; Bradbury et al. 2002, Carter et al. 2008, Tester and Howland 2008). Use of the enzyme has two main consequences for the injured spinal cord. CSPGs in astrocytic scar tissue are degraded, promoting axon regeneration across the lesion. CSPG axon growth-inhibition is also diminished in perineuronal nets, aggregations of dense organized extracellular matrix that surround many CNS neurons (Deepa et al. 2006), thereby activating neuronal plasticity (Pizzorusso et al. 2002). Both of these actions have been shown to promote substantial recovery of function after SCI in rodents (Bradbury et al. 2002), particularly when recovery is driven by rehabilitation (García-Alías et al. 2009). There is also evidence that chondroitinase has a neuroprotective effect (Carter et al. 2008) and promotes target reinnervation (Massey et al. 2008).

An important question concerns the mechanism of CSPG-based axon growth-inhibition and its amelioration by chondroitinase. Repair may follow disruption of receptor-mediated growth-inhibitory signalling caused by CSPGs. For example, a transmembrane receptor tyrosine phosphatase (RPTPσ) activated by CSPGs has recently been identified that contributes to axon growth-inhibition in the injured adult rat spinal cord (Duan and Giger 2010). Other possible mechanisms include reduced calcium entry into neurons, unmasking of axon growth-promoting molecules in the glial scar such as laminin and β-integrins, or dissipation of matrix-associated growth-inhibitory molecules such as secreted semaphorins (Bradbury and Carter 2011). There is also evidence that the enzyme may act by modulating the immune/inflammatory responses that follow SCI (Bradbury and Carter 2011), and it remains to be determined which of these several mechanisms predominates in vivo.

The independent verification of chondroitinase efficacy by many different laboratories using a variety of experimental models indicates that chondroitinase treatment is a promising strategy for clinical translation. So far no adverse effects have been noted in smaller mammals, but the means of administration needs to be optimized for use in humans. Animal studies have suggested that multiple injections of the bacterial enzyme are necessary, increasing the risk of infection and further trauma. The recent development of an engineered form of chondroitinase that can be synthesized by mammalian cells overcomes this difficulty (Muir et al. 2010), making it possible to deliver the enzyme by gene therapy or cell transplants. The timing of treatment may also be critical, as there is now evidence that CSPGs may be required during the acute recovery stage to modulate activity of infiltrating myeloid cells and microglia. Inhibition of CSPG synthesis immediately after injury has been found to impair motor recovery and to increase tissue loss (Rolls et al. 2009), and an optimal outcome may require chondroitinase delivery to be delayed by a few days after initial trauma.

Chondroitinase may also have advantages as part of a combination therapy. For example, when using cellular bridge grafts (see also below), CSPGs build up at the interface of the graft and host tissue, preventing regenerating axons from exiting the graft to make connections with host neurons. Chondroitinase treatment has been shown to facilitate the exit of such axons (Fouad et al. 2005). It has also been shown to promote survival and migration of neural progenitor cells transplanted into the chronically injured rat spinal cord. This enhances plasticity of descending serotonergic pathways, and is associated with significantly improved behavioural recovery (Karimi-Abdolrezaee et al. 2010).

In summary, an increasing number of preclinical studies have reported beneficial effects of chondroitinase for experimental acute SCI, and there are reports of efficacy in animal models of chronic SCI. Taken together, these support the use of chondroitinase as a component of future strategies to treat SCI.

OTHER INHIBITORY MOLECULES
As noted above, two major families of repulsive axon guidance molecules, the semaphorins and ephrins, have also been implicated in experimental SCI. Both secreted and transmembrane semaphorins are expressed after SCI; for example Sema3A is secreted by meningeal fibroblasts (Pasterkamp and Verhaagen 2006, Giger et al. 2010). The net contribution of

semaphorin-based growth inhibition after SCI remains uncertain at present, for a recent study in the mouse has shown that combined genetic deletion of two receptors for class 3 (secreted) semaphorins, plexinA3 and plexinA4, does not enhance serotonergic axon regeneration (Lee et al. 2010). On the other hand, genetic deletion of the EphA4 tyrosine kinase receptor, which is expressed by glial scar astrocytes after SCI, does lead to significant axon regeneration (Goldshmit et al. 2004, Afshari et al. 2009, Giger et al. 2010).

THE RHO FAMILY OF SMALL GTPASES

Many ligands involved in axon growth-inhibition, including myelin proteins (Filbin 2003, Schwab 2010), CSPGs (Monnier et al. 2003), semaphorins (Giger et al. 2010), and Eph/ephrins (Shamah et al. 2001), have been shown to inhibit axon growth cones by signalling through the small GTPase Rho and its associated serine/threonine kinase ROCK. Rho inhibition therefore provides another strategy for therapeutic intervention, and clinical trials testing the efficacy of a RhoA antagonist have been initiated (by BioAxone Therapeutic, Cambridge, MA, USA; see also Baptiste et al. 2009).

GROWTH FACTORS AND CELL ADHESION MOLECULES

Another approach to promoting axon regeneration concerns the secreted neurotrophic factors that regulate growth and survival of diverse neuronal populations during development (Reichardt 2006), and the cell adhesion molecules that are permissive for axon outgrowth (Giger et al. 2010).

It is noteworthy that neurotrophin expression persists widely into adulthood in many CNS regions associated with functional plasticity (Maisonpierre et al. 1990), and neurotrophins promote extensive axon outgrowth from several axonal populations after SCI. For example, BDNF promotes outgrowth of lesioned raphespinal, coerulospinal, rubrospinal, and reticulospinal axons into permissive growth matrices placed in sites of SCI, and prevents corticospinal neuronal death after axotomy (Giger et al. 2010). NT3 has been shown to promote regeneration of lesioned dorsal column proprioceptive sensory axons (Taylor et al. 2006). Using this injury model, lentiviral-induced NT3 expression in the gracile nucleus also promotes morphological synapse formation (Alto et al. 2009). Although the reconstituted neural circuitry was not electrophysiologically active, probably because of the absence of remyelination after injury (Alto et al. 2009), these findings are encouraging in confirming that regenerating axons can be guided to their correct targets to form synapses in the mature CNS (see also Carter et al. 1989).

Several cell surface molecules other than neurotrophin receptors are well known to promote axon outgrowth, including laminin, NCAM and L1, and upregulation of α_5- and α_7-integrins promotes robust regeneration after SCI after a conditioning sciatic nerve crush (Afshari et al. 2009). Similar results have also been reported for L1, which is expressed on neurons and Schwann cells and promotes axon outgrowth and myelination during development and regeneration (Chen et al. 2007). In a recent study (Lavdas et al. 2010), after a compression-SCI in adult mice, L1-expressing Schwann cells were grafted rostral to the lesion site. This promoted motor recovery, enhanced myelination, and increased growth of serotonergic fibers across the lesion site. The combination of cell grafting with increased expression of adhesion molecules permissive to axon outgrowth is therefore another plausible option for therapeutic intervention.

CELL TRANSPLANTATION

A key factor in the failure of CNS axon regeneration after injury is the absence of aligned glial pathways that regenerating axons require for optimal long-distance elongation (Raisman and Li 2007), and such pathways may be provided by implanting a cellular scaffold to bridge the lesion site. A variety of tissues, cell types, and matrices have been tested, including grafts of peripheral nerve (Schwann cells and associated extracellular matrix), fetal CNS tissue, fibroblasts engineered to secrete growth factors, embryonic stem cells, bone marrow stromal cells, neural progenitor cells, and olfactory ensheathing cells (OECs) (for review see Bunge 2008). Schwann cells and OECs have been used most extensively and will be discussed further here.

Following Cajal's original insights it is widely accepted that Schwann cells promote axon regeneration in peripheral nerve by producing a variety of growth-promoting molecules. A particular advantage is that they can be easily grown in large quantities for autologous transplantation. They can also be engineered to overexpress growth factors (Bunge 2008) and therefore provide an excellent candidate for bridge-grafting in the clinical setting.

Transplantation of Schwann cells to bridge the severed stumps of thoracic rat spinal cord allows regenerating axons to enter the bridge, but axons do not leave it to enter the host cord. This correlates with the accumulation of inhibitory molecules/CSPGs at the interface with the spinal cord. As noted above, the outcome is enhanced, including functional recovery, by combining Schwann cell grafts with bacterial chondroitinase (Bunge 2008).

Studies of Schwann cell grafts using a rat contusion injury model are highly relevant to the human injury state. Large cavities are generated but some axons are spared, and sprouting/plasticity of these spared axons may contribute to functional recovery. In rat contusion SCI, cavity size is significantly reduced by transplantation of Schwann cell grafts into the contusion site at 7 days after injury, and a higher number of myelinated axons is observed in the implant. This is matched by increased axon growth beyond the graft, accompanied by a modest improvement in locomotor function (Bunge 2008). The outcome can be augmented by combining Schwann cell transplantation with rolipram administration to increase ambient cAMP levels in spinal cord cells, resulting in a significant recovery of hind-limb function (Pearse et al. 2004).

OECs are located in the olfactory neuroepithelium, in the olfactory nerves extending into the CNS and in the olfactory bulb, regions where axon outgrowth from newborn primary olfactory neurons continues throughout life (for review see Raisman and Li 2007). Similar to Schwann cell grafts, OEC grafts in experimental SCI have been shown to reduce scar formation and contusion-induced cavitation, and to promote axon regeneration and myelination. They also improve functional recovery after partial and complete spinal cord lesions (Li et al. 1997, Ramón-Cueto et al. 1998, Santos-Benito and Ramón-Cueto 2003), although the outcome depends on the injury model and the timing of transplantation after injury (Franssen et al. 2007). Unlike Schwann cell grafts, axons may grow more readily from the OEC graft into the host neuropil (Raisman and Li 2007). Optimizing the clinical benefits of OEC transplants may require combination with other synergistic therapies (Barnett and Riddel 2007). Further issues include collecting sufficient cell numbers for use in humans, and identifying the most suitable source of cells (Raisman and Li 2007). Although the olfactory bulb is clearly a less practicable site for human biopsy than the olfactory mucosa, the latter furnishes a variety of other cell types (Mackay-Sim 2005), making interpretation of the role of OECs from this source more problematic. It is possible that future advances in reprogramming of patient-derived stem cells will overcome these problems.

CLINICAL TRIALS USING CELL TRANSPLANTS

Trials using human OECs have been initiated, and have shown the method to be technically feasible without significant disadvantages so far (Lima et al. 2006, Mackay-Sim et al. 2008). A recent randomized, blinded, and placebo-controlled trial of OECs in spinal-injured dogs has shown promising results, with improved motor coordination suggestive of altered function of intraspinal circuits, albeit without evidence of significant long tract regeneration in the spinal cord (Granger et al. 2012).

The US Federal Drug Authority recently approved the first clinical trial of a human embryonic stem cell-based therapy (Geron Corporation), aimed at remyelinating spinal cord axons after injury. Geron has developed lines of oligodendrocyte progenitor cells derived from human embryonic stem cells for use in the phase 1 trial. Previous rodent studies have shown that transplanted oligodendrocyte progenitor cells remyelinate spinal axons, restoring a limited amount of motor and sensory function, and that they express neurotrophic factors (Zhang et al. 2006). Although eight to ten patients with thoracic contusion SCI were scheduled to receive a single injection of oligodendrocyte progenitor cells from 1 to 2 weeks after injury, regrettably the trial was subsequently halted (for financial reasons; see *New York Times*, 14 November 2011).

Concluding remarks

During the past three decades important advances have been made towards the treatment of human SCI. Experiments using animal models have elucidated some of the mechanisms that are responsible for the regenerative failure of CNS axons. These include reduced cAMP levels and a decrease in mTOR activity in mature neurons. Major players responsible for blocking axon regeneration and plasticity have been identified as the myelin-derived inhibitors and the CSPGs, as well as several axon guidance molecules, and promising approaches to overcome these inhibitors have been devised. It is encouraging that cell-based treatment strategies have at last reached the stage of clinical trial in humans. To reach full potential, cell transplantation will probably need to be combined with other regeneration-promoting strategies, as outlined above and summarized in Figure 9.1. Convincing evidence that such treatment combinations actually work in clinical practice may be forthcoming in the near future, and whether or not specifically identified mechanisms will be responsible, this would be a transformative change of the therapeutic horizon.

REFERENCES

Afshari FT, Kappagantula S, Fawcett JW. Extrinsic and intrinsic factors controlling axonal regeneration after spinal cord injury. *Expert Rev Mol Med* 2009; **11**: e37.

Alto LT, Havton LA, Conner JM, Hollis Ii ER, Blesch A, Tuszynski MH. Chemotropic guidance facilitates axonal regeneration and synapse formation after spinal cord injury. *Nat Neurosci* 2009; **12**: 1106–1113.

Atwal JK, Pinkston-Gosse J, Syken J, et al. PirB is a functional receptor for myelin inhibitors of axonal regeneration. *Science* 2008; **322**: 967–970.

Baptiste DC, Fehlings MG. Pharmacological approaches to repair the injured spinal cord. *J Neurotrauma* 2006; **23**: 318–334.

Baptiste DC, Tighe A, Fehlings MG. Spinal cord injury and neural repair: focus on neuroregenerative approaches for spinal cord injury. *Expert Opin Investig Drugs* 2009; **18**: 663–673.

Barnett SC, Riddell JS. Olfactory ensheathing cell transplantation as a strategy for spinal cord repair—what can it achieve? *Nat Clin Pract Neurol* 2007; **3**: 152–161.

Berry M. Post-injury myelin-breakdown products inhibit axonal growth: an hypothesis to explain the failure of axonal regeneration in the mammalian central nervous system. *Bibl Anat* 1982; **23**: 1–11.

Bradbury EJ, Carter LM. Manipulating the glial scar: chondroitinase ABC as a therapy for spinal cord injury. *Brain Res Bull* 2011; **84**: 306–316.

Bradbury EJ, Moon LDF, Popat RJ, et al. Chondroitinase ABC promotes functional recovery after spinal cord injury. *Nature* 2002; **416**: 636–640.

Bunge MB. Novel combination strategies to repair the injured mammalian spinal cord. *J Spinal Cord Med* 2008; **31**: 262–269.

Cafferty WBJ, Duffy P, Huebner E, Strittmatter SM. MAG and OMgp synergize with Nogo-A to restrict axonal growth and neurological recovery after spinal cord trauma. *J Neurosci* 2010; **30**: 6825–6837.

Cai D, Shen Y, De Bellard M, Tang S, Filbin MT. Prior exposure to neurotrophins blocks inhibition of axonal regeneration by MAG and myelin via a cAMP-dependent mechanism. *Neuron* 1999; **22**: 89–101.

Cajal S. Degeneration and Regeneration of the Nervous System. Oxford University Press, 1928.

Carter DA, Bray GM, Aguayo AJ. Regenerated retinal ganglion cell axons can form well-differentiated synapses in the superior colliculus of adult hamsters. *J Neurosci* 1989; **9**: 4042–4050.

Carter LM, Starkey ML, Akrimi SF, Davies M, McMahon SB, Bradbury EJ. The yellow fluorescent protein (YFP-H) mouse reveals neuroprotection as a novel mechanism underlying chondroitinase ABC-mediated repair after spinal cord injury. *J Neurosci* 2008; **28**: 14107–14120.

Chen J, Wu J, Apostolova I, et al. Adeno-associated virus-mediated L1 expression promotes functional recovery after spinal cord injury. *Brain* 2007; **130**: 954–969.

Chen MS, Huber AB, van der Haar ME, et al. Nogo-A is a myelin-associated neurite outgrowth inhibitor and an antigen for monoclonal antibody IN-1. *Nature* 2000; **403**: 434–439.

David S, Aguayo AJ. Axonal elongation into peripheral nervous system 'bridges' after central nervous system injury in adult rats. *Science* 1981; **214**: 931–933.

Deepa SS, Carulli D, Galtrey C, et al. Composition of perineuronal net extracellular matrix in rat brain: a different disaccharide composition for the net-associated proteoglycans. *J Biol Chem* 2006; **281**: 17789–17800.

Duan Y, Giger RJ. A new role for RPTPsigma in spinal cord injury: signaling chondroitin sulfate proteoglycan inhibition. *Sci Signal* 2010; **3**: pe6.

Fabes J, Anderson P, Brennan C, Bolsover S. Regeneration-enhancing effects of EphA4 blocking peptide following corticospinal tract injury in adult rat spinal cord. *Eur J Neurosci* 2007; **26**: 2496–2505.

Fawcett JW, Asher RA. The glial scar and central nervous system repair. *Brain Res Bull* 1999; **49**: 377–391.

Filbin MT. Myelin-associated inhibitors of axonal regeneration in the adult mammalian CNS. *Nat Rev Neurosci* 2003; **4**: 703–713.

Fouad K, Schnell L, Bunge MB, Schwab ME, Liebscher T, Pearse DD. Combining Schwann cell bridges and olfactory-ensheathing glia grafts with chondroitinase promotes locomotor recovery after complete transection of the spinal cord. *J Neurosci* 2005; **25**: 1169–1178.

Franssen EHP, de Bree FM, Verhaagen J. Olfactory ensheathing glia: their contribution to primary olfactory nervous system regeneration and their regenerative potential following transplantation into the injured spinal cord. *Brain Res Rev* 2007; **56**: 236–258.

García-Alías G, Barkhuysen S, Buckle M, Fawcett JW. Chondroitinase ABC treatment opens a window of opportunity for task-specific rehabilitation. *Nat Neurosci* 2009; **12**: 1145–1151.

Ghasemlou N, Bouhy D, Yang J, et al. Beneficial effects of secretory leukocyte protease inhibitor after spinal cord injury. *Brain* 2010; **133**: 126–138.

Giger RJ, Hollis ER, Tuszynski MH. Guidance molecules in axon regeneration. *Cold Spring Harb Perspect Biol* 2010; **2**: a001867.

Goldshmit Y, Galea MP, Wise G, Bartlett PF, Turnley AM. Axonal regeneration and lack of astrocytic gliosis in EphA4-deficient mice. *J Neurosci* 2004; **24**: 10064–10073.

Granger N, Blamires H, Franklin RJM, Jeffery ND. Autologous olfactory mucosal cell transplants in clinical spinal cord injury: a randomized, double-blinded trial in a canine translational model. *Brain* 2012; **135**: 3227–3237.

Han S, Arnold SA, Sithu SD, et al. Rescuing vasculature with intravenous angiopoietin-1 and αvβ3 integrin peptide is protective after spinal cord injury. *Brain* 2010; **133**: 1026–1042.

Hendriks WTJ, Eggers R, Ruitenberg MJ, et al. Profound differences in spontaneous long-term functional recovery after defined spinal tract lesions in the rat. *J Neurotrauma* 2006; **23**: 18–35.

Jones LL, Tuszynski MH. Spinal cord injury elicits expression of keratan sulfate proteoglycans by macrophages, reactive microglia, and oligodendrocyte progenitors. *J Neurosci* 2002; **22**: 4611–4624.

Karimi-Abdolrezaee S, Eftekharpour E, Wang J, Schut D, Fehlings MG. Synergistic effects of transplanted adult neural stem/progenitor cells, chondroitinase, and growth factors promote functional repair and plasticity of the chronically injured spinal cord. *J Neurosci* 2010; **30**: 1657–1676.

Lavdas AA, Chen J, Papastefanaki F, et al. Schwann cells engineered to express the cell adhesion molecule L1 accelerate myelination and motor recovery after spinal cord injury. *Exp Neurol* 2010; **221**: 206–216.

Lee JK, Geoffroy CG, Chan AF, et al. Assessing spinal axon regeneration and sprouting in Nogo-, MAG-, and OMgp-deficient mice. *Neuron* 2010; **66**: 663–670.

Lees KR, Zivin JA, Ashwood T, et al. NXY-059 for acute ischemic stroke. *N Engl J Med* 2006; **354**: 588–600.

Li Y, Field PM, Raisman G. Repair of adult rat corticospinal tract by transplants of olfactory ensheathing cells. *Science* 1997; **277**: 2000–2002.

Lima C, Pratas-Vital J, Escada P, Hasse-Ferreira A, Capucho C, Peduzzi JD. Olfactory mucosa autografts in human spinal cord injury: a pilot clinical study. *J Spinal Cord Med* 2006; **29**: 191–203.

Liu K, Lu Y, Lee JK, Samara R, et al. PTEN deletion enhances the regenerative ability of adult corticospinal neurons. *Nat Neurosci* 2010; **13**: 1075–1081.

Mackay-Sim A. Olfactory ensheathing cells and spinal cord repair. *Keio J Med* 2005; **54**: 8–14.

Mackay-Sim A, Féron F, Cochrane J, et al. Autologous olfactory ensheathing cell transplantation in human paraplegia: a 3-year clinical trial. *Brain* 2008; **131**: 2376–2386.

Maisonpierre PC, Belluscio L, Friedman B, et al. NT-3, BDNF, and NGF in the developing rat nervous system: parallel as well as reciprocal patterns of expression. *Neuron* 1990; **5**: 501–509.

Massey JM, Amps J, Viapiano MS, et al. Increased chondroitin sulfate proteoglycan expression in denervated brainstem targets following spinal cord injury creates a barrier to axonal regeneration overcome by chondroitinase ABC and neurotrophin-3. *Exp Neurol* 2008; **209**: 426–445.

Monnier PP, Sierra A, Schwab JM, Henke-Fahle S, Mueller BK. The Rho/ROCK pathway mediates neurite growth-inhibitory activity associated with the chondroitin sulfate proteoglycans of the CNS glial scar. *Mol Cell Neurosci* 2003; **22**: 319–330.

Mueller BK, Yamashita T, Schaffar G, Mueller R. The role of repulsive guidance molecules in the embryonic and adult vertebrate central nervous system. *Philos Trans R Soc Lond B Biol Sci* 2006; **361**: 1513–1529.

Muir EM, Fyfe I, Gardiner S, et al. Modification of N-glycosylation sites allows secretion of bacterial chondroitinase ABC from mammalian cells. *J Biotechnol* 2010; **145**: 103–110.

Murray AJ, Tucker SJ, Shewan DA. cAMP-dependent axon guidance is distinctly regulated by Epac and protein kinase A. *J Neurosci* 2009; **29**: 15434–15444.

Nesathurai S. Steroids and spinal cord injury: revisiting the NASCIS 2 and NASCIS 3 trials. *J Trauma* 1998; **45**: 1088–1093.

Neumann S, Bradke F, Tessier-Lavigne M, Basbaum A. Regeneration of sensory axons within the injured spinal cord induced by intraganglionic cAMP elevation. *Neuron* 2002; **34**: 885–893.

Niclou SP, Franssen EH, Ehlert EM, Taniguchi M, Verhaagen J. Meningeal cell-derived semaphorin 3A inhibits neurite outgrowth. *Mol Cell Neurosci* 2003; **24**: 902–912.

Omoto S, Ueno M, Mochio S, Takai T, Yamashita T. Genetic deletion of paired immunoglobulin-like receptor B does not promote axonal plasticity or functional recovery after traumatic brain injury. *J Neurosci* 2010; **30**: 13045–13052.

Park KK, Liu K, Hu Y, Smith PD, et al. Promoting axon regeneration in the adult CNS by modulation of the PTEN/mTOR pathway. *Science* 2008; **322**: 963–966.

Pasterkamp RJ, Verhaagen J. Semaphorins in axon regeneration: developmental guidance molecules gone wrong? *Philos Trans R Soc Lond B Biol Sci* 2006; **361**: 1499–1511.

Peace AG, Shewan DA. New perspectives in cyclic AMP-mediated axon growth and guidance: The emerging epoch of Epac. *Brain Res Bull* 2011; **84**: 280–288.

Pearse DD, Pereira FC, Marcillo AE, Bates ML, Berrocal YA, Filbin MT, Bunge MB. cAMP and Schwann cells promote axonal growth and functional recovery after spinal cord injury. *Nat Med* 2004; **10**: 610–616.

Pizzorusso T, Medini P, Berardi N, Chierzi S, Fawcett JW, Maffei L. Reactivation of ocular dominance plasticity in the adult visual cortex. *Science* 2002; **298**: 1248–1251.

Qiu J, Cai D, Dai H, et al. Spinal axon regeneration induced by elevation of cyclic AMP. *Neuron* 2002; **34**: 895–903.

Raisman G, Li Y. Repair of neural pathways by olfactory ensheathing cells. *Nat Rev Neurosci* 2007; **8**: 312–319.

Ramón-Cueto A, Plant GW, Avila J, Bunge MB. Long-distance axonal regeneration in the transected adult rat spinal cord is promoted by olfactory ensheathing glia transplants. *J Neurosci* 1998; **18**: 3803–3815.

Reichardt LF. Neurotrophin-regulated signalling pathways. *Philos Trans R Soc Lond B Biol Sci* 2006; **361**: 1545–1564.

Rolls A, Shechter R, Schwartz M. The bright side of the glial scar in CNS repair. *Nat Rev Neurosci* 2009; **10**: 235–241.

Rossi F, Gianola S, Corvetti L. The strange case of Purkinje axon regeneration and plasticity. *Cerebellum* **5**: 2006; 174–182.

Santos-Benito FF, Ramón-Cueto A. Olfactory ensheathing glia transplantation: a therapy to promote repair in the mammalian central nervous system. *Anat Rec B New Anat* 2003; **271**: 77–85.

Schültke E, Griebel RW, Juurlink BHJ. Quercetin attenuates inflammatory processes after spinal cord injury in an animal model. *Spinal Cord* 2010; **48**: 857–861.

Schwab ME, Kapfhammer JP, Bandtlow CE. Inhibitors of neurite growth. *Annu Rev Neurosci* 1993; **16**: 565–595.

Schwab M. Functions of Nogo proteins and their receptors in the nervous sytem. *Nature Rev Neurosci* 2010; **11**: 799–811.

Schwartz M. 'Tissue-repairing' blood-derived macrophages are essential for healing of the injured spinal cord: from skin-activated macrophages to infiltrating blood-derived cells? *Brain Behav Immun* 2010; **24**: 1054–1057.

Shamah SM, Lin MZ, Goldberg JL, et al. EphA receptors regulate growth cone dynamics through the novel guanine nucleotide exchange factor ephexin. *Cell* 2001; **105**: 233–244.

Shechter R, London A, Varol C, et al. Infiltrating blood-derived macrophages are vital cells playing an anti-inflammatory role in recovery from spinal cord injury in mice. *PLoS Med* 2009; **6**: e1000113.

Shewan D, Berry M, Cohen J. Extensive regeneration in vitro by early embryonic neurons on immature and adult CNS tissue. *J Neurosci* 1995; **15**: 2057–2062.

Silver J. Much ado about nogo. *Neuron* 2010; **66**: 619–621.

Steward O, Zheng B, Banos K, Yee KM. Response to: Kim et al. 'Axon regeneration in young adult mice lacking Nogo-A/B.' *Neuron* 2007; **38**: 187–199. *Neuron* 54: 191–195.

Taylor L, Jones L, Tuszynski MH, Blesch A. Neurotrophin-3 gradients established by lentiviral gene delivery promote short-distance axonal bridging beyond cellular grafts in the injured spinal cord. *J Neurosci* 2006; **26**: 9713–9721.

Tester NJ, Howland DR. Chondroitinase ABC improves basic and skilled locomotion in spinal cord injured cats. *Exp Neurol* 2008; **209**: 483–496.

Yiu G, He Z. Glial inhibition of CNS axon regeneration. *Nat Rev Neurosci* 2006; **7**: 617–627.

Zhang YW, Denham J, Thies RS. Oligodendrocyte progenitor cells derived from human embryonic stem cells express neurotrophic factors. *Stem Cells Dev* 2006; **15**: 943–952.

Zheng B, Ho C, Li S, Keirstead H, Steward O, Tessier-Lavigne M. Lack of enhanced spinal regeneration in Nogo-deficient mice. *Neuron* 2003; **38**: 213–224.

Zheng B, Atwal J, Ho C, et al. Genetic deletion of the Nogo receptor does not reduce neurite inhibition in vitro or promote corticospinal tract regeneration in vivo. *Proc Natl Acad Sci U S A* 2005; **102**: 1205–1210.

Zörner B, Schwab ME. Anti-Nogo on the go: from animal models to a clinical trial. *Ann N Y Acad Sci* 2010; **1198** (Suppl 1): E22–E34.

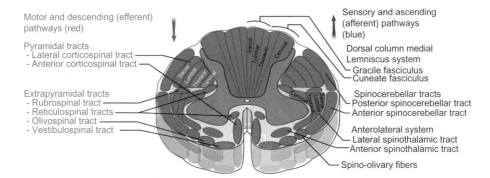

Motor and descending (efferent)
pathways (red)

Pyramidal tracts
 - Lateral corticospinal tract
 - Anterior corticospinal tract

Extrapyramidal tracts
 - Rubrospinal tract
 - Reticulospinal tracts
 - Olivospinal tract
 - Vestibulospinal tract

Sensory and ascending
(afferent) pathways
(blue)

Dorsal column medial
Lemniscus system
 - Gracile fasciculus
 - Cuneate fasciculus

Spinocerebellar tracts
 - Posterior spinocerebellar tract
 - Anterior spinocerebellar tract

Anterolateral system
 - Lateral spinothalamic tract
 - Anterior spinothalamic tract

Spino-olivary fibers

Fig. 1.4. Cross-sectional anatomy of spinal cord showing tracts within spinal cord.

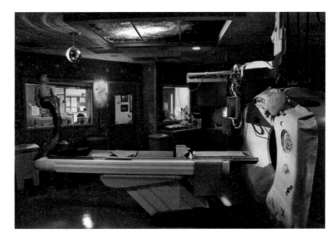

Fig. 2.1. An example of a child-focused computed tomography (CT) scanning suite with appropriate modifications, including 'disguise' of the gantry and a ceiling-mounted fixture of the galaxy (Google Images). Reproduced with permission from the Children's Hospital Pittsburgh.

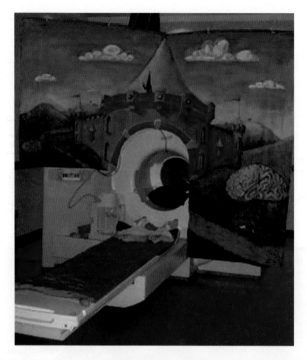

Fig. 2.2. A child-focused magnetic resonance imaging (MRI) scanner with brightly coloured mural and display. Internet picture from University of Oregon.

INDEX

Other titles from Mac Keith Press www.mackeith.co.uk

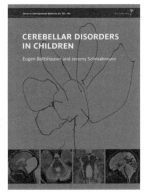

Cerebellar Disorders in Children
Eugen Boltshauser and Jeremy Schmahmann (Eds)

Clinics in Developmental Medicine no. 191-192
2012 ▪ 456pp ▪ hardback ▪ 978-1-907655-01-2
£125.00 / €150.00 / $200.00

This clinically orientated text by an international group of experts is the first definitive reference book on disorders of the cerebellum in children. It presents a wealth of practical clinical experience backed up by a strong scientific basis for the information and guidance given. This book will be an invaluable resource for all those caring for children affected by cerebellar disorders, including malformations, genetic and metabolic disorders, acquired cerebellar damage, vascular disorders and acute ataxias.

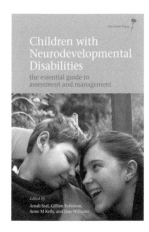

Children with Neurodevelopmental Disabilities: the essential guide to assessment and management
Arnab Seal, Gillian Robinson, Anne M. Kelly and Jane Williams (Eds)

2013 ▪ 744pp ▪ softback ▪ 978-1-908316-62-2
£65.00 / €78.00 / $154.95

A comprehensive textbook on the practice of paediatric neurodisability, written by practitioners and experts in the field. Using a problem-oriented approach, the authors give best-practice guidance, and centre on the needs of the child and family, working in partnership with multi-disciplinary, multi-agency teams. Drawing on evidence-based practice, the authors provide a ready reference for managing common problems encountered in the paediatric clinic.

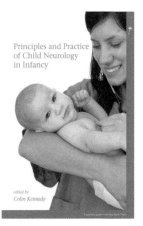

Principles and Practice of Child Neurology in Infancy
Colin Kennedy (Ed)

A practical guide from Mac Keith Press
2012 ▪ 384pp ▪ softback ▪ 978-1-908316-35-6
£29.95 / €38.10 / $49.50

This handbook of neurological practice in infants is designed to be of practical use to all clinicians, but particularly those in under-resourced locations. Seventy per cent of children with disabilities live in resource-poor countries and most of these children have neurological impairments. This book presents recommendations for investigations and treatments based on internationally accepted good practice that can be implemented in most settings.

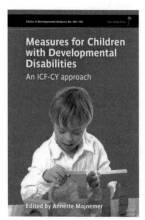

Measures for Children with Developmental Disabilities
An ICF-CY approach
Annette Majnemer (Ed)

Clinics in Developmental Medicine No. 194-195
2012 ▪ 552pp ▪ hardback ▪ 978-1-908316-45-5
£150.00 / €186.00 / $235.00

This title presents and reviews outcome measures across a wide range of attributes that are applicable to children and adolescents with developmental disabilities. It uses the children and youth version of the International Classification of Functioning, Disability and Health (ICF-CY) as a framework for organizing the various measures into sections and chapters. Each chapter coincides with domains within the WHO framework of Body Functions, Activities and Participation and Personal and Environmental Factors.

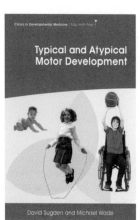

Typical and Atypical Motor Development
David Sugden and Michael Wade

Clinics in Developmental Medicine
2013 ▪ 400pp ▪ hardback ▪ 978-1-908316-55-4
£145.00 / €180.00 / $234.95

Sugden and Wade, leading authors in this area, comprehensively cover motor development and motor impairment, drawing on sources in medicine and health-related studies, motor learning and developmental psychology. A theme that runs through the book is that movement outcomes are a complex transaction of child resources, the context in which movement takes place, and the manner in which tasks are presented.

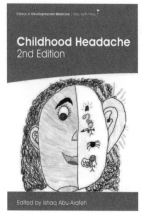

Childhood Headache, 2nd Edition
Ishaq Abu-Arafeh (Ed)

Clinics in Developmental Medicine
2013 ▪ 362pp ▪ hardback ▪ 978-1-908316-75-2
£95.00 / €115.20 / $154.95

Childhood Headache is a comprehensive source of knowledge and guidance for practising clinicians looking after children with headache. It includes many clinical examples to illustrate the difficulties in diagnosis or options for treatment. The scientific basis of headache and migraine is clearly presented and simplified in the chapter of pathophysiology. Headache classification and common headache disorders (migraine and tension-type headache) are fully discussed. It is also a resource for researchers who are looking for a full analysis of the published studies.

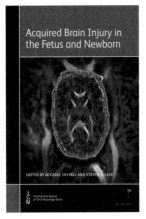

Acquired Brain Injury in the Fetus and Newborn
Michael Shevell and Steven Miller (Eds)

International Review of Child Neurology Series
2012 ▪ 330pp ▪ hardback ▪ 978-1-907655-02-9
£125.00 / €155.00 / $195.00

Given the tremendous advances in the understanding of acquired neonatal brain injury, this book provides a timely review for the practising neurologist, neonatologist and paediatrician. The editors take a pragmatic approach, focusing on specific populations encountered regularly by the clinician. They offer a 'bench to bedside' approach to acquired brain injury in the preterm and term newborn infant. The contributors, all internationally recognized neurologists and scientists, provide readers with a state-of-the art review in their area of expertise.

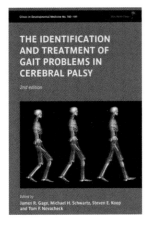

The Identification and Treatment of Gait Problems in Cerebral Palsy, 2nd edition
James R. Gage, Michael H. Schwartz, Steven E. Koop and Tom F. Novacheck (Eds)

Clinics in Developmental Medicine No. 180-181
2009 ▪ 660pp ▪ hardback ▪ 978-1-898683-65-0
£125.00 / €150.00 / $209.00

The only book to deal specifically with the treatment of gait problems in cerebral palsy, this comprehensive, multi-disciplinary volume will be invaluable for all those working in the field of cerebral palsy and gait. The book is accompanied by a DVD containing a teaching video on normal gait and a CD-ROM containing videos of all case examples used in the book.

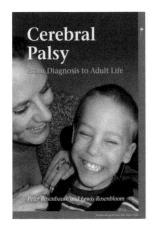

Cerebral Palsy: From Diagnosis to Adult Life
Peter Rosenbaum and Lewis Rosenbloom

A practical guide from Mac Keith Press
2012 ▪ 224pp ▪ softback ▪ 978-1-908316-50-9
£29.95 / €36.10 / $50.00

This book has been designed to provide readers with an understanding of cerebral palsy as a developmental as well as a neurological condition. It details the nature of cerebral palsy, its causes and its clinical manifestations. Using clear, accessible language (supported by an extensive glossary) the authors have blended current science with metaphor to explain the biomedical underpinnings of cerebral palsy.

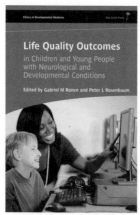

Life Quality Outcomes in Children and Young People with Neurological and Developmental Conditions
Gabriel M. Ronen and Peter L. Rosenbaum (Eds)

Clinics in Developmental Medicine
2013 ▪ 394pp ▪ hardback ▪ 978-1-908316-58-5
£95.00 / €120.70 / $149.95

Healthcare professionals need to understand their patients' views of their condition and its affects on their health and well-being. This book builds on the World Health Organization's concepts of 'health', 'functioning' and 'quality of life' for young people with neurodisabilities: it emphasises the importance of engaging with patients in the identification of both treatment goals and their evaluation. Uniquely, it enables healthcare professionals to find critically reviewed outcomes-related information.

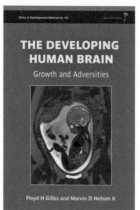

The Developing Human Brain
Floyd H. Gilles and Marvin D. Nelson Jr

Clinics in Developmental Medicine No. 193
2012 ▪ 416pp ▪ hardback ▪ 978-1-908316-41-7
£110.00 / €132.00 / $170.50

This book treats the embryonic and fetal brain as an exciting way to explore growth and aberrations of the most complicated structure in the human body, focusing on the second half of gestation and the neonatal period. It is a unique resource, with its emphasis on quantitative methods and more than 200 pathological and radiological images.

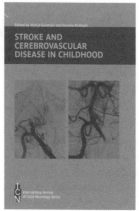

Stroke and Cerebrovascular Disease in Childhood
Vijeya Ganesan, Fenella Kirkham (Eds)

International Review of Child Neurology Series
2011 ▪ 248pp ▪ hardback ▪ 978-1-898683-34-6
£145.00 / €174.00 / $199.95

The field of stroke and cerebrovascular disease in children is one in which there has been much recent research activity, leading to new clinical perspectives. This book for the first time summarizes the state of the art in this field. A team of eminent clinicians, neurologists and researchers provide an up-to-the-minute account of all aspects of stroke and cerebrovascular disease in children, ranging from a historical perspective to future directions, through epidemiology, the latest neuroimaging techniques, neurodevelopment, comorbidities, diagnosis, and treatment.